P9-DGJ-623

THE Wellness Workbook

Watkins

THE Wellness Workbook

· ·

Second Edition

· ·

John W. Travis, M.D.

AND

Regina Sara Ryan

TEN SPEED PRESS

Copyright © 1981, 1988 by John W. Travis

All rights reserved. No part of this book may be reproduced in any form, except for brief reviews, without the written permission of the publisher.

Published 1981. Revised Edition 1988.

🌱

Ten Speed Press
P O Box 7123
Berkeley, California 94707

Book Design by Paula Schlosser
Cover Design by Brenton Beck

Illustrations on pages xvii, xix, xxiii, 1, 15, 16, 26, 48, 52, 93 and 100 by Ellen Sasaki
Illustrations on pages xxiv, xxv, xxvi, xxvii and xxx by Kurt West
Illustrations on pages 96, 97, 98 and 99 by Pedro Gonzales
Illustration on page 110 by Bruce Mills

Library of Congress Cataloging-in-Publication Data

Travis, John W., 1943- .
    The wellness workbook.
    Includes bibliographies and index.
    1. Health. I. Ryan, Regina Sara
II. Title.
RA776.R94   1988   613   86-6052
ISBN 0-89815-179-1

Printed in the United States of America

2 3 4 5 — 90 89 88

The authors gratefully acknowledge the kindness of the following authors, illustrators, publishers and groups in giving permission to reprint from their copyrighted material:

Nutrition Action, a monthly publication of the Center for Science in the Public Interest, 1755 S Street NW, Washington, DC 20009, for permission to reprint the editorial "Stamp Out Food Faddism."

The International Transactional Analysis Association, for permission to reprint the diagram from Stephen B. Karpman's article entitled "Fairy Tales and Script Drama Analysis," from *TAB* 7:26 (April 1968).

John O. Stevens and Real People Press, for permission to reprint from *Notes to Myself* by Hugh Prather, © 1970, Real People Press, Box F., Moab, UT 84532.

Concern for Dying, 250 W. 57th St., New York, NY 10701, for permission to reprint the *Living Will*.

Mrs. E. L. Masters, for permission to reprint "George Gray" and "Lucinda Matlock" from *Spoon River Anthology* by Edgar Lee Masters, © 1976, New York: MacMillan Publishing Co. pp. 65, 229.

Liveright Publishing Corporation, 550 Fifth Ave., New York, NY 10036, for permission to reprint the first four lines from the poem "since feeling is first" from *IS 5* by E. E. Cummings, © 1926 by Horace Liveright; © renewed 1953 by E. E. Cummings.

Harper and Row, Publishers, Inc., for permission to reprint "Balloon Walk" from *Water in the Lake: Real Events for the Imagination* by Kenneth Maue, ©1979 by Kenneth G. Maue.

Charles E. Fleishman, Box 527, San Anselmo, CA 94960, and the *Pacific Sun*, Mill Valley, CA, for permission to reprint *Dag's Bag* cartoon.

Susan Stewart, R. N., Calabasas Park Center for Cervical and TMJ/Cranio-mandibular Orthomedics, 4766 Park Granada, Calabasas, CA 91302, for permission to reprint material on aerobic exercise.

The Hanuman Foundation, Box 478, Santa Fe, NM 87501, for permission to reprint selections from *Be Here Now* by Ram Dass, New York: Crown Publishing Co.; New Mexico: The Lama Foundation, 1971.

Van Nostrand Reinhold Co., for permission to quote from *The Transparent Self* by Sidney Jourard, second edition, © 1971 by Litton Educational Publishing, Inc.

Lloyd Barde, Backroads Distributors, 417 Tamal Plaza, Corte Madera, CA 94925, for the Music Appendix.

The New England Journal of Medicine, from permission to reprint from the editorial by F. J. Ingelfinger, M.D., vol. 293 (18 December 1975), p. 1320.

Ashleigh Brilliant for permission to reprint *Pot Shot Postcards* from a catalog of 1400 selections, Brilliant Enterprises, 117 W. Valerio St., Santa Barbara, CA 93101 ($1 for catalog and five postcards); and also from his books, *I May Not Be Totally Perfect, but Parts of Me Are Excellent* © 1979, and *I Have Abandoned My Search for Truth, and Am Now Looking for a Good Fantasy* © 1980, Woodbridge Press Publishing Co., Box 6189, Santa Barbara, CA 93111.

Celestial Arts, Berkeley, CA for permission to reprint from *The Magical Child Within You* by Bruce Davis, © 1977 by Celestial Arts.

Simon and Schuster, a Division of Gulf and Western, for permission to reprint directions for yoga postures from *Yoga For All Ages* by Rachel E. Carr, © 1972.

Harcourt Brace Jovanovich, Inc., for permission to reprint the poem "i thank You God for most this amazing" by E. E. Cummings, in *Complete Poems 1913-1962* © 1975 by Nancy T. Andrews.

Gerald G. Jampolsky, M.D., of the Center for Attitudinal Healing, 21 Main St., Tiburon, CA 94920, for permission to reprint from the *Minicourse for Healing Relationships and Bringing About Peace of Mind.*

The Art of Listening by Jud Morris, originally published by Industrial Education Institute, 1968 (out of print). At time of publication, address unknown.

Warner Bros. Music, for permission to quote from Bob Dylan's "It's Alright Ma (I'm Only Bleeding)." © 1965 WARNER BROS. INC. All Rights Reserved. Used by Permission.

For Jere Pramuk, my partner and friend.
                                    —R.S.R.

For Meryn Callander-Travis.
                                    —J.W.T.

Contents

...... Introduction ......
xv

.....Wellness Index.....
xvi

.... One ....
Wellness, Self–Responsibility, and Love
1
The Problems with Illness-Care
Self-Responsibility
Love and Compassion

.... Two ....
Wellness and Breathing
25
The Process of Breathing
Problems in the System
A Metaphor for Life
Breathing for Awareness
Breathing and Relaxing
Breathing for Work and Play
Breathing for Healing
The Person Breathes/
The Planet Breathes

..........Three..........
Wellness and Sensing
41
The Sense of Touch
Why We Don't Touch
Creative Uses of Touch
A Sense of Temperature
The Sense of Sight
The Sense of Smell
The Sense of Hearing

.... Four ....

Wellness and Eating
64

The Food Story—Back to Basics
The "Why" Behind the Problems
The Problems With What We Eat
Eating for High Level Wellness
Explore Your Own Uniqueness
Awareness and Self-Trust
Love and Compassion
Growing Your Own
Feeding Our Planet

.... Five ....

Wellness and Moving
91

Exercise—The New National Craze
Types of Exercise
What Movement Does for the Mind and Emotions
And It's Good for the Soul
On Behalf of Trust and Compassion . . . or Why Jerry Doesn't Run
Eleven Easy Steps
Moving on the Planet

............Six............

Wellness and Feeling
109

Sensing . . . Feeling . . . Thinking
Primer of Transactional Analysis
Are Feelings Good or Bad?
The Basic Emotions
Developing Awareness and Support
Love

.........Seven..........

Wellness and Thinking
128

Thinking Molds Reality
Thinking Changes the Body
Beware of Your Hypnotists
GIGO
Right Brain—Left Brain
Whole Brain Wellness
Creative Thinking and Wellness
Brainstorming a Big Question

..........Eight..........

Wellness and Playing/Working
148

Redefining Play
Our Children—The Natural and the Adapted
The Natural Child Plays
Self-Nourishment: The Healing Qualities of Play
Healing Laughter
Defining Work
The Problems with Work
Working Well
The Planet At Play

.... Nine ....

Wellness and Communicating
165

Talking to Yourself—Intrapersonal Communication
Rescuing
Listening
Beyond Human Communication
Communication and the Planet

............Ten............

Wellness and Sex
185

"Well-Sex"
Sex and Love

.... Eleven ....

Wellness and Finding Meaning
196

Where Do Meanings Come From Anyway?
On Goals and Meaning

.... Twelve ....

Wellness and Transcending
209

Peeking Through the Cracks
Transpersonal Psychology and Wellness

...... Appendix A ......
228

.... Appendix B.......
231

..........Index..........
233

... Beyond This Book ...
238

..... Preface to the Second Edition .....

. . . .

I T IS A PLEASURE to have been invited to write the preface for this new edition of the *Wellness Workbook.* In 1981 I heartily endorsed it and with 75,000 copies sold at this writing, it has proved to be a major contribution to the field of health and human understanding.

In 1981 when I mentioned "wellness" to many people, I also had to spell it. "What-ness?" No more. Today, with a cursory glance at popular magazines, a look at a list of workshop topics being offered to corporate executives, or a visit to a community gym or health club, you are apt to encounter it several times. Wellness is "in," and consequently, wellness is big business.

Concern for greater vitality in all aspects of life has resulted in a fitness revolution/craze, stress-management seminars for everyone, and "million-seller" books on life extension possibilities. All of these are impacting the culture

at large, and touching nearly every segment of the population from children to older adults. Wellness was rolling in 1981. In 1988, particularly in the U.S, it is an avalanche.

Or is it?

While the "trappings" or practices associated with wellness are gaining in popularity, I believe that the understanding of it is still extremely limited. The concept is more often than not much too narrowly defined. Often only one component, such as diet, exercise, or stress reduction is emphasized, and sometimes to the point of frustration and distortion. Perfect bodies, impeccable diets, are unrealistic goals for most people. When not met, they easily leave individuals feeling guilty and bad.

So many books or programs today, which identify themselves as having a "wellness" approach, simply deal with symptomatic relief strategies: hypertension screening, smoking cessation,

weight reduction, alcohol/drug dependency treatment. All of these efforts are excellent but their primary goal is early detection and treatment of disease with the goal being an "average" state of health. For many people, this is simply inadequate.

Halbert Dunn, M.D., who first used the word wellness in the 1950s, wrote in his book *High Level Wellness,* a much broader definition. His view encompassed the physical, emotional, psychological, and spiritual aspects of being and their interrelation. It was this book that moved a young doctor, John Travis, to leave the formal practice of medicine and devote his life to education. Instead of focusing on treatment or the alleviation of symptoms, which John saw as only the tip of an iceberg, he focused his career on self-responsibility and prevention.

I first met John in 1974 while researching Health Hazard Appraisals for my book *Mind as*

Healer, Mind as Slayer. A year later, John moved from Baltimore to California to found the first wellness center, as far as I know. Together with his staff, he developed many of the practical approaches that became a part of this *Wellness Workbook.*

When he met his friend, and future co-author, Regina Ryan, who had been teaching courses in holistic health since the early 70s, he was inspired to "go public" with his beliefs that love, compassion, forgiveness, self-acceptance and other "romantic notions" were actually the key elements necessary for the full understanding of wellness. So, this book was born. Here it is again, seven years older, wiser, and I think, more lively and relevant than ever.

The *Wellness Workbook* provides today, as it did in 1981, a bold new model that suggests alternative ways of living, primarily through self-responsibility and self-appreciation, whereby difficulties are resolved when more basic human needs are addressed. Instead of the typical problem-illness orientation, it offers what I would call a possibility orientation. What if, as Regina and John suggest, you put yourself to the task of self-awareness and sensitivity; what if you laughed more; what if you really understood that the way you communicate with other people, the way you breathe, the way you express feelings, make love, pray, and especially think, all were contributing factors to your state of illness or wellness? These are among the questions raised, and the very real possibilities offered, by the *Wellness Workbook.*

The Wellness Energy System, which is explained in the introductory chapter, serves as the unifying principle of the rest of the book. This orientation is their special contribution to a truly holistic view of the human being. Not that they were the first, or only ones, to express the phenomenon of illness or health in terms of energy flow, or energy usage. In fact, the ancient Chinese science of *Chi,* demonstrated in the technique of acupuncture, preceded them by just a few centuries. But, John and Regina have put this understanding together in such a clean and workable way as to make it irresistible. They have introduced to the public at large a profound wisdom in a form that even a child can appreciate. In John Travis' terms, "The process [of how human beings serve as energy channelling systems] may be compared to the movement of water through a pipe." Illness is explained graphically as a "problem in the pipe . . . a leak, a blockage, a contamination . . . ," or an inadequate supply of water, or a wasteful use of it at the other end. We learn that every aspect of life, from breathing through dying, may be considered an input or an output process. How efficiently we, as the channels, interact in that process, and how our lifestyles affect the quality of the energy (the air and water, our food, etc.) being channelled in the first place, will determine whether we live ill or well. Simple, but not easy to actually live day by day. Wellness is aptly defined as a "way of life."

Most of all, I am particularly impressed by the "big picture" the book takes, in establishing a person/planet connection throughout the chapters. No longer can we, as global citizens, consider our cancers, or even our colds, as solely our own private concerns. Our health is tied, inextricably, with the health of our environment. No longer can we neglect to examine the impact that everything—from the chair we sit in at work to the conversations we engage in over dinner—is having on our life and health. While we may not be able to act upon such an awareness, it is this goal of total consciousness or enlightenment which has been the state advocated by all systems of meditation for thousands upon thousands of years. John and Regina remind and gently urge us to wake up to all of it. That's the real power of wellness as far as I'm concerned.

The *Wellness Workbook* in its first edition was enthusiastically received. Currently, it is being used throughout the United States, Canada, Europe, Australia, and New Zealand by educators, medical personnel, and health-conscious individuals from all walks of life. This new edition is even better. It is my hope that it will be even more widely read and used within different segments of the population, the business community, and among the general public. It is the most accessible, comprehensive, and certainly the most "heartful" book of its kind on the market today.

Dr. Kenneth R. Pelletier,
San Francisco, California.

Dr. Pelletier is Associate Clinical Professor, Department of Medicine and Department of Psychiatry, at the University of California School of Medicine, San Francisco, California.

.... Preface to the First Edition ....

M Y OWN SEARCH for wellness has been a long path of learning. Originally I, like many of my brothers and sisters, thought someone "out there" would tell me what was wrong and what I needed to do. Some "educated" person held the power, knew the answers, had the authority to intervene on behalf of my health. The Parent to Child stance somehow seemed acceptable.

However, it was only when I took responsibility for my health, when I acknowledged my own power, when I learned to trust my own answers, when I recognized that *I* was the real authority about my own body, that my search for wellness brightened.

As a consequence, rather than the accepted Parent to Child relationship, which of course is appropriate to many circumstances, I sought interactions which were more Adult to Adult in their essence. This perception freed me to view health care professionals as resource people, to explore alternative approaches, to read, listen,

learn and grow in my own confidence, My search was a long one of many years. It is not over.

The Wellness Workbook would have been (and still is) a marvelous asset to me. It would have shortened my quest and given me a whole view illuminating the narrow focus on disease and prescription.

Travis' and Ryan's book not only gives practical information on nutrition, exercise, attitudes, etc., but happily it also acknowledges the human spirit. After an age of directing our attention and energy to technology, including medical technology, we are recognizing that it is a mixed blessing. However, it holds immeasurable and still unperceived value if we use it to enhance the unfolding of the Universe and to unleash human potential, freeing us to be more of our possible selves.

We appear to be standing on the edge of a spiritual renaissance ready to weld scientific knowledge and spiritual growth. The contribution of our values, our sense of mission, and

our purpose in life to our health and sense of well-being can no longer be denied as a factor underpinning our wellness. Health comes when we are total, whole people; when we have achieved a level of integration between the mind, body, emotions, and spirit; when we allow ourselves to balance.

The Wellness Workbook holds the potential to build the confidence and to support the intelligent choices of any person on the path toward wellness. It is an act of love and caring.

—Dorothy Jongeward, Ph.D.
Orinda, CA
February, 1981

Dr. Jongeward is president of Dorothy Jongeward Associates, Inc., a management consulting firm in Orinda, California, and she coauthored, among other books, *Born to Win: Transactional Analysis with Gestalt Experiments; Women as Winners: Transactional Analysis for Personal Growth; Choosing Success: Transactional Analysis on the Job;* and *Winning Ways in Health Care: Transactional Analysis for Effective Communication.*

......Acknowledgments ......

A FEW OF those who made it possible for me to write this book are:

My parents, Boyd and Eloise Travis, who encouraged me to "do my own thing," and backed me financially;

Rev. Jack Hannum, Wilford Geiger and the Triplett families in Bluffton, Ohio, who were sources of stimulation during my years of high school;

Drs. Ted Williams and J. Garber Drushal, "Mom" Quigley and Diana Moseson Brown who both challenged and supported me in my years at the College of Wooster in Ohio;

Sara Winkler Barnes, my former wife, who supported me through medical training and helped me in developing my early thinking about wellness;

Drs. Halbert Dunn, Lawrence Green, Richard Hsieh, and Lewis Robbins whose innovations in preventive medicine were sources of inspiration to me during my Johns Hopkins years;

Anne Baird, Charles Elias, the Koinonia Community, Valerie Lankford, Kim Muller-Thym, Harry Rose, Ruth and Tony Zyna who helped me get my act together during the transition years in Baltimore;

Mikal Baker, Marina Delfino, Joy Holloway, Kate Lynch, Barbara McNeill (a.k.a. Bobbie Salzer-Rae), Kenneth Maue, Annie Styron Leonard, and Jerry Wylie— the former staff of Wellness Resource Center—for their hugs and hassling and heartfulness;

Marty Albert, Bob Allen, Skip Andrew, Don Ardell, Pam Blackwell, Denny Bullens, George and Julia Cagwin, Elliott Dacher, Fran DuBois, Tom Ferguson, Terry Graves, Jutta Hagner, Chuck Hess, Dorothy Jongeward, Marc Kasky, Cissa Kelley, George Leonard, Floyd Mann, Emmett Miller, Russ Munsell, Jeff Patterson, Kent and Ginny Peterson, Gaye and Roy Raymond, Dean and Cheryl Radetsky, Jo Sherrill, Elaine Sullivan,

Bob Tollaksen, Dave Travis, Marie-Francis Vance, and Tara White, a few of the inner circle of Wonderful Persons who've made Wellness Resource Center and Wellness Associates so real and dear to me; David Isaacs and Lance Hays who pulled and pushed, humored and harassed me until I agreed to write this book;

Linda Berzow who researched the Wellness Index;

Bonnie Callander, the best mother-in-law a man could have;

My trusty Kaypro II and Perfect Writer which made the second edition possible;

Regina, who so bravely wrestled and wrought with both me and herself, to make manifest in printed form our ideas;

And Hannelore Travis, my daughter, who proudly carried her own copy of the early 3-ring binder edition of the *Wellness Workbook* to 2nd grade almost every day.

—JWT

Heartful thanks go to:

My parents, Bernard and Helene Ryan, who have always held the crazy notion that their kids were smart and powerful, and could do anything they put their minds to;

My beautiful friend Ruth Sharon who so gently encouraged me to trust my feminine energy and to share it with my readers.

Liz Campbell and my AHP friends who loved and supported me, and held doors open all along the way;

Anita Jordan who celebrated my joy and pain throughout; Mike Richards and Don Barley who encouraged simple, straight talk about wellness and sex;

Barbara, Joy, and Annie of Wellness Associates who motivated us to hurry up and get the word out;

Lloyd Barde for musical inspiration and friendship all along the way;

Greg Pickernell, Jim Sharon, Jim Wing, Benjamin Marstellar, and especially Darla Grace for their assistance in research and the infinite details;

Terry Knob who typed the manuscript and was always so pleasant and available;

John Travis, my friend and co-author, who wouldn't let me give up;

George Young of Ten Speed Press, who believed in us; Jackie Wan, our amazing editor who never failed to find the needle in the haystack; Hal Hershey, our production coordinator; and Brenton Beck of Fifth Street Design Associates, who all labored with us through the birthing of our book;

Meryn Callander, who served us so generously in the work, and cared about me, personally;

My friends and students at Aims College, Greeley, Colorado, who taught me how to make wellness fun;

My teachers, Bhagwan Shree Rajneesh, Barry Tellman, and Lee Lozowick, who inspire me to caution that everything in this book may be wrong.

—RSR

. . . .

Wellness is a choice—a decision you make to move toward optimal health.

Wellness is a way of life—a lifestyle you design to achieve your highest potential for well-being.

Wellness is a process—a developing awareness that there is no end point, but that health and happiness are possible in each moment, here and now.

Wellness is an efficient channelling of energy—energy received from the environment, transformed within you, and sent on to affect the world outside.

Wellness is the integration of body, mind and spirit—the appreciation that everything you do, and think, and feel, and believe has an impact on your state of health.

Wellness is the loving acceptance of yourself.

. . . .

This book is about learning to love your whole self. It is about assuming charge of your own life, living in process, and channelling life energy. It is about choices. It is about the ONE WAY to wellness—YOUR WAY. This book is about you.

Introduction

What is Wellness?

WELLNESS IS THE right and privilege of everyone. There is no prerequisite for it other than your free choice. The "well" being is not necessarily the strong, the brave, the successful, the young, the whole, or even the illness-free being. A person can be living a process of wellness and yet be physically handicapped, aged, scared in the face of challenge, in pain, imperfect. No matter what your current state of health, you can begin to appreciate yourself as a growing, changing person and allow yourself to move toward a happier life and positive health.

Wellness is never a static state. You don't just get well or stay well. There are many degrees or levels of wellness, just as there are degrees of illness. Nor is wellness simply the absence of disease. While people often lack physical symptoms, they may still be bored, depressed, tense, anxious, or generally un-

He not busy being born is busy dying.

—BOB DYLAN

happy with their lives. These emotional states often set the stage for physical disease through the lowering of the body's resistance. The same feelings can also lead to abuses like smoking, drinking, and overeating. But these symptoms and behaviors represent only the tip of the iceberg. They are the surface indication of underlying human needs such as recognition from others, a stimulating environment, caring and affection from friends, and self-acceptance.

Diseases and symptoms are not really the problem. They are actually the body-mind's attempt to solve a problem—a message from the subconscious to the conscious.

Much of traditional medical practice is involved with chipping away at surface needs. Its orientation is toward the treatment and elimination of the evidence of disease, and this is important. But it is not enough. It is essential to look below the surface signs to address the real needs. Wellness extends the definition of health to encompass a process of awareness, education, and growth.

The Illness/Wellness Continuum (next page) illustrates the relationship between the traditional medical model (or any other symptom-treatment system) and the wellness model, which is based on self-responsibility.

Moving toward high-level wellness will involve the three steps of awareness, education, and growth (p. xviii). This book is designed to get you moving. In each chapter, there are exercises to help you in self-evaluation, in the awareness of what is working, or not working, in your life right now. Then there is material offered to assist you in your self-education. Some of it comes from others who have studied, and lived it for a time. Much of

Key Concept #1:

Wellness is a process,
never a static state.

Illness/Wellness Continuum

Wellness Model

PRE-
MATURE   Disability Symptoms Signs   Awareness Education Growth   HIGH
DEATH   LEVEL
                                                                       WELLNESS

Treatment Model

Neutral Point
(No discernible illness or wellness)

©1972 John W. Travis, M.D.

Moving from the center to the left shows a progressively worsening state of health. Moving to the right of center indicates increasing levels of health and well-being. The treatment model can bring you to the neutral point, where the symptoms of disease have been alleviated. The wellness model, which can be utilized at any point, directs you beyond neutral, and encourages you to move as far to the right as possible. It is not meant to replace the treatment model on the left side of the continuum, but to work in harmony with it. If you are ill, then treatment is important, but don't stop there.

The Illness/Wellness Continuum pictured here was first developed by John in 1972. It was an immediate success, an easy way to illustrate what this newly emerging "wellness concept" was all about. Health practitioners and educators began using it and soon it was appearing in books, journals, and slide presentations everywhere. We naturally included it in the first edition of this book, and will continue to do so because of its representational value.

However, a simple model cannot always convey a complex concept. And for a number of years we have recognized that this continuum could be misleading in one very significant area. Namely, we think it is quite possible to be physically ill and still be oriented towards

ILLNESS/WELLNESS CONTINUUM

wellness, or physically healthy and still be functioning from an illness mentality. Yet the model didn't immediately allow for this distinction. For example, imagine a disabled, sick, or dying person who is taking responsibility for his/her life and is consciously engaged in the experience. While they would fall on the left side of the continuum if only the physical dimension were considered, they would definitely be on the right side if emotional, intellec-tual, spiritual dimensions were fully taken into account. It then occurred to us that regardless of what point on the continuum a person might assign to them-selves, *what mattered most was which direction they were facing* —towards High Level Wellness, or towards Premature Death.

Think of the continuum as a pathway. People can be walking in either direction on the path. A person who is physically in good health, but always com-plaining or worrying might be standing to the right of the neu-tral point, but definitely facing towards the left—towards Pre-mature Death. Similarly, an-other person whose body is in pain, or who is handicapped physically or mentally, can still have a genuinely positive/ opti-mistic outlook, be cultivating love instead of fear, and conse-quently would be facing to the right in the direction of High Level Wellness.

it is a reminder of what you already know, but may have avoided or forgotten. In addition each chapter includes growth options—suggestions of alternatives, invitations to stretch your limits, permission to risk, encouragement to change.

The *Wellness Workbook* is an invitation to you to consider illness and health in a bigger context, that of your connection with other people, as well as with the entire planet. As we understand it, health is a result of a dynamic energy exchange between the individual and everything in creation. People cannot live well while remaining isolated from other people and things around them. We are interdependent elements in a living system. When any part is ill or healthy, it necessarily affects the energy, and changes the health, of the whole.

We think this understanding is so basic to an appreciation of wellness that we've built the entire structure and content of this book on it. So let's begin by exploring our foundation. Let's talk about energy.

About Energy

Life is a continual dance of energy. Literally everything that we know, including this realization itself, is

- - - - - - - - - - - - - - - - - - -

No Fascism Please!

I'm sometimes alarmed by a kind of "neo-fascism" that I see in the holistic health movement. Peer pressure and covert or overt means are applied to get people to adhere to a particular lifestyle. There are "nutrition nuts" who want everyone to take high doses of a particular supplement or go on a certain diet. There are runners who want to make marathoners out of everyone. There are meditators who want everyone to meditate their way. Health becomes equated with a certain set of behaviors or practice, and pressure is applied to make people conform to the group norm.

While I want to get my message across, I do not want to be looked on as the expert dictating the one true way; I do not want to become part of the neo-fascism. The wellness paradigm calls for options, individuality, and choices freely made.

—J.W.T.

- - - - - - - - - - - - - - - - - - -

energy in one of its many forms and expressions.

Nearly all of our physical energy comes to us from the sun. Follow a bundle of sunbeams from their source across 93 million miles of space until they reach the earth's atmosphere. Observe their progress when they get here and you'll have a better idea of what energy transformation is all about.

As they near the surface of the earth, sunbeams warm the atmosphere, and weather is born. Winds are created, waters move, and the planet is sculpted. This is only the beginning.

Some of our sunbeams are captured by hungry green plants and put to work to grow new shoots or leaves. Carbohydrates—food—ready to satisfy the first lucky cow who happens along. The process continues. Cow eats grass and manufactures milk. Child drinks milk, grows big and strong. Big, strong adult takes a walk, or dreams a dream, cries over a silly movie, builds a monument, or makes a baby . . . and all essentially powered by sunbeams. Amazing! This is the simple magic that creates life as we know it. It's all energy dancing!

Key Concept #2:

Illness and health are only the tip of an iceberg.
To understand their causes, you must look below the surface.

The Iceberg Model

ICEBERGS ARE INTERESTING! They reveal only about one-tenth of their mass above the water. The remaining nine-tenths remain submerged. This is why they are such a nightmare in navigation; and why they make such an appropriate metaphor in considering your state of wellness.

Your current state of health—be it one of disease, or vitality—is just like the tip of the iceberg. This is the apparent part—what shows. If you don't like it, you can attempt to change it, "do things" to it, chisel away at an unwanted condition. But, whenever you knock some off, more of the same comes up to take its place.

To understand all that creates and supports your current state of health, you have to look "underwater." The first level you encounter is the Lifestyle/Behavioral level—what you eat, how you use and exercise your body, how you relax and let go of stress, and how you safeguard yourself from the hazards around you.

Many of us follow lifestyles that we know are destructive, both to our own well-being and to that of our planet. Yet, we may feel powerless to change them. To understand why, we must look still deeper, to the Psychological/Motivational level. Here we find what moves us to lead the lifestyle we've chosen. We can learn, for example, what payoffs we get from being overweight, smoking, driving recklessly, or from eating well, being considerate of others, and getting regular exercise.

Exploring below the Psychological/ Motivational level, we encounter the Spiritual/Being/Meaning level. Other descriptors here may include: transpersonal, philosophical, or metaphysical. Actually, we prefer to call it a realm rather than a level because it has no clear boundaries. It includes the mystical and mysterious, and everything else in the unconscious mind, and concerns such issues as your reason for being, the real meaning of your life, or your place in the universe. How you address these questions, and the answers you choose, underlie and permeate all of the layers above. Ultimately, this realm determines whether the tip of the iceberg, representing your state of health, is one of disease or wellness.

Cultural Norms and the Iceberg Model

Robert F. Allen, Ph.D., the founder of the Human Resources Institute in Morristown, New Jersey, pioneered an approach to wellness (long before the word was in common use) through the identification of *cultural norms*.

Norms are beliefs and values generally accepted as true by the population as a whole. Mainstream thinking in Western medicine has traditionally considered the state of personal health (the area above the water in the Iceberg Model) as independent of the deeper levels. We disagree entirely.

You get sick, you go to the doctor and you get fixed—has long been the "American (Canadian, English, Australian…) Way." How you live your life before and after your bout with illness has little or nothing to do with your state of health. At least that's the illusion we've believed.

Many people now know that smoking, drinking alcohol, and other abusive behaviors affect their health. But the norms that condone public smoking or the use of a wide range of less-than-healthy products have been slow to change. You need only watch an hour of television, or peruse a single issue of a popular magazine, noting the types of products advertised, to verify this incongruency. Just try it, and then ask yourself: How many products are really necessities? How many are downright unhealthy? What lifestyles do these commercials or ads presume and promote? Do they fit my pictures of how life realistically is, or should be?

These advertisements are good indicators of our cultural norms.

The state of Florida recently enacted a law that establishes "nonsmoking" as the norm for all restaurants unless they specifically indicate that smoking areas are available. The positive implications of this legislation should not be underestimated. A precedent is being set for the entire country. A significant "illness norm" has been turned around. Cities and towns across the nation are taking similar action. Some, like Fort Collins, Colorado, are banning smoking in nearly all public places, unless special smoking sections are provided. Hopefully, by the time you read this, the shift will be even more widely observable.

The overwhelming power of advertising notwithstanding, greater and greater numbers of us are taking a stand and making a change. Since the mid-1970s, running and other forms of exercise and fitness have risen in popularity to the point of becoming something of a national obsession. Other behavior-change indicators, such as greater public awareness of food addictions and eating disorders, and a massive campaign against drinking and driving, are evident everywhere. We are, at long last, recognizing the implications that our lifestyle activities (the Behavioral level of the Iceberg Model) have on our overall state of health. As a culture, we are finally admitting that there just may be something "below the surface."

Turning to the Psychological/Motivational level (one layer deeper in the Iceberg Model), we also find a number of very positive signs that this level is being connected with our state of health. Witness the discussion topics on the extremely popular Phil Donahue Show, for example, or the bulging shelves in the Psychology or Self-Help sections of your local bookstore. We need less convincing that our feelings and thoughts are making us sick at least as often as germs are. We're not so dumb!

Those who study the culture, as Bob Allen and his associates do, generally agree that the norms themselves usually lag years behind what the majority of people secretly think. This "lowest common denominator" effect serves to maintain the "public mind" at a level which is acceptable to everyone, even if most of us actually think it is outmoded and inadequate. Fear is often the motivator here. Quite commonly people do not realize that their progressive beliefs are also shared by a wider segment of society. Coming together in settings like seminars and workshops on wellness, where it is acceptable to discuss such values openly, has served to amaze participants and professionals alike. When people discover just how widespread their "unconventional beliefs" about illness truly are, they are relieved and positively empowered. In the political arena, the same effect is often demonstrable. Major segments of the population in countries throughout the world are opposed to nuclear arms buildup, and the insane policies of Mutually Assured Destruction, which nuclear war guarantees. Yet, leaders of government are often afraid even to speak out, let alone act, against the supposed lowest common denominator of the cultural norm.

The last major area to achieve cultural acceptability, especially in Western societies where science and technology are revered as the gods of progress, is the Spiritual/Being/Meaning level of the Iceberg. Even this is changing. When we wrote the first edition of the *Wellness Workbook* in 1980, we were hesitant to use the word "spiritual." Instead, we opted for "philosophical" and "transpersonal" in labeling this portion of our model. The term "spiritual" was, we thought, too often confused with either the hocus pocus of occultism, or with formal religion, and we meant neither. To us, "spirit" is something much deeper and all-pervasive, and certainly not confined to one set of doctrines, experiences, or forms. Spirit, for us, means a connection with everything in creation; an animating force; the principle of unification; the shared consciousness of the one body of life. Religion, we believe, is simply one form of expressing this awareness. As such, its importance must not be undervalued.

Our experience is that we are far from alone in "coming out of the closet" with our acknowldgement of the spiritual nature of being. We feel a growing hunger in ourselves, and sense the same in the people we encounter in our work, for understanding and expression of this level of reality. No longer satisfied with the testimony of professional witnesses, like priests, ministers, and rabbis, we want to experience the spirit first hand, and integrate it into all aspects of our lives. Perhaps there is a peaceful revolution in the making. Perhaps, even sooner than we think, we will see the upgrading of the lowest common denominator in this area as well.

Within or without formal religion, we believe that attunement to "spirit" (the foundational level in the Iceberg Model) is the ultimate source of well-being. Furthermore, we suggest that wellness as a way of life orients one toward greater awareness of communion with this source. These are assertions not easily explainable with words or grasped by the rational mind. In the realm of the spirit, one must read and lead more often with the heart. (See chapter 11, Finding Meaning, and chapter 12, Transcending.)

. . . . *Exercise* . . . .

Questioning Your Cultural Norms

(from Dr. Robert Allen's *Cultural Norm Indicator*)

Respond to these questions here, or in your journal.

It is a norm in one or more groups that I belong to:

1. For people to use their cars to go short distances even when there is no need to do so;

2. For people to be surprised when someone uses the stairs instead of the elevator or escalator;

3. For people not to mention it if someone else's smoking bothers them;

4. For people to take on more responsibility than they can handle;

5. For people to look at being slightly overweight as "natural," particularly among older people;

6. For people to drink a great many coffee and cola drinks and other caffeine-based beverages;

7. To persuade guests to stay for one more round of drinks or "one more for the road";

8. For waiters and waitresses and others in restaurants to "expect" that people will be having a drink before or during dinner;

9. For people not to see themselves as being as capable as they really are.

Used With Permission: from *Lifegain*, by Robert F. Allen with Shirley Linde, Human Resources Institute, Morristown, NJ, 1981.

. . . .

The Wellness Energy System

In 1977, Ilya Prigogene won a Nobel Prize for his theory of dissipative structures.[1] Dissipative structures are open systems in which energy is taken in, modified (transformed), and then returned (dissipated) to the environment. A rock or a cold cup of coffee are closed systems because they do not channel and transform energy in this way. A seed, which constructs a plant from soil, air, and light, is an open system. So is a town, one of Prigogene's favorite examples. Raw materials are sent to factories where they are shaped. Manufactured goods are then sent out into the world. Information is sent into schools; "educated minds" are released to make their impact on the world.

A human being is an open system, too. We take in energy from all the sources around us, organize it, transform it, and return (dissipate) it to the environment around us. The underlying theory in this book is that *efficient flow of energy is essential to wellness; disease is the result of any interference with this flow*. This is true of energy usage in all life processes, from breathing to dying.

Think of yourself as a conduit of energy—energy flowing in, coursing around, and flowing out. And because you are different from every other "channel" walking around, it goes without saying that your condition (physical, emotional, mental, spiritual) is going to determine how much you take in, what it feels like inside, and how it moves out into the environment. When the flow is balanced and smooth, you feel good. When there is interference at any point—the input, the output, or in-between—you can feel empty, pressured, or blocked. Illness is often the result.

The process may be compared to the movement of water through a pipe (Fig. 1). The source of the water, the reservoir, constitutes the *input*. The size and condition of the pipe will determine the *flow-through*. The water that emerges at the other end, from your faucet for instance, is the *output*. Ideally, it looks like this.

Experience tells us, however, that many things could go wrong. There could be problems at the source—the reservoir may be dry because of a long drought (Fig. 2); the water might be poisoned by industrial wastes (Fig. 3).

There may be problems in the pipe itself. There could be a leak; the pipe might be blocked by accumulated debris (Fig. 4); it could be rusty. Whatever the problem, it is obvious that the amount and the quality of water at the faucet, the *output*, will be seriously affected. Overuse, due to extreme need, such as putting out a huge fire, may quickly deplete the input source. Lack of use, on the other hand, may cause the water in the pipes to freeze in cold weather, or stagnate and discolor as it sits in the channel. These examples highlight interdependent systems in which changes in one part impact the other parts in some way, and affect the operation of the whole system in general.

Keep these realizations in mind now as we look at an Energy System for wellness of the human being. You have at least three major sources for *input* around you all the time (Fig. 5). These are: (1) oxygen, (2) food, (3) sensory stimulation such as physical touch, heat, light, sound, and other forms of electromagnetic radiation. In addition there are the less tangible inputs: emotional/spiritual energy such as attention, caring, love, enthusiasm, and extra-sensory data.

You are the *conduit,* or the transformer of these energy sources. In the waterpipe analogy, the flow-through is dependent on the shape, diameter, and composi-

Fig. 1. *Normal Conduit for Water (Representing Energy)*

Fig. 2. *Dry Reservoir*

Fig. 3. *Contaminated Water*

Fig. 4. *Blocked Conduit*

tion of the pipe. For the human organism the list of modifiers of energy is much greater. Your sex, blood type, the pigmentation of your skin, and other racial characteristics are your genetic inheritance and there isn't much you can do about them. Over other conditions, however, you have much more voluntary control. These include: education and beliefs, previous experience, the activity of your nervous system, flexibility, strength, body weight, emotional development, muscle tension, general state of health, and functioning of organs. The less measurable

factors of sensitivity, open-mindedness, and self-love are also up to you.

We use part of the energy we take in to maintain the pathway—to build and repair the body itself. This is the *internal-output*. At the most elementary level we use energy to maintain a narrow, internal temperature range (around 98.6° F/ 37° C), as circulating blood brings heat to cold areas. We secrete digestive juices for breakdown and absorption of food. We synthesize chemicals which are sent to many different organs. We produce electrochemical impulses which travel

throughout the nervous system. Taking a step up in this energy transformation process, we replace worn tissue and blood cells—repairing cuts and scratches, and mending bones. We move muscles which control digestion, respiration, elimination, and reproduction. And don't forget those less tangible expressions of energy—the generation of emotions, the internal dialogue of your thinking processes, your intuition, dreams, and the creation of what may be spiritual insights and altered states of consciousness.

Fig. 5.   Wellness Energy System (Input)

The outside world will also be affected by the ways you transform and return energy to it (Fig. 6). This is the external output. You radiate heat, eliminate waste products in the form of urine, perspiration, carbon dioxide, and the shedding of dead skin. The rest of us will be affected by your touching, your physical work and play, your laughter and tears. We will learn about you, and ourselves, through communication, the sharing of intellectual pursuits, and the expression of creativity. You can't help but influence the planet by your interaction with the environment. Less understood energy communications such as intuition, telepathy, and other psychic phenomena may be taking place as well. And there is no doubt that your loving energy will change us all.

Fig. 6.   Wellness Energy System (Output)

Key Concept #3:

We are energy transformers, connected with the whole universe. All our life processes, including illness depend on how we manage energy.

Putting together the input and output we have the complete Wellness Energy System of a human being (Fig. 7).

Fig. 7. Wellness Energy System (Complete)

Please note that each arrow corresponds to an entire chapter of this book.

Since there are many of us, and we are all interacting and exchanging energy with each other and everything else in our environment, the picture gets more complex (Fig. 8). Try looking at the world around you as composed not of separate fixed *things,* but as structures reflecting the energy which creates them—a vast dance with myriads of participants.

Fig. 8. Wellness Energy System (Individual and Environment Interacting)

We have shown an idealized model of wellness based on a balanced exchange of energy. But the world is not a perfect place. Like the clogged, contaminated or empty pipes above, we have distortions which lead to imbalances in the ways we process energy. Fig. 9 shows six possible distortions of energy which human beings might develop: 1) Insufficient intake of energy; for example, denying acknowledgment or compliments from other people. 2) Too much of one form of energy; for example, too much food and not enough breathing. 3) An intermingling, contamination or substitution of one form of energy with another; for example, an attempt to use sex to satisfy a spiritual hunger. 4) Blockage causing an internal buildup of unprocessed energy; for example, fear of open communication with others leading to a censoring of one's behavior out of fear about what others might be thinking (co-dependency). 5) Too strong an interface with the environment; for example, an abrasive, explosive way of relating to people, which discourages further interaction. 6) Too weak an interface with the environment; for example, an unfocused diffusion of energy, which shows up as a wishy-washy approach to people and commitments.

These six examples do not cover all the possibilities, but they do graphically show some of the possible distortions of energy that can lead to illness.

A simpler way of representing how well your energy is balanced is the Wellness Wheel (Fig. 10), which you shortly will complete as a part of the Wellness Index (next section). Each of the twelve sections of the wheel corresponds to one of the arrows in the Wellness Energy System (and to one of the remaining chapters of this book). Each section

Fig. 9. Wellness Energy System (Distortions)

1) Insufficient Flow of Energy
2) Too Much of One Type of Energy
3) Contamination—Intermingling of Energy
4) Blockage of Energy
5) Poor Interface of Energy with Environment (Explosive)
6) Poor Interface of Energy with Environment (Ineffective)

represents one slice of this whole pie called wellness.

Your complete wheel will allow you to see which areas of your life are in need of attention. This simpler representation of your personal energy system does not show as graphically as Fig. 9 what specific problems you may encounter in your own energy economy. It does, however, give a good overall picture of how balanced or unbalanced your system is. For a deeper understanding of any problems, you will need to look back at the questions in the Wellness Index whose low or high scores led to the imbalanced-looking summary.

In the five hypothetical examples which follow we have attempted to show some of the practical applications of using the Wellness Energy System to assess and help guide us in directions we may want to take in our lives. To test your understanding of the concept, imagine how the actual distortions of each person's arrows might look.

In summary, we have shown how the Wellness Energy System is our alternative to the usual piecemeal way of looking at health. We offer an integrated overview of all human life functions, seeing them as various forms of energy. The har-

monious balancing of these life functions results in good health and well-being.

The Wellness Energy System is our alternative to the usual piecemeal way of looking at health. We offer an integrated overview of all human life functions, seeing them as various forms of energy. The harmonious balancing of these life functions results in good health and well-being.

Taken together as a whole, our picture can be no smaller than the whole planet (Fig. 11).

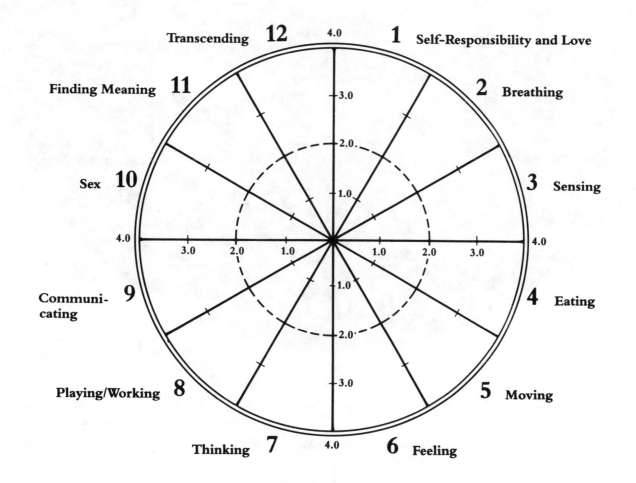

Fig. 10. Wellness Energy System Represented as Wellness Wheel

Fig. 11. Wellness Energy System (Global)

Here are some hypothetical examples of people we, as wellness facilitators, might encounter, and how we use the Wellness Energy System as a guide to understanding their lives.

Example #1—Homer:

"My job as an accountant is a sedentary one, and I am not inclined to exercise. Thus the low score on the movement dimension. Since I was a kid I have always been the fat guy, and now I am about forty pounds over-weight, and I hate it. No matter how much I eat, I never really feel satisfied. But I feel so guilty when I eat because I hate being so fat. I know people make jokes about me when I walk down the street, and even the people in my office aren't inclined to include me in things. I think they're joking about me too. Sometimes I try to join the joke by making fun of myself, but actually it hurts me a lot. I don't have many friends, and don't think I'll ever find a woman who would want to be with me."

Our Comments: Since Homer has gotten very little positive attention in his life, he has a very low self-esteem. He is generally acknowledged by others in negative ways because of his appearance, and he attempts unsuccessfully to fill his inner void by over-eating for which he subsequently feels guilty. This provides him with a continuous built-in source of negative self-talk. He discourages people from reaching out to him, and puts down any positive strokes offered because he doesn't believe he is worthy of them. This further discourages people from exchanging good energy with him because it seems to disappear into a black hole. He is probably headed for diabetes or heart disease and will die a lonely man unless he chooses to take charge of his life.

Recommendations: Working on a diet would only be the tip of the iceberg for Homer. More than anything he needs a support system, and a heightened awareness of communication skills, both intrapersonal and

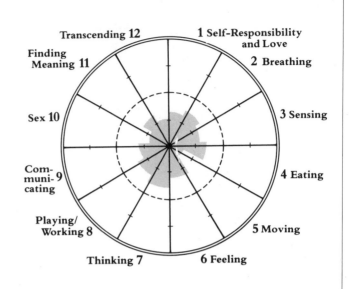

Example #1 — *Homer*

interpersonal. It is essential for him to get the connection between his negative self-talk and the results created in his life. An abundance of positive attention is available from other people in his environment if only he did not exclude that possibility. Homer would profit from a weight control group that deals with deeper issues, or another type of support group that encourages self-appreciation and allows him the opportunity to receive from others. The wellness dimensions that should be addressed first and most strongly are: Self-Responsibility and Love, and Communicating.

Example #2—Kathryn:

"I see from my chart what I've already known too well. I am unhappy in working/playing basically because I don't do either one to my satisfaction. I am a homemaker, and most of the time I feel overwhelmed by that, so there's little energy for anything else. My mood swings are outrageous. Often I get nearly hysterical over the slightest thing, but when it comes to telling other people what I want or even what I think, I can't open my mouth. My relationship with my husband Chuck is the greatest thing in my life, but

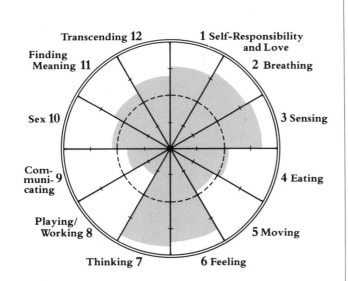

Example #2 — *Kathryn*

lately I lie awake at night worrying about what I would ever do if he died. Doing the Transcending and Finding Meaning sections of this evaluation I recall how hungry I am for a deeper understanding of God in my life."

Our Comments: Kathryn's overdeveloped emotional responses are largely a result of a small "backyard"—her unwillingness to extend herself beyond a very limited range of activities. She rarely exercises, and consequently her energy fails to circulate in a balanced way. Also, her diet includes much caffeine and sugar, both of which contribute to mood swings. Failure to ask for what she wants and needs only bottles up anger and sets the stage for more serious depression and physical disease (like arthritis or cancer). Her excessive dependence on her relationship with her husband serves to keep her from developing herself in many ways. She is a bright and gifted woman who undervalues herself greatly. Her desire for God may partially be another way of letting somebody else be responsible for her.

Recommendations: Kathryn's initial wellness endeavors should focus on the Feel-

ing and Moving domains. She needs to learn healthy ways to express her angers and fears, and to develop more outlets for her energy. Dance, really energetic dance, would be a good start. She is a strong and powerful being, and anything that would remind her of this should be advantageous. An assertiveness training course, and other adult education courses would be important vehicles to expand her "backyard."

Example #3—Bob:

"I am forty-five years old and beating guys ten years younger than me. I run at least six miles a day, take long-distance bicycle trips on the weekends, and am building strength and endurance. My work is so stressful that if I didn't do this much exercise I'd be dead. I lost one job in the past year, and now have to work three times as hard, for less pay, to create a space for myself in this new company. I still make a good salary but like everyone else, always want more. My marriage is tolerable, although we don't really communicate with each other. We love our son very much.

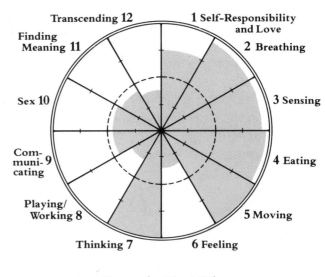

Example #3 — *Bob*

Sex is a joke. My wife has to get drunk before she'll let me touch her. She goes to counseling about this, but it doesn't help much. I know we should go together for help, but I simply do not have the time."

Our Comments: Bob's Wellness Wheel is so imbalanced that one would think he was actually two people. He scores "off the charts" in the Moving section, and his diet is an exceptionally healthy one, although his eating habits are poor. His motivation at work, and his drive for success are phenomenal, but the cost is very high. Bob is almost dead in so many other arenas of life because he has "put all his eggs" so completely into one basket. Bob can probably maintain this imbalanced life-style almost indefinitely if his wife stays around. He is emotionally unavailable to her as well as to himself. His only outlet for the expression of love is towards his son, but even here he has not allowed himself to admit how important this relationship is. Bob admits to a *belief* in self-responsibility but *feels* that his emotional needs are not being met because of his wife's sexual hang-ups.

Recommendations: Bob's first order of business involves looking at Self-Responsibility with ruthless honesty, and then moving on to the exploration of Finding Meaning. He is running himself out-of-control because of misaligned priorities. He talks one thing, and walks another. Although his body is strong, it is also tremendously rigid due to years of emotional denial which have created a solid armor. We recommend weekly massage at least, or deeper body work (such as Rolfing) to help him realize some breakthroughs in his body. Bob needs to start seeing a counselor, with his wife, or alone, and the two need to share their emotional lives immediately. Unless he makes some serious decisions soon, Bob is setting a course towards a major crisis, probably the breakup of his marriage and loss of his son, in order to "wake himself up."

Example #4—Rebecca:

"I'm surprised and pleased at how much I have handled about my life, my wellness. What I see from my Wellness Wheel is that my work is still the area of greatest dissatisfaction. If only I didn't have to "make a living" I would be ecstatic. I can get by with very little, and like contributing my life in worthwhile ways with others. The future doesn't mean much to me. I think God will provide. But I do get scared now and again, when I think about getting old and not having support of some kind."

Our Comments: Rebecca knows exactly what she needs to do to develop herself work-wise, but her deeper questions are whether or not it's worth doing. Her attitudes are generally positive and her health reflects it. She struggles to understand her ultimate meaning and how to live with that, and this openness to the mystery keeps her flexible. She is extremely likeable because she gives others so much permission to be themselves. However, she is a perfectionist with herself, and this creates much of her insecurity and fear.

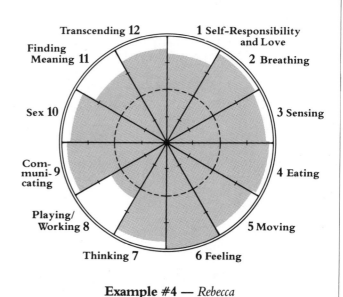

Example #4 — *Rebecca*

Recommendations: Because of her tendency to be ungrounded in practical concerns, Rebecca needs to develop working partnerships with people who will demand the focusing of her creative energy. Rebecca needs to see that even though she can do it all alone, and very well if she chooses to, she will have so much more fun investing the help of others. If she is not already doing so, Rebecca should be encouraged to do much more self-exploration through writing, perhaps keeping a journal. Since she is generally clear and honest about herself, this practice would be extremely valuable.

Example #5—Ramon:

"I just turned sixty this year and have never felt better. As you can see, however, my diet and eating habits are still not to my satisfaction. I want to be able to lose about fifteen pounds and keep it off, but all that sweating and aerobic stuff is not my thing either."

Our Comments: Like so many other people, Ramon knows what he should work on, but lacks the motivation to change because he is basically feeling good. He operates under the mistaken notion that exercise has to be painful if it is to be effective. Ramon is a well-balanced human being, despite a few slight problem areas.

Recommendations: The movement from awareness to action in any domain requires forgiveness of the past. Ramon is still holding

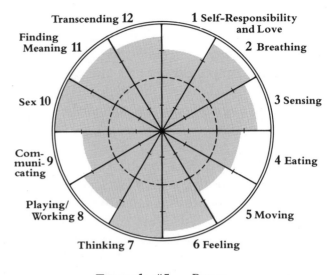

Example #5 — *Ramon*

his eating habits and lack of exercise as "bad." If he can see this, and live with an intention of self-acceptance for a while, without trying to change anything, it is very likely that the motivation he wants will begin to grow very naturally. He also ought to know that there are many ways to exercise besides jogging or similarly taxing sports. We suggest he start with a morning walk, while listening to music or inspiring talks on a tape recorder. The focus of his walk should be enjoyment only. With time, his desire to increase the exercise for conditioning value may emerge. Gentleness and self-appreciation will be his way through the initial resistance.

In oneself lies the whole world and if you know how to look and learn, then the door is there and the key is in your hand. Nobody on earth can give you either the key or the door to open except yourself.

—KRISHNAMURTI.

How Best to Use This Book

Now you are ready to study each of the twelve areas in greater depth. First we suggest you complete the *Wellness Index* which follows. It will help you assess how well you are balancing the twelve expressions of energy and raise questions for you to explore in your reading.

The twelve chapters of the book correspond to the twelve forms of energy. The sequence of chapters approximates the order in which these forms of energy develop in human beings. In each chapter we will discuss some possible problems and diseases caused by mismanaging that form of energy. We also suggest ways to optimize the expression of each form of energy. There is overlap, of course, and it is also fine to follow your strongest interests and read the chapters in any order you wish.

This book is not "nice." It does not provide ready answers. It takes you into unexpected places. It leaves you there. For logical thinkers, and that includes most of us, it will be a challenge. You may be surprised that the pages are not "neat." We have interspersed the factual text with exercises and personal examples. This may be upsetting to some people, but we think it's necessary. Our intent is to address the logical, verbal parts of you, as well as to invite your participation in nonlogical processes like intuition, creativity, and feelings. This book is addressed to the whole of you—whole-brain, whole-heart, whole-body, whole-soul. So, we want you to be prepared. We want you to put the *Wellness Workbook* to the best possible use for yourself, and have a great time doing so. Here are a few suggestions:

- Master the three keys. This sounds like a riddle. If you've read this far, the three keys are already in your hands. It remains for you to keep them and use them as you continue exploring the chapters that follow. The keys are the three graphic illustrations of wellness that have been elaborated upon in this chapter: 1) The Illness/Wellness Continuum, 2) The Iceberg Model, and most important of all, 3) The Wellness Energy System. If you don't clearly understand them, please refer back to them now.

- Expect more questions than answers. Alfred North White-

. . . . . .

Be patient toward all that is unsolved in your heart and try to love the questions themselves like locked rooms and like books that are written in a very foreign tongue . . . And the point is, to live everything. Live the questions now. Perhaps you will then gradually, without noticing it, live along some distant day into the answer.

—RAINER MARIA RILKE

. . . . . .

head, the philosopher, once said: "This generation has all the answers. It's the questions that we seek." We agree. If you finish reading a chapter and find yourself with more "whys" and "hows" than when you started, we will have done our job. The *Wellness Workbook* is not about herbal prescriptions, or vegetarian diets, or aerobic exercise regimens, even though some of these things are considered. Wellness is so much more. Wellness is about you, trusting your energy, and creating your unique and vibrant life in your own way. And that may take some serious question-asking.

- Stay active in the process. This is a workbook to be played with, not a novel to get lost in. Stay wide awake as you read by actively participating with us. Do the exercises. Keep lists of questions. Develop a personal Wellness Journal to chart your progress. Argue when you want to and write us a letter. We invite your interaction, your energy, your insights. It is important to

remember that wellness is a *process* and that once begun, this exploration is a lifelong adventure.

- Don't do it right. If there is one way to discourage learning of any kind it is to consciously attempt to avoid mistakes. We would like you to welcome them. If you're not making any in your life now, it's probably because you aren't taking any risks. It's time to venture forth. Use the *Wellness Workbook* as a jumping-off point for some new experimentation, self-reflection, reeducation, and let false starts and dead-ends be your friends and teachers. Expect nothing, but anticipate miracles.

Suggested Reading

Capra, F. *The Tao of Physics*. Boston, MA: Shambhala Press, 1975.

Ferguson, M. *The Aquarian Conspiracy*. Los Angeles, CA: J.P. Tarcher, 1980.

Russell, P. *Global Brain: Speculations on the Evolutionary Leap to Planetary Consciousness*. Los Angeles, CA: J.P. Tarcher, 1983.

Wolfe, F.A. *Taking the Quantum Leap*. New York, NY: Harper and Row, 1981.

Young, A. *The Reflexive Universe*. New York, NY: Delacorte Press, 1976.

Zukav, G. *The Dancing Wu Li Masters*. New York, NY: William Morrow and Co., 1979.

Notes

1. See: Ferguson, M. *The Aquarian Conspiracy*. Los Angeles, CA: J.P. Tarcher, 1980, pp. 163-69.

WELLNESS INDEX

We suggest that before proceeding any further with the book, you take time to complete the Wellness Index. It may raise many questions for you, and make the remaining chapters more meaningful.

We also suggest that you use one color of pen to record your answers as they are now, and then six months after completing the book, take the Index again using another color. Notice any changes that have occurred.

Individual copies of the *Wellness Index* may be obtained from the publisher:
Ten Speed Press, P.O. Box 7123, Berkeley, CA 94707
An abridged version and an interactive computer version are available from:
Wellness Associates, P.O. Box 5433, Mill Valley, CA 94942

Instructions:

Set aside time for yourself in a quiet place where you will not be disturbed while taking the Index. Allow one to two hours. Record your responses to each statement in the columns to the left where:

4 = Yes, always, or usually
3 = Often
2 = Sometimes, maybe
1 = Occasionally, rarely
0 = No, never, or hardly ever

Select the answer which best indicates how true the statement is for you at *this time*.

After you have responded to all the appropriate statements in each section, compute an average score from that section using the formula provided at the end of each section. Then transfer your average score from each section to the corresponding box provided around the Wellness Index Wheel at the end of the questionnaire.

Your completed wheel will give you a clear presentation of the balance you have given to the many dimensions of your life. If your wheel is not well balanced, or small in size, we urge you to study the corresponding areas in the *Wellness Workbook*. Begin with those that in-terest you most and take your wellness journey at a gradual pace. We caution against undertaking massive and sweeping life changes. Gentle, steady progress is much longer lasting.

You will find some of the statements are really two in one. We do this to show an important relationship between the two parts— usually an awareness of an issue, combined with an action based on that awareness:

I am aware of the importance of good nutrition, and eat accordingly.

If only one part of the statement is true, mentally average the sum of your answers to the two parts of the question and record that score. This way you won't get high scores for being aware of something, but doing nothing about it.

Many of the statements have further explanation in a footnote (marked with an asterisk). Where possible we have cited a page in the Wellness Workbook where more information can be found on the subject. (Due to space limitations, not every question is directly addressed in the text.)

Each statement describes what we believe to be a wellness attribute. Because much wellness information is subjective and "un-provable" by current scientific methods, you, (and possibly other authorities as well) may not agree with our conclusions. If an idea sounds strange to you, read any footnotes or page reference in the Wellness Workbook. We ask only that you keep an open mind until you have studied available information, then make up your mind.

This questionnaire was designed to educate more than to test. All statements are worded so that you can easily tell what we think are wellness attributes (which also makes it easy to "cheat" on your score). This means there can be no trick questions to test your honesty or consistency—the higher your score, the greater you believe your wellness to be. Full responsibility is placed on you to answer each statement as honestly as possible. It's not your score, but what you learn about yourself that counts in the end.

If you decide that a statement does not apply to you, or you don't want to answer it, you can skip it and not be penalized in your score.

The sentence completion portions at the end of some of the sections are optional, and your responses to them are not scored.

Example:

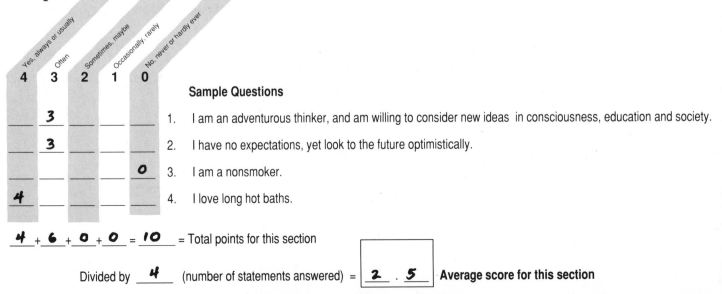

4	3	2	1	0	**Sample Questions**
	3				1. I am an adventurous thinker, and am willing to consider new ideas in consciousness, education and society.
	3				2. I have no expectations, yet look to the future optimistically.
				0	3. I am a nonsmoker.
4					4. I love long hot baths.

4 + **6** + **0** + **0** = **10** = Total points for this section

Divided by **4** (number of statements answered) = **2** . **5** **Average score for this section**

© 1975, 1981, 1988, John W. Travis, MD, not to be copied. (Bulk copies available)

4	3	2	1	0
Yes, always or usually	Often	Sometimes, maybe	Occasionally, rarely	No, never or hardly ever

Section 1—Wellness, Self-Responsibility and Love

1. I believe how I live my life is an important factor in determining my state of health, and I live it in a manner consistent with that belief.

2. I feel as though I am in charge of my life.*

3. I vote regularly.*

4. I take an active interest in community, national and world events.

5. I contribute time/money to support organizations, issues and people of my choice.

6. I know my neighbors.*

7. When I see a broken bottle or other hazard on a pathway or in the street, I remove it.

8. If I saw a crime being committed, or an emergency situation, I would do what I could to help.

9. When I see a car with faulty lights, leaking fuel, or other dangerous condition, I attempt to tell the driver.

10. I am an active member of community organizations, ie. social change group, singing group, church or political group.

11. I feel financially secure.

12. I use public transportation or car pools when possible.

13. I turn off unused lights and appliances.

14. I recycle paper, glass, aluminum, clothes, books, and organic waste.

15. I keep my living space at 68 F. (20 C.) or cooler in winter.

16. In summer I use air conditioning only when necessary and keep the temperature at 77 F. (25 C.) or higher.

17. I conserve materials/energy at home and at work.

18. My car gets at least 30 miles per gallon (13km/liter).

19. My house has adequate insulation, and if I live in a cold climate, storm windows. (Skip this question if you live in climates which require minimal heating or cooling.)

20. I use a humidifier with my home heating (skip if you don't have central heating.)*

21. I protect my living area from fire and safety hazards.

22. I keep a dry chemical fire extinguisher in my kitchen and at least one other extinguisher elsewhere in my living quarters.

23. I generate less than one garbage can full of trash per month.*

24. My domestic energy use (electricity, gas, fuel oil, kerosene, wood and/or coal) costs on the average less than $50/month *per person.**

25. I use dental floss and a soft toothbrush daily.

26. I smoke fewer than 1 pack of cigarettes or 5 cigars/10 pipes per week (nonsmokers take 4 points on this and the next question).

27. I am a nonsmoker.

28. I am always sober when driving or operating dangerous machinery.

4	3	2	1	0

Yes, always or usually — 4
Often — 3
Sometimes, maybe — 2
Occasionally, rarely — 1
No, never or hardly ever — 0

29. I abstain from drugs (prescription or non-prescription) that affect my mental alertness, when driving or operating dangerous machinery.

30. I wear a safety belt when I ride in a vehicle.

31. I maintain any smog equipment or safety devices installed on my car.

32. I stay within 5 miles (or 10 km) per hour of the speed limit.

33. I regularly inspect my automobile's tires, lights, brake fluid level, etc., and keep it well serviced.

34. I drive on belted radial tires.

35. I carry emergency flares/reflectors, and a dry chemical fire extinguisher in my car.

36. I stop on yellow when a traffic light is changing.

37. For every 10 miles per hour (15 km/hr) I maintain at least one car length of distance from any vehicle ahead.

38. I have fewer than three colds per year.

39. I avoid exposure to sprays, chemical fumes, or exhaust gases.

40. I purchase cleaning products and cosmetics only from manufacturers that do not test them for toxicity on animals in cruel ways.*

41. I am aware of any changes which occur in my physical or emotional state and would seek professional advice about any problems which seem unusual.

42. I can strongly influence my rate of recovery from an illness or injury.

43. I understand the difference between blaming myself for a problem and simply taking responsibility (ability to respond) for that problem.

44. I use any physical symptoms I might experience as messages to alter my behavior/attitude.

45. If the above is true, I do so without feeling guilt for "causing" the problem.

46. I believe I am responsible (able to respond) for every aspect of my life, even if I am not aware of how I may have created a problem.

47. I experience love for many people and aspects of my life.

48. I try out and evaluate new or different methods of self care.

49. When seeking help with a health problem, I work with physicians or healers as consultants rather than unquestioningly following their instructions.

50. I exercise compassion towards myself when I fall short of my own expectations.*

51. Rather than hold a grudge, I do my best to thoughtfully communicate my feelings and forgive those whom I feel may have wronged me in some way.*

52. I make efforts towards reconciliation with those from whom I feel estranged.*

Women only:

53. I check my breasts for unusual lumps each month.

54. I have a pap test at intervals appropriate for my age.*

Men only:

55. If over 45, I have my prostate checked annually.

©1975, 1981, 1988, John W. Travis, MD. Not to be copied. (Bulk copies available)

© 1975, 1981, 1988, John W. Travis, MD, Not to be copied. (Bulk copies available)

4	3	2	1	0
Yes, always or usually	Often	Sometimes, maybe	Occasionally, rarely	No, never or hardly ever

Parents: *(skip those that are not appropriate for the age of your children):*

56. When riding in a car, I make certain that any child weighing *fewer* than 50 pounds, (23 kg.) is secured in an approved child's safety seat or safety harness.*

57. When riding in a car, I make certain that any child weighing *greater* than 50 pounds, (23 kg.) is wearing an adult seatbelt.*

58. I store cleaning products/toxic products in locked cabinets or out of the possible reach of small children.

59. When leaving my child(ren) in another's care, I make certain their safety standards meet mine, and that they have emergency telephone numbers readily available.

60. I keep any medications, firearms, or other dangerous equipment locked in compartments away from childrens' reach.

61. My children wear firm shoes with laces tied snugly when riding on escalators.*

62. I prepare my own baby food (with a blender, etc.) rather than use commercially sold products high in salt, sugar, and preservatives.

63. I am aware of the benefits of breast feeding and am breastfeeding any infant I currently have.

64. I seek out useful parenting information and continuously increase my parenting skills.

65. I frequently touch or hold my children.

66. I feed my children fruits or healthy snacks instead of high-sugar/overprocessed junk foods.

67. My child is physically fit.

68. I encourage my child to explore the world and exercise his/her creativity.

69. My children freely talk with me about sex, drugs and other intimate issues.

70. My children respect the limits/guidelines I set for them (hours away from home, quality of study time, etc.)

71. I respect my child as a complete human being at all stages of her/his growth.

____ + ____ + ____ + ____ = _____ = Total points for this section

Divided by _____ (number of statements answered) = |___ . ___| **Average score for this section**
(Transfer to the Wellness Index Wheel on summary page)

Notes: Section 1 (For more information see Chapter 1, *Wellness Workbook*)

2. If you experience assistance from a source beyond yourself, so much the better!

3. Voting is a simple measure of your willingness to participate in the social system which ultimately impacts your state of health.

6. A sense of belonging to your community is an important aspect of wellness, and as Neighborhood Watch programs have shown, can be a deterrent to crime as well.

20. You will feel warmer in humidified air even at lower temperatures. Higher humidity also prevents many respiratory illnesses, and you don't have to water your plants as much.

23. Besides recycling glass, paper, aluminum, etc, if you purchase products which are reusable rather than disposable, and are packaged with a minimum of material, you will reduce the drain of resources and the toxic load on the environment caused by the disposal of these wastes.

24. Becoming conscious of your personal energy useage can reduce the amount of waste and offset the present negative planetary energy balance. The figure suggested is only approximate because of the differences in climate and energy cost in different areas.

25. After age 12, most teeth are lost, not from decay, but from periodontal disease—easily prevented by proper flossing and using a soft brush with rounded tip bristles.

40. Most testing is no longer necessary, as data on basic ingredients are readily available. Many companies, recognizing the rights of others species, now use only these ingredients, thereby avoiding the torture of countless laboratory animals.

50, 51, 52. There is growing evidence that the inability to forgive yourself or others leads to a higher incidence of cancer.

54. Most sources recommend every five years between age 25-55; more often if 1) history of herpes or venereal warts, 2) mother who took DES, 3) smoking more than 12 pack-yrs 4) intercourse before age 17, or with more than 3 partners. Consult your physician.

56, 57. In the US over 1000 children a year are killed by careless parents who do not use adequate safety restraints. Adult seatbelts are lethal to children under 50 lbs.

61. Every year escalators mangle the feet of thousands of bare footed children, or injure them by cutting through canvas shoes when loosely tied laces get caught at the end of the escalator.

4	3	2	1	0	
Yes, always or usually	Often	Sometimes, maybe	Occasionally, rarely	No, never or hardly ever	

Section 2—Wellness and Breathing

1. I stop during the day to become aware of the way I am breathing.

2. My normal breathing is deep and regular rather than shallow and erratic.

3. I wear comfortable clothing which does not bind my waist, chest, or throat.

4. I sit in a relaxed, upright position with my spine relatively straight.

5. When ill, I pay special attention to breathing and to visualizing healing of the problem area of my body.

6. I meditate or relax myself for at least 15 (to 20) minutes each day.

7. I am limber when I awaken in the morning.

8. I can easily touch my hands to my toes when standing with knees straight.*

9. My *hands* are free of perspiration or clamminess except during hot weather or strenuous work.*

10. My *feet* are free of perspiration or clamminess except during hot weather or strenuous work.*

11. In temperatures over 70 F. (21 C.), my **fingers** feel warm when I touch my lips.*

12. In temperatures over 70 F. (21 C.), my **feet** feel warm to the touch.*

13. I am satisfied with my abilities to relax.

14. If under 45 years of age, my forehead does not have deep wrinkles.*

15. My nails are healthy and I do not bite or pick at them.

16. I enjoy my work and do not find it overly stressful.

17. My personal relationships are satisfying.

18. I take time out for deep breathing several times a day.

19. I have plenty of energy.

20. I enjoy what I do to manage my stress.

21. I am at peace with myself.

22. I get adequate sleep and awake refreshed.

23. When I am tense, angry, or upset I take several deep breaths and feel myself relax.

____ + ____ + ____ + ____ = _____ = Total points for this section

Divided by _____ (number of statements answered) = ____ . ____ **Average score for this section**
(Transfer to the Wellness Index Wheel on summary page)

Notes: Section 2 (For more information see Chapter 2, *Wellness Workbook*)

8. A lack of spinal flexibility is usually a symptom of chronic muscle tension as well as indicative of a poor balance of physical activities.

9, 10. Constantly moist hands or feet often indicate excessive anxiety manifesting through your sympathetic nervous system.

11, 12. If hand or foot temperature is below 85 F. (30 C.) in a warm room, you're cutting off circulation to them via an overactive sympathetic nervous system. You can learn to warm your hands with biofeedback and to thereby better relax.

14. With age (accelerated by cigarette smoking) your skin reveals any constant stresses on it from tense muscles. To learn what anxiety creates the wrinkle patterns, make the wrinkles while looking in a mirror and notice what you feel.

©1975, 1981, 1988, John W. Travis, MD. Not to be copied. (Bulk copies available)

Yes, always or usually
Often
Sometimes, maybe
Occasionally, rarely
No, never or hardly ever

4	3	2	1	0

Section 3—Wellness and Sensing

1. My place of work has largely natural lighting or full spectrum fluorescent lighting.*

2. I avoid using sunglasses except in extreme glare.*

3. If I wear glasses, my lenses are the special full-spectrum type and not tinted.*

4. I avoid extremely noisy areas or wear protective ear covers.*

5. I take long walks, hikes or other outings to actively explore my surroundings.

6. I give myself presents, treats or nurture myself in other ways.

7. I enjoy getting, and can acknowledge, compliments and recognition from others.

8. It is easy for me to give sincere compliments and recognition to other people.

9. At times I like to be alone.

10. I enjoy touching or hugging other people.*

11. I enjoy being touched or hugged by others.*

12. I get and enjoy backrubs or massages.

13. I honor the changes of the seasons by listening to my body's response to temperature, varying lengths of daylight, changes in vegetation, etc.*

14. I am aware of what quarter (phase) the moon is in today.*

For the next statements, quickly complete the sentence with the first thoughts/feelings which come to mind.

15. Sights in my environment are _____.

16. Sounds in my environment are _____.

17. Smells in my environment are _____.

18. Touching is _____.

19. I nurture myself by _____.

20. I am critical of myself when _____.

21. I am pleased with myself when _____.

22. I like the way I _____.

____+____+____+____ = _____ = Total points for this section

Divided by _____ (number of statements answered) = |____ . ____| **Average score for this section**
(Transfer to the Wellness Index Wheel on summary page)

Notes: Section 3 (For more information see Chapter 3, *Wellness Workbook*)

1, 2, 3. Full-spectrum light, like sunlight, contains many different wavelengths. Most eye-glasses, and the glass windows in your home or car, block the "near" ultra violet light needed by your body. Special bulbs and lenses are available.

4. Loud noises that leave your ears ringing cause irreversible and cumulative nerve damage over time. Ear plugs/muffs, obtained in sporting goods stores, should be worn around power saws, heavy equipment, and rock concerts!

10. Touch is one of the most unrecognized human needs for sensory input. However, insincere touching or "plastic" hugging may be worse than none at all.

11. Long recognized by hospitals as therapeutic, nurturing touch can be a powerful preventative as well.

13. The changing number of daylight hours throughout the year establishes rhythms in our bodies. You may feel less stressed if you do more inner directed work when the days are short with a more outwardly directed focus on the longer days.

14. The moon has been scientifically shown to strongly influence many biological organisms including humans. Urban people are often oblivious to the natural forces surrounding them and can benefit from paying attention to such processes as the changing effects of the moon, etc.

© 1975, 1981, 1988, John W. Travis, MD, Not to be copied. (Bulk copies available)

©1975, 1981, 1988, John W. Travis, MD. Not to be copied. (Bulk copies available)

4	3	2	1	0

Yes, always or usually — 4
Often — 3
Sometimes, maybe — 2
Occasionally, rarely — 1
No, never or hardly ever — 0

Section 4—Wellness and Eating

1. I pay attention to the quality and quantity of foods I eat.

2. I am aware of the difference between refined carbohydrates and complex carbohydrates and eat a majority of the latter.*

3. I avoid fast foods and greasy, overcooked restaurant meals.

4. I am aware that I feel different when I eat different foods and chose foods that help me feel good.

5. I think my diet is well balanced and wholesome.

6. I minimize my intake of fats.

7. I drink fewer than 5 alcoholic drinks per week.

8. I drink fewer than 2 cups of coffee or black (non-herbal) tea per day.*

9. I have no need for medications or drugs (including prescription drugs).*

10. I drink fewer than 5 soft drinks per week.*

11. I add little or no salt to my food.*

12. I read the labels for the ingredients of all processed foods I buy and I inquire as to the level of toxic chemicals used in production of fresh foods—choosing the purest available to me.

13. I eat at least two raw fruits or vegetables each day.

14. I am aware of the benefits of fasting and fast regularly (with either water or juice).*

15. I have a good appetite and am within 15% of my ideal weight.

16. I enjoy eating and take time for leisurely, relaxing meals.

17. I can tell the difference between "stomach hunger" and "mouth hunger," and I don't stuff myself when I am experiencing only "mouth hunger." *

18. I have a well-stocked, well-equipped kitchen and I enjoy cooking.

19. I chew my food thoroughly.

20. If my diet contains largely processed foods, I add unprocessed bran to my diet to provide roughage.*

21. I steam or stir-fry my vegetables (instead of boiling them).*

22. I eat whole (unrefined) grains and stoneground 100% whole wheat bread.*

23. I minimize my intake of red meats.

24. I have a bowel movement each day.

25. My bowel movements are bulky and float.*

26. I feel good about how I eat and avoid using food as a reward, escape, or punishment.

27. I avoid dieting and if my weight is an issue, work with the underlying causes.*

28. If most of my food is processed or commercially grown, I take mineral and vitamin supplements.*

29. The water I drink and cook with either comes from a certified pure source or I pass it through a well maintained, up-to-date filter.*

30. I eat as low on the food chain as possible.*

31. I am aware of the symptoms of eating disorders and am not overly compulsive about what I do or don't eat.

If weight is not an issue for you skip the next group of statements; otherwise quickly complete the sentence with the first thoughts which come to mind.

32. When I binge, I feel _____ .

33. Aspects of my regular diet that I would like to change are _____

_____ .

34. Food habits which contribute to my weight issues are _____

_____ .

35. Diets are _____ .

36. When I want to lose/gain weight, I _____

_____ .

____ + ____ + ____ + ____ = _____ = Total points for this section

Divided by _____ (number of statements answered) = | ____ . ____ | **Average score for this section**
(Transfer to the Wellness Index Wheel on summary page)

Notes: Section 4   (For more information see Chapter 4, *Wellness Workbook*)

2. Refined carbohydrates (white flour, sugar, white rice, alcohol, etc.) are burned up by the body very quickly and contain no minerals or vitamins. Complex carbohydrates (fruits and vegetables) burn evenly and provide the bulk of dietary nutrients.

8. Coffee and non-herbal teas contain stimulants which, when over-used, abuse your body's adrenal glands.

9. With a healthy lifestyle, we can live a normal life with far fewer drugs than many modern people think is possible.

10. Besides caffeine, the empty calories in these chemical brews may cause a sugar "crash" shortly after drinking. Artificially sweetened ones may be worse. Consider the other nutrients you won't be getting, and the prices!

11. In addition to a presumed connection with high blood pressure, salting of foods during cooking draws out minerals which are then usually lost when the water is poured off.

14. Fasting, once commonplace as a result of early humans' unsteady supply of food, allows the body to metabolically flush out toxic substances ingested and stored in fat cells. Often part of spiritual rituals, along with deep breathing, it is one of the most effective natural "highs" for self exploration. *NOTE: Fasting is not effective for long term weight loss and should be done only under supervision and in moderation, and always with plenty of pure water.*

17. Stomach hunger is a signal that your body needs food. Mouth hunger is a signal that it needs something else (attention/acknowledgement), which you are not getting, so it asks for food, a readily available "substitute."

20. Raw bran flakes can supplant some of the bulk missing in most people's diets and needed by the colon. Bran is inexpensive, a byproduct of flour mills and looks like fluffy sawdust. It should not be confused with commercial cereals.

21. Boiling draws out most of the minerals and vitamins to the water which is usually poured down the drain.

22. "Wheat Flour" or enriched flour, is really white flour with a few nutrients put back—look for the words "100% whole wheat". The steel (vs. stone) milling of wheat creates high temperatures destroying nutrients in the wheat.

25. Diets with adequate fiber produce large quantities of bulky stools which usually float in the toilet—an excellent measure as to whether you are getting enough bulk.

27. Dieting rarely works. Starving your body only causes it to extract nutrients from food more efficiently. Unless your "set point" is lowered, lasting weight changes are unlikely. It is more important to meet your underlying needs, for which food is often a substitute. Weight (fat) is stored (withheld) energy or power, (both biochemically and psychologically). Learning how to focus energy or express personal power directly is a more satisfying alternative than storing it in your body.

28. The mineral content of most commercial croplands is severely depleted from chemicals used instead of properly rotating crops. Long shipping times account for decreases in vitamin content. Beware of high pesticide levels also.

29. US Government regulations on tap water and bottled water alike are not current with technology, so much drinking water contains toxic levels of industrial/agricultural residues. Most tap water filters are ineffective. Do your research carefully!

30. To produce a 1 lb. feedlot steak costs the world 5 lbs. of grain, 2,500 gal. of water, 1 gal. of gasoline, and 35 lbs. of eroded topsoil (Worldwatch Institute). Eating lower on the food chain conserves our rapidly depleting resources.

©1975, 1981, 1988, John W. Travis, MD, Not to be copied. (Bulk copies available)

4	3	2	1	0
Yes, always or usually	Often	Sometimes, maybe	Occasionally, rarely	No, never or hardly ever

Section 5—Wellness and Moving

1. I climb stairs rather than ride elevators.*

2. My daily activities include **moderate** physical effort.*

3. My daily activities include **vigorous** physical effort.*

4. I run at least **one** mile three times a week (or equivalent aerobic exercise).*

5. I run at least **three** miles three times a week (or equivalent aerobic exercise).

6. I do some form of stretching/limbering exercise for 10 to 20 minutes at least **three** times per week.*

7. I do some form of stretching/limbering exercise for 10 to 20 minutes at least **six** times per week.

8. I enjoy exploring new and effective ways of caring for myself through the movement of my body.

9. I enjoy stretching, moving, and exerting my body.

10. I am aware of and respond to messages from my body about its needs for movement.

11. I know how to calculate my recommended training heart rate.*

12. I know how to take my pulse during exercise.*

13. When exercising aerobically I keep at or below my recommended training heart rate.

14. I enjoy dancing and/or moving my body in rhythm with music.

15. I try out new forms of physical activity so there will be less likelihood of my getting bored and discontinuing my regular exercise program.

16. I am aware that exercise alters brain chemistry and use it to feel better when depressed, anxious, or overstressed.

17. I use exercise as a metaphor or tool to break through self-imposed limitations.

For the next statements, quickly complete the sentence with the first thoughts/feelings which come to mind.

18. I usually do the following physical activities during the week. _____

19. I am satisfied/dissatisfied with my physical activities because _____

_____ .

20. Exercise is _____ .

21. I would like to change the following things regarding my body's fitness _____

_____ .

22. After a day of little physical movement I _____ .

23. After a day of much physical movement I _____ .

24. My childhood experience of exercise/sports was _____ .

____ + ____ + ____ + ____ = _____ = Total points for this section

Divided by _____ (number of statements answered) = ____ . ____ Average score for this section

(Transfer to the Wellness Index Wheel on summary page)

1. If a long elevator ride is necessary, try getting off five flights below your destination. Urge building managers to keep stair doors unlocked.

2. Moderate = rearing young children, gardening, scrubbing floors, brisk walking, etc.

3. Vigorous = heavy construction work, farming, moving heavy objects by hand, etc.

4. An aerobic exercise (like running) should keep your heart rate at about 60% of its maximum, (120-150 bpm) for 12-20 minutes. Less vigorous exercise will also produce the "training effect", but takes a much longer period of time.

6. The stretching of muscles is important to maintaining maximum flexibility of joints and ligaments, etc. It feels good, too.

11, 12. See Chapter 5, *Wellness Workbook* or any reference book on aerobic conditioning.

Yes, always or usually	Often	Sometimes, maybe	Occasionally, rarely	No, never or hardly ever
4	3	2	1	0

Section 6—Wellness and Feeling

1. I am able to feel and express my anger in ways that solve problems, rather than swallow anger or store it up.*

2. I allow myself to experience a full range of emotions and find constructive ways to express them.

3. I am able to say "no" to people without feeling guilty.

4. In addition to feeling other emotions, I experience happiness.

5. I laugh often and easily.

6. I feel OK about crying and allow myself to do so when appropriate.*

7. I listen to and consider other's criticisms of me rather than react defensively.

8. I have at least five close friends.

9. I like myself and look forward to the rest of my life.

10. I easily express concern, love and warmth to those I care about.

11. I can ask for help when needed.

12. I seek help from professional counselors if needed.

13. I understand the importance of grieving after a loss, and allow myself to do so.

14. I meet several people a month whom I would like to get to know better, and I get to know some of them.

15. When I'm angry, I look into the source of it rather than just continuing to feel angry.

16. I see conflict as a necessary and important part of being alive and do not confuse it with violence (physical or mental) against myself of others.*

17. I am willing to take important risks, and do so.

18. I am aware that feelings provide me with information about myself and use them accordingly.

19. I am aware of the power contained in so called negative feelings and draw on that power to achieve greater self-understanding instead of denying these feelings or unquestioningly trying to turn them into "joy".

20. I am able to measure my own worth/adequacy without comparing myself to others.

4   **3**   **2**   **1**   **0**

Yes, always or usually / Often / Sometimes, maybe / Occasionally, rarely / No, never or hardly ever

For the next statements, quickly complete the sentence with the first thoughts/feelings which come to mind.

21. When I am angry, I _____ .

22. Being angry _____ .

23. When I feel sad _____ .

24. Crying _____ .

26. Laughing out loud _____ .

27. My life is full of _____ .

28. Taking risks can lead to _____ .

29. In order to take important risks, I _____ .

30. I resolve conflict by _____ .

____ + ____ + ____ + ____ = _____ = Total points for this section

Divided by _____ (number of statements answered) = | ____ . ____ | **Average score for this section**

(Transfer to the Wellness Index Wheel on summary page)

Notes: Section 6   (For more information see Chapter 6, *Wellness Workbook*)

1. Learning to take charge of your emotions and using them to solve problems can prevent disease, improve communications, and increase your self awareness. Suppressing emotions or using them to manipulate others is destructive to all.

6. Crying over a loss relieves the body of pent-up feelings. In our culture males often have a difficult time allowing themselves to cry, while females may have learned to cry when angry, using tears as a means of manipulation.

16. Many people confuse conflict with the violence (emotional or physical) often used to "resolve" conflict. Thus they seek to avoid conflict, suppressing many feelings rather than learning how to creatively grow from conflict.

Section 7—Wellness and Thinking

1. I am in charge of the subject matter and the emotional content of my thoughts; and am satisfied with what I choose to think about.*

2. I am aware that I make judgements wherein I think I am "right" and others are "wrong".*

3. It is easy for me to concentrate.

4. I am conscious of changes (such as breathing pattern, muscle tension, skin moisture, etc.) in my body in response to certain thoughts.*

5. When "accidents" "happen", I am aware of the thoughts which preceded them and learn from my experience.*

6. I am aware when I take an action seemingly independent of my conscious will.*

7. I use this awareness to further my growth.

8. I am aware of internal contradictions among my thoughts/beliefs.*

9. I notice my perceptions of the world are colored by my thoughts at the time.*

10. I am aware that my thoughts are influenced by my environment.

11. I use my thoughts and attitudes to make my reality more life-affirming.*

©1975, 1981, 1988, John W. Travis, MD. Not to be copied. (Bulk copies available)

12. Rather than worry about a problem when I can do nothing about it, I temporarily shelve it and get on with the matters at hand.

13. I approach life with the attitude that no problem is too big to confront, and some mysteries aren't meant to be solved.

14. I can let go of repetitive thoughts.

15. Before going to sleep I can set my "internal clock" and wake up at a specific time.*

16. I use my creative powers in many aspects of my life.

17. I can solve problems through the use of my dreams or unconscious mind.

18. I remember what I read and hear.

19. I know the difference between linear, verbal ("left-brain") thinking and pattern-oriented, integrative, holistic ("right-brain") thinking and am able to use both.

____ + ____ + ____ + ____ = _____ = Total points for this section

Divided by _____ (number of statements answered) = |____ . ____| **Average score for this section**

(Transfer to the Wellness Index Wheel on summary page)

Notes: Section 7 (For more information see Chapter 7, *Wellness Workbook*)

1. When you are unconscious of the content of your thoughts, they are more likely to control you. Observing them objectively develops self awareness and strengthens your ability to take charge.

2. Rather than trying to completely stop yourself from judging, you can observe your judgements as efforts by your ego to avoid getting on with life and hiding behind "right/wrong" game playing.

4. Both biofeedback and the field of psycho-neuro-immunology have shown the connections between the mind, nervous system and body. The more you become consciously aware of that connection, the greater degree of control you have of your health.

5. Those who hold a world-view that there are no "accidents" are usually aware of how they unconsciously create "unexpected" events, either for their good ("miracles") or to their detriment.

8. For most of us, even though we may not be consciously aware of it, our mind is filled

with contradictions, because we are really many people living inside one skin. The more you become aware of these contradictions, the less likely they are to cause you pain.

9. Being aware of your internal distortion of perceptions can allow you to step back and re-assess a situation more objectively when it is important to do so.

11. Honesty, tempered with care and concern, clears out many negative thoughts which can clutter up your mind and make your reality more fun. "Positive thinking" without honesty and truthfulness can backfire by suppressing valid concerns.

15. This is an example of one aspect of using the power of your mind.

19. The two halves of our brains seem to be specialized in their method of processing information. Western culture (especially through its school systems) almost exclusively rewards only "left-brain" thinking, leaving vast untapped potentials for creativity.

Section 8—Wellness and Playing/Working

1. I enjoy expressing myself through art, dance, music, drama, sports, etc., and make time to do so.

2. I regularly exercise my creativity "muscles".

3. I enjoy spending time without planned or structured activities and make the effort to do so.

4. I enjoy playing with other people and make time to do so.*

5. I enjoy playing on my own and make time to do so.

6. I can readily think of five people with whom I can play.

7. When appropriate, I can play before all my work is done, and feel good about it.

8. I can make much of my work into play.

9. I approach tasks from a playful point of view.

10. I readily shift from a goal-oriented frame of mind to a "purposeless" activity when it is appropriate to do so.*

11. At times I allow myself to do nothing.*

12. At times I can sleep late without feeling guilty.

13. The work I do is rewarding to me.

14. I am proud of my accomplishments.

15. I am playful and the people around me support my playfulness.

16. I have at least one activity (hobby, sport etc.) that I enjoy regularly but do not feel compelled to do.

17. I am a good worker.

18. I am a good player.

19. The work I do enhances the well-being of others and the planet without taking away from anyone.

20. I am more than my work.

21. I make opportunities for my "inner child" to play and be heard.

22. I do not turn play activities into work by feeling compelled to win.

On the four lines below, list four of the activities which you most enjoy doing above anything else in your life.

23a. _____ .

23b. _____ .

23c. _____ .

23d. _____ .

24. Work is _____ .

25. For fun I _____ .

26. I spend my leisure time.

27. I allow myself to experience the activity listed in 23a above.

28. I allow myself to experience the activity listed in 23b above.

29. I allow myself to experience the activity listed in 23c above.

30. I allow myself to experience the activity listed in 23d above.

____ + ____ + ____ + ____ = _____ = Total points for this section

Divided by _____ (number of statements answered) = ____ . ____ **Average score for this section**

(Transfer to the Wellness Index Wheel on summary page)

Notes: Section 8 (For more information see Chapter 8, *Wellness Workbook*)

4. Play and laughter allow the more creative self-renewing parts of our being to re-emerge. Engaging in play can reveal the limitations we chose to develop in our childhood to defend us from our fears.

10. Purposeless activity (play) allows us to relax from one mode (rational thinking) and open up to our creative impulses.

11. Doing "nothing" can give us access to the more creative and non-verbal aspects of our being, so from another perspective, doing nothing becomes doing much more.

©1975, 1981, 1988, John W. Travis, MD. Not to be copied. (Bulk copies available)

© 1975, 1981, 1988, John W. Travis, MD, not to be copied. (Bulk copies available)

4	3	2	1	0
Yes, always or usually	Often	Sometimes, maybe	Occasionally, rarely	No, never or hardly ever

Section 9—Wellness and Communicating

1. I inititate conversation on my own.

2. I am able to communicate with strangers easily.

3. In conversation I can introduce a difficult topic and stay with it until I've gotten a satisfactory response from the other person.

4. I enjoy communicating and am interested in what others have to say.

5. I enjoy silence.

6. I have at least three friends with whom I can communicate intimately.

7. I can communicate my limitations to others when appropriate.*

8. I consider how other people are likely to react before I initiate a difficult communication.*

9. I am truthful and caring in my communications with others.

10. I am aware of how I communicate with others non-verbally.*

11. I am aware when I'm responding to my internal "tapes" rather than acting or thinking independently.*.

12. I communicate clearly with friends and family.

13. I speak loudly enough so that others don't ask me to repeat myself.*

14. Instructions I give to others are carried out properly.*

15. I assert myself (in a non-attacking manner) in an effort to be heard, rather than be passively resentful of others with whom I don't agree.*

16. I am aware of situations when I blame others rather than accept that I may be in error.

17. I do not try to cover up my mistakes and apologize for them if appropriate.

18. I am aware of my negative judgements of others and accept them as simply judgements—not necessarily truth.*

19. I am aware of my defense mechanisms and can set them aside when appropriate.*

20. I am able to listen to and objectively consider opposing viewpoints.*

21. I am a good listener.

22. I don't try to change the subject in a conversation in order to win "points" for myself.

23. I am aware of my own and others' tones of voice, facial expression and body language when communicating.

24. I like myself and accept my "shortcomings" rather than get down on myself because I think I should be "better".

25. I am able to listen to people without interrupting them or finishing their sentences for them.

26. I am not responsible for keeping (making) other people happy.*

27. I take charge and manage a situation when it is appropriate for me to do so.*

28. I let others take charge and manage a situation when it is appropriate for them to do so.*

29. I cooperate with others when it is necessary for several people to take charge of a situation.*

30. I am able to let go of control and allow a situation to work itself out through means I may not fully understand.*

4	3	2	1	0	
Yes, always or usually	Often	Sometimes, maybe	Occasionally, rarely	No, never or hardly ever	

____ ____ ____ ____   31. I can let go of my mental "labels" (ie. this is good, that is wrong) and judgemental attitudes about events in my life and see them in the light of what they offer me.

____ ____ ____ ____   32. I am aware when I play psychological "games" with those around me and work to be truthful and direct in my communications.*

____ ____ ____ ____   33. I clearly express my thoughts/feelings rather than assume others can read my mind.*

____ + ____ + ____ + ____ = _____ = Total points for this section

Divided by _____ (number of statements answered) = | ____ . ____ | **Average score for this section**

(Transfer to the Wellness Index Wheel on summary page)

Notes: Section 9   (For more information see Chapter 9, *Wellness Workbook*)

7. Trust is more readily established when we are open about our limitations.

8. This does not mean you let others control your behavior, but that you initiate a communication in a way that is likely to accomplish its goal.

10. If you pay attention to only your words, you may be missing strong messages your unconscious mind is sending, often contrary to what your words are saying.

11. Our self chosen "tapes" (ie. internal conversations like "you should feel guilty for not working all the time") can be hard to turn off, but being aware of when they are trying to control us can give us more choice in a situation.

13, 14. If many people don't understand you or follow your instructions, consider the possiblity that you may not be communicating clearly.

15. Attacking others rarely accomplishes your goals in the long run. Persisting in your convictions without using force is more effective and usually solves the problem without creating new ones.

18. It is important to recognize that our internal judgements of others are based on personal biases that often have little objective basis.

19, 20. Defense mechanisms (phobias, over-reacting, not listening, changing the subject, etc.) allow us to keep our world view intact. Letting go of outmoded beliefs can be painful but rewarding for the growth it produces.

26. Each of us, regardless of how inadequate we may make ourselves appear, is ultimately responsible for our own happiness. Co-dependency, a disease of lost selfhood, causes suffering from focusing on the needs and behavior of others more than ourself.

27, 28, 29, 30. Control of, and management of situations is an important form of communication. Being able to deal with it in a balanced way provides us with more options.

32. Psychological games, defined by Eric Berne in *Games People Play*, are complex unconscious manipulations which result in their players getting negative attention and feeling bad about themselves.

33. Another symptom of co-dependency (an addiction to other people and what you think they think about you) is believing that they know what you are thinking without telling them.

©1975, 1981, 1988, John W. Travis, MD, Not to be copied. (Bulk copies available)

©1975, 1981, 1988, John W. Travis, MD, Not to be copied. (Bulk copies available)

4	3	2	1	0	
Yes, always or usually	Often	Sometimes, maybe	Occasionally, rarely	No, never or hardly ever	

Section 10—Wellness and Sex

1. I feel comfortable touching and exploring my body.

2. I think it's OK to masturbate if one chooses to do so.

3. My sexual education is adequate.

4. I feel good about the degree of closeness I have with men in my life.

5. I feel good about the degree of closeness I have with women in my life.

6. I am content with my level of sexual activity.*

7. I feel good about my body.

8. I fully experience the many stages of lovemaking rather than focus only on orgasm.*

9. I express myself directly rather than use sexual energy as a covert means of communication.*

10. I feel comfortable touching persons of my own sex.*

11. I am informed on issues of birth control.

12. I am familiar with methods of preventing venereal disease, and use them if appropriate.

13. I communicate any upset feelings with my partner rather than withhold sex as "punishment".

14. When I'm upset with my partner, I resolve the problem before making love.

15. I feel comfortable looking at myself nude in a mirror.

16. I love myself unconditionally, even when I'm upset with some of my behaviors.*

17. I desire to grow closer to some other people.

18. I am aware of the difference between needing someone and loving someone.

19. I am able to love others without dominating or being dominated by them.

20. I am able to love others unconditionally.*

21. I am comfortable in consciously abstaining from sexual activity as a way of learning more about myself.

For the next statements, quickly complete the sentence with the first thoughts/feelings which come to mind.

22. When I want to initiate love making_____.

23. My favorite erogenous zones are _____.

24. Making love is _____.

25. After lovemaking I feel _____.

26. My sexual behavior is _____.

27. To me a heterosexual lifestyle is _____.

28. To me a homosexual lifestyle _____.

29. To me a bisexual lifestyle is _____.

30. Oral sex is _____.

31. Orgasm _____.

32. Love involves _____.

33. Loving someone means _____.

____+____+____+____ = _____ = Total points for this section

Divided by _____ (number of statements answered) = |____ . ____| **Average score for this section**

(Transfer to the Wellness Index Wheel on summary page)

Notes: Section 10 (For more information see Chapter 10, *Wellness Workbook*)

6. Including the choice to have no sexual activity.

8. A common problem for many people is an overemphasis on performance and orgasm, rather than on enjoying a close sensual feeling with their partner, regardless of their having an orgasm.

9. Flirting and using sex playfully can be fun and healthy if balanced with direct communication.

10. An especially difficult barrier for men because of cultural norms which indiscriminately link touch with sexual desire.

16, 20. Unconditional love does not depend on previous accomplishments or performance, but is based on the belief that all entities are a part of "the plan." It is a non-controlling/non-manipulative form of love and is not "earned".

Section 11—Wellness and Finding Meaning

1. I believe my life to have direction and meaning (although I may not always be able to see either).

2. My life is exciting and challenging.

3. I have goals in my life.

4. I am achieving my goals.

5. I look forward to the future as an opportunity for further growth.

6. I am able to talk about the death of someone close to me.

7. I am able to talk about my own death with family and friends.

8. I am prepared for my death.

9. I see my death as a step in my evolution.*

10. My daily life is a source of pleasure to me.

11. I am satisfied with any counseling and/or growth-related processes in which I am involved.

12. I live primarily in the here and now rather than in the past or future.*

13. My life has purpose.

14. I let my "inner voice" guide me rather than the expectations of others.

15. I place importance on achieving both outward (material) *and* inward (spiritual) goals.

©1975, 1981, 1988, John W. Travis, MD, Not to be copied. (Bulk copies available)

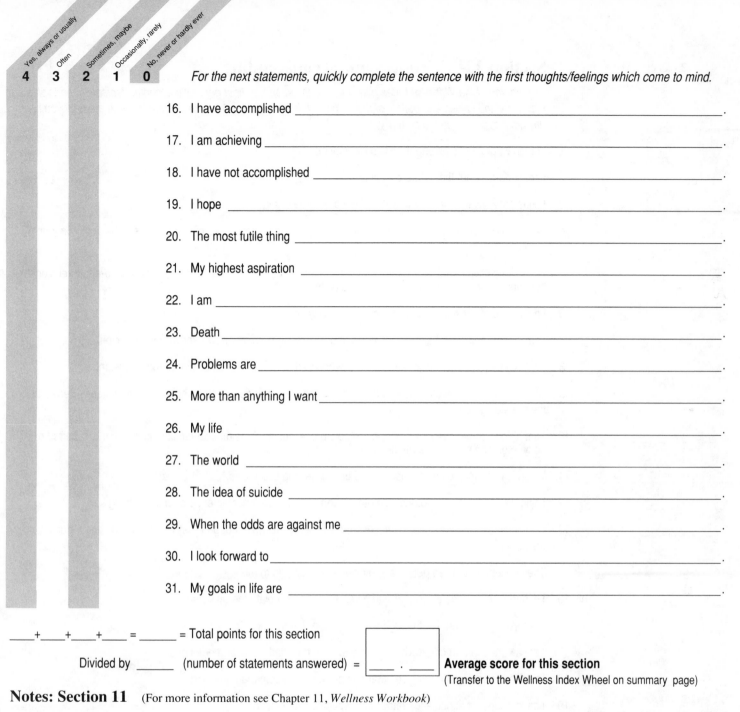

| 4 | 3 | 2 | 1 | 0 |

Yes, always or usually — 4
Often — 3
Sometimes, maybe — 2
Occasionally, rarely — 1
No, never or hardly ever — 0

For the next statements, quickly complete the sentence with the first thoughts/feelings which come to mind.

16. I have accomplished _____.

17. I am achieving _____.

18. I have not accomplished _____.

19. I hope _____.

20. The most futile thing _____.

21. My highest aspiration _____.

22. I am _____.

23. Death _____.

24. Problems are _____.

25. More than anything I want _____.

26. My life _____.

27. The world _____.

28. The idea of suicide _____.

29. When the odds are against me _____.

30. I look forward to _____.

31. My goals in life are _____.

____ + ____ + ____ + ____ = _____ = Total points for this section

Divided by _____ (number of statements answered) = | ____ . ____ | **Average score for this section**
(Transfer to the Wellness Index Wheel on summary page)

Notes: Section 11   (For more information see Chapter 11, *Wellness Workbook*)

9. Seeing your death as a stage of growth and preparing yourself consciously is an important part of finding meaning in your life.

12. This does not imply that you disregard either past or future, but see both in the context of your present reality. Many people live in memories of the past or in fantasies of the future at the expense of being in present time.

©1975, 1981, 1988, John W. Travis, MD, Not to be copied. (Bulk copies available)

Yes, always or usually	Often	Sometimes, maybe	Occasionally, rarely	No, never or hardly ever
4	**3**	**2**	**1**	**0**

Section 12—Wellness and Transcending

This portion of the Wellness Index goes beyond the scope of most generally accepted "scientific" principles and expresses the values and beliefs of the authors. It is intended to stimulate interest in these areas. If you have any beliefs strongly to the contrary, feel free to skip the questions or make up your own.

1. I perceive problems as opportunities for growth.

2. I am curious about the nature of reality.*

3. I consider myself to be an integral part of some greater plan.*

4. I am comfortable with and excited by the seemingly mysterious nature of what seems to be going on in the universe.*

5. I experience synchronistic events in my life ("coincidences" which appear to have no cause-effect relationship but happen more often than chance would dictate).*

6. I am aware of experiencing "miracles" in my daily life.*

7. I am comfortable about knowing things without knowing precisely how I know them (intuition).

8. I believe there are dimensions of reality beyond verbal description or human comprehension.

9. At times I experience confusion and paradox in my search for understanding of the dimensions referred to in the preceding question.

10. I am able to consciously alter my physiologic processes such as muscle tension, circulation to a part of my body, etc., and so improve my health.*

11. When ill I am able to consciously speed up my healing processes.*

12. I sing, pray, chant, or meditate with other people, and experience a sense of unity in doing so.

13. Confusion and paradox seem a necessary part of my growth although I may not always be comfortable with them.

14. The concept of god has personal definition and meaning to me.

15. I experience a sense of wonder and awe when I contemplate the universe.

16. It is OK with me if certain things are unknowable to the mind.

17. I am aware of a part of me which is greater than my mind, body and emotions.

18. I trust and use the part of myself that has a greater wisdom than my mind.

19. I have abundant expectancy rather than specific expectations.

20. I experience a merging of my consciousness with a larger sense of consciousness (universal mind).

21. I do not pressure others to accept my beliefs.

22. I remember my dreams.

23. I interpret the symbols in my dreams.

24. I use the messages interpreted from my dreams to better live my waking life.

©1975, 1981, 1988. John W. Travis, MD. Not to be copied. (Bulk copies available)

4	3	2	1	0
Yes, always or usually	Often	Sometimes, maybe	Occasionally, rarely	No, never or hardly ever

_____ _____ _____ _____ _____ 25. I enjoy practicing a spiritual discipline or allowing time to sense the presence of a greater force in guiding my passage through life.

_____ _____ _____ _____ _____ 26. I believe that how I think, and correspondingly act, contributes to the well being of the planet.

____+____+____+____ = _____ = Total points for this section

Divided by _____ (number of statements answered) = |____ . ____| **Average score for this section**

(Transfer to the Wellness Index Wheel on summary page)

Notes: Section 12 (For more information see Chapter 12, *Wellness Workbook*)

2, 3, 4. Exploration of your views about the universe have considerable impact on how you live your life and hence your personal wellness.

5. Modern physics reveals that the idea of cause and effect may be as limited as Newton's theory of a mechanical universe. It suggests that we must expand our view to see that everything in the universe is connected to everything else. (Synchronicity describes that experience.)

6. Occurrences which seem to fall outside the realm of causality may be experienced as miraculous, but may just indicate our ignorance of the way things are. They can become everyday phenomena when accepted as a normal part of life.

10. Evidence from biofeedback research shows that most physiologic processes, previously thought to be outside conscious control, are accessible to the conscious mind.

11. Healing processes are also physiologic processes and can be controlled by conscious intention.

©1975, 1981, 1988, John W. Travis, MD. Not to be copied. (Bulk copies available)

The Wellness Index Wheel

Transfer your average score from each section to the corresponding box around the wheel below. Then graph your score by drawing a curved line between the "spokes" that define each segment. (Use the scale provided—beginning at the center with 0.0 and reaching 4.0 at the circumference.) Lastly, fill in the corresponding amount of each wedge-shaped segment, using different colors if possible.

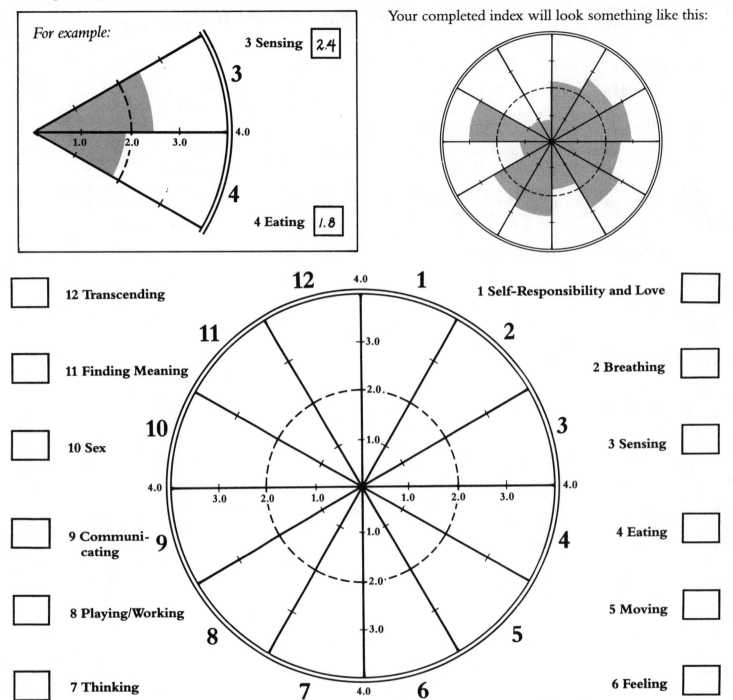

For example:

Your completed index will look something like this:

Now that you have completed the Wellness Index, study the wheel's shape and balance. How smoothly would it roll? What does it tell you? Are there any surprises in it? How does it feel to you? What don't you like about it? What do you like about it?

You may first want to work on the sections where you scored lowest, or you may want to address a section that you can more easily handle. (Keep in mind our caution against undertaking massive and sweeping life changes all at once.) We also recommend that you go back over the questions using colored pens to note the ones that you are interested in working on versus those of lower priority to you now. Remember that you can use the *Wellness Workbook* page references to aid you in your study.

©1975, 1981, 1988, John W. Travis, MD, Not to be copied. (Bulk copies available)

Wellness,
Self-Responsibility,
and Love

WELLNESS IS LIKE a bridge supported by two piers. Each pier is crucial to the bridge's integrity just as the two principles of self-responsibility and love are fundamental to the process of wellness. In each case, the piers support a connection between two distant points, allowing for movement back and forth. This freedom to move between different places or attitudes, rather than rigid attach-

Self-responsibility, with love and compassion, are the forms of energy we will address first in the Wellness Energy System. They are choices which create an environment, or context, within which all other energy expressions can be considered. Self-responsibility and love flow from the appreciation that we are not separate and individual entities, nor are we made up of separate parts. Rather, we are united in one energy system with everything else in creation.

ment to any particular one, is the hallmark of wellness.

Self-responsibility and love establish a life-context in which freedom and flexibility are natural. They are primary expressions of life energy. Self-responsibility and love together form the foundations of wellness, and encourage the free flow of all other types of energy. If either principle (or pier) is weakened, living harmoniously (or tra-

THE WELLNESS BRIDGE

SELF RESPONSIBILITY

LOVE

versing the bridge) becomes more difficult. When both are strong, energy dances back and forth, and the crossing is easy.

Self-Responsibility Means:
- Developing awareness of your own processes and patterns—physical, mental, emotional, and spiritual

- Discovering your real needs, and finding ways to meet them directly

- Realizing that you are unique and *the* expert about yourself

- Making choices and living courageously in the midst of uncertainty

- Creating the life you want, rather than just reacting to whatever comes along

- Asking simply and directly for what you need and want from others

- Expressing yourself, both your ideas and feelings, in ways that effectively communicate to other people who you are, and what you know

- Respecting your body through nutrition, exercise, and personal safety

- Creating and nourishing close relationships with others

- Engaging in projects that are meaningful to you; being supportive of others; and respecting your environment.

Love Means:
- Honoring your uniqueness, and enjoying the uniqueness of others

- Listening to your own heart—

treasuring your inner wisdom

- Responding to life's challenges as opportunities for growth, rather than as problems

- Caring for all aspects of yourself—body, mind, emotions, spirit—and sharing your caring with others

- Exercising compassion for your weaknesses, and forgiving yourself and others

- Experiencing yourself as your own best friend, and remaining faithful to yourself, especially in the rough times

- Realizing your connectedness with all things

- Being truthful with yourself and others

- Celebrating the irrepressible process of life.

With love and self-responsibility as our foundations and supports, living and wellness are synonymous.

Wellness, like life, is always a question of balance. It is a dynamic process because there are seeming contradictions to be resolved, apparent oppositions to be integrated, infinite shades of grey from which to choose. In considering the subject of health, for instance, you just don't find absolute answers to questions like: What should I eat? How should I exercise? What form of treatment is best? Rather, you must learn to balance what *you* know and what the "experts" tell you. Even though you are connected with me and everyone else, you are also very much alone, and singularly must make your own life and death decisions. (Sounds

. . . .
Do I contradict myself?
Very well then
I contradict myself,
I am large, I contain
multitudes.

—WALT WHITMAN
. . . .

serious. And it is!) But, if you make your life about self-responsibility and love, then the burden can be transformed into the opportunity, and the questions can become the impetus for experimentation, for learning, for trusting, for loving this magnificent and paradoxical creation—yourself.

Illness is created when we resist the movement and flexibility which characterize life and change. Wellness offers us a bridge to cross over into new territory, to explore different possibilities, to understand the other side of any situation. When we resign ourselves to being helpless victims of disease, when we give up on ourselves, when we hold on to one system and refuse to question it even when it fails to meet our needs, we encourage sickness and death.

Wellness allows us to integrate contradictions like illness and health. It appreciates these as complementary parts of one life process. It is open to new ideas, courageous, and noncompulsive. Wellness means that we can move freely between seeming opposites, learning from each, growing from both.

The traditional treatment model of medicine, which most of us have come to accept as the norm, is actually only one way of dealing with illness. Because we have lived with it for so long, we

. . . . *Exercise* . . . .

Remembering What You Already Know

I. As quickly as you can, list the words, phrases or images that come to mind when you thing of illness.

Now do the same for wellness.

Look back over what you have recorded.

II. Go on now to recall what you know about encouraging wellness.

What supports my well-being: What discourages my well-being:

Look back over what you have written.

III. What is one step you can take today to encourage what you feel good about?

I will . . .

What is one step you can take today to eliminate what doesn't support you?

I will . . .

IV. Congratulate yourself.

. . . .

may never have learned that there are alternatives. Sometimes, even though it may have failed us, we have dismissed its shortcomings. Because the treatment model is such familiar territory, the "home field" so to speak, we are strongly encouraged to stay there.

The Problems with Illness-Care

The practice of medicine in the world today is often labeled "health care." Actually, it should be described as "illness care." It is built upon diagnosis of disease, the repair of injury, and the treatment of symptoms—all of which are necessary and valuable services.

. . . .

Patients must begin to change from passive recipients of medical care to active, self-responsible participants; otherwise our goal of developing an adequate national health system cannot be realized.

—ELMER E.
GREEN, PH.D.
MENNINGER
FOUNDATION

. . . .

Sometimes, it delivers just what we ask for. Oftentimes, however, we get more than we bargained for.

We've asked our medical professionals to take care of us, to be responsible for our lives. The demands come in a variety of questions and prayers:

"What's wrong, Doc?"

"Will you fix me up?"

"Just tell me I'm going to be all right!"

"I want relief now!"

"Please Doc, just let me live!"

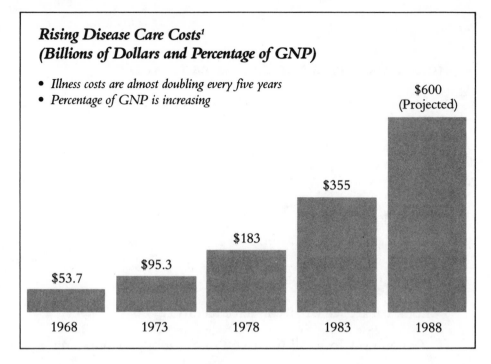

Rising Disease Care Costs[1]
(Billions of Dollars and Percentage of GNP)

- *Illness costs are almost doubling every five years*
- *Percentage of GNP is increasing*

$53.7	$95.3	$183	$355	$600 (Projected)
1968	1973	1978	1983	1988

At the same time, we've become dissatisfied with the doctor's inability to play God, threatening lawsuit or censure should treatment prove inadequate. This system also operates at an ever-increasing financial cost to the consumer and is running wildly out of control. Each of us now spends on the average $1,000 per year for such services. As the chart indicates, the cost of illness-care is nearly doubling every five years.

Our resistance to footing such an expensive bill might not be so great if we were getting *only* what we paid for. The fact is we're getting more than we can handle. The term for these unasked for benefits is "iatrogenesis." It means a condition created by the doctor's treatment. Prescription drugs, for example, have become one of the leading causes of death. In the U.S., drug-related deaths rank number eleven on the list of killers, following closely behind bronchitis, emphysema, and asthma. A World Health Organization study estimated that one of every four peo-

. . . .

. . . until the 1850s only half of all the children born in the United States reached the age of five. Today, almost 98% make it to that age. In 1790, a sixty-year old veteran of the American Revolution had a life expectancy of around fifteen more years. Incredibly, in 1970, his sixty-year-old counterpart had almost the same number of years to live.

. . . .

ple who die in hospitals is killed by drugs. At a 1974 U.S. Senate hearing it was reported that 30,000 people annually die from misuse of drugs. Moreover, the misuse and overuse of antibiotics have contributed to the development of treatment-resistant bacteria which kill 50,000–100,000 Americans every year.[2]

The illness-care system, moreover, is often overrated. If you examine the list of the ten most frequent causes of death among the

When the cost of health care in America has risen to $140 billion a year, with most of this going for after-the-fact attempts at treatment and cure, it is obvious that we need to reorder our national and individual priorities. How much more health effective and cost-effective it would be if more emphasis were placed on prevention—on keeping harmful materials out of the air, water, and soil—and out of our people.

—DOUGLAS M. COSTLE ADMINISTRATOR, E.P.A.

U.S. population in the early 1900s, you see that we have made great strides in controlling the infectious killers: T.B., diphtheria, and influenza. But in their place today we find cancer, heart-disease, and stroke. We have merely substituted one set of killers for another.

Actually, medical science has done little to increase the potential life span of the American adult. Figures quoted about average life expectancy show an increase since the introduction of antibiotics in the 1940s. But this supposed increase is due mainly to a lower infant and childhood mortality rate. More children living a normal life span radically affect the statistics. We are really not living any longer than did people 60 years ago. In fact, it may be that our potential life span is being shortened by increased stresses, and by poisons in the environment.[3]

Much about the illness-care system de-emphasizes the role played by lifestyle in determining the state of health. Most illness results from choices about lifestyle, not from lack of access to health services. The excessive strains of sedentary work can encourage obesity and cigarette smoking, for example. It can foster depression and anxiety. These conditions are common among the white collar middle class in the U.S. And the mortality rates of this group during mid-life (45–64) are substantially higher than those of the population at large—particularly from such conditions as cancer, heart disease, and stroke.[4]

The cost of illness-care in terms of emotional drain on the provider (the doctor) and the consumer (you) is also great. Treatment fosters dependency of the patient

Leading Causes of Death in the United States, 1985

Cause	Annual Deaths Per 100,000 Population
Heart disease	424.2
Malignancies/Cancer	184.0
Accidents	43.9
Asthma/Bronchitis/ Emphysema	25.7
Pneumonia/Influenza	23.4
Diabetes mellitus	15.1
Chronic liver disease and cirrhosis	12.8
Suicide	12.0
Homicide	10.3
Diseases of early infancy	9.4
Kidney diseases	7.5
Congenital anomalies	6.0

Source: Statistical Abstract of the United States, 1985, p.75. U.S. Department of Commerce, Bureau of the Census.

on the professional. The public demands a pill for every ill, and it wants relief now! The doctor (or other health professional) is cast in the role of the "Pill Fairy," a character who must possess both omnipotence and infallibility. When the pressures of this game become too great over time, professional "burn out" — a whole range of attitudes and behaviors from ill-temper to suicide—is the common result. The statistics for suicide, drug abuse, and heart attack among physicians reflect the dangers in this kind of situation.

The interaction between the professional and the patient often looks like the relationship between a parent and a child. Parents have power, and answers, and prescriptions. They are nurturing ("Here, let me help"), and demanding ("You should do this"), and judgmental ("That's wrong"). Children have questions, feelings and needs, and compelling desires to please. They are compliant sometimes, downright stubborn and rebellious at others, and looking for both help and approval. And while this situation may be natural and necessary when one person is two years old and the other is forty, it is far from desirable, for instance, when you are fifty and your doctor is thirty.

Our current system for personal health may not be a system after all. Its orientation is toward treatment of an ailing part, a particular disease or set of symptoms, or the physical body alone. But most forms of treatment neglect to take into account that it is not a stomach which gets sick, but rather a whole person who doesn't feel well. And that human beings also have intellects, emotions, and souls, besides physical bodies. When was the last time your doctor asked you about your ability to express personal creativity in your job, your reluctance to cry or express anger, your sense of meaning and purpose in life, your awareness of the connectedness of all things in the universe?

The current illness-care system is expensive; it is risky; it discourages adults from taking charge of their own lives; it causes doctors and other "helpers" to burn out. It is limited in its perspective of life and health, and in acceptance of its own inadequacy. What it does well can be appreciated, and used. What it fails to do must be assumed by another system.

This whole situation may be likened to your dealings with your automobile. You can find the best mechanics in town to fix the vehicle each time it breaks down, but they can never prevent you from abusing it and causing the next problem. A great deal of expense and effort might be saved were you to practice preventive maintenance more consistently, and exercise more care in the way you drive. There are two separate systems at work here: one for automobile repair (acute care/crisis intervention) and one for driver's education (prevention/education). Both are necessary for assuring maximum efficiency and long-term dependability of your car. The former bears a strong resemblance to the operation of our traditional medical model; the latter represents the neglected component of wellness education. It is the happy occurrence when one institution can perform both of these functions, but to demand this of our medical professionals, in most cases, may

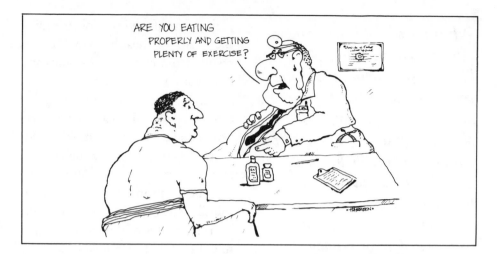

simply serve to increase the frustrations all around. In any case, the responsibility for prevention lies not with the doctor, it lies within each of us. It is long overdue that we recognize this and start reclaiming our personal power.

Self-Responsibility

Human beings continually persist in looking "out there" for answers, formulas, and fortunes, only to discover that they had them within themselves all along. Many fables recount the adventures of a young seeker who travels the world in search of a noble truth or a priceless treasure. After years of weary searching, pain, and hardship, the aged pilgrim finally returns home only to find the object of the search in his/her own backyard.

This story applies equally to our desires for health and wholeness, as it does to the finding of treasures. Attempts to find the doctor, or the therapy, or the book, which contains the magical solutions to all our problems and questions will end in frustration. Looking within, and assuming responsibility for what you find there, is a necessary condition for wellness.

This may be hard for many to

accomplish since from our earliest years we have accepted that somebody else knows what is best for us. As a society we have given up our personal power in many ways. To the teachers in our schools, we give the responsibility for telling us what we need to learn, and when and how to learn it; to professional mechanics—the decisions about the upkeep of our cars; to our professional politicians—the right to use our money and direct the military power of our country. Even in the area of spirituality, many people continue to allow their professional "holy one" to tell them what God demands. Likewise, we have entrusted our medical professionals with the responsibility for our health, giving them, and only them, the power to determine what our minds and bodies need.

．．．．．．．

The next major advances in health of the American people will come from the assumption of individual responsibility for one's own health and a necessary change in lifestyle for the majority of Americans.

—JOHN H. KNOWLES, M.D., FORMER PRESIDENT, ROCKEFELLER FOUNDATION

．．．．．．．

The Pill Fairy

A LONG, LONG TIME ago, when Life was still very young, the blessed Pill Fairy arrived on her first official visit to the people of planet Earth. And she came on an errand of mercy. Her job was to end the reign of pain and suffering that had kept our ancestors from enjoying the full fruits of their labors. And so she set to work.

Assuming many disguises and dispensing her gifts in various forms—sometimes as magical chants accompanied by shaking rattles, often as strong smelling brews, concocted from the herbs and roots of fields and forest, frequently as salves spread lavishly over the body—there seemed no end to the ways of her magic. She was honored, and sought after everywhere.

Slowly, however, the people began to suspect that hers was a temporary power. Her offerings brought only a short-lived release. Though sometimes lasting for many weeks, more often relief was brief, and soon they had to seek her out again, queuing up on longer and longer lines to receive her healing potions. But what else were they to do?

Time passed. And some of the people began to question, to voice their doubts. "Is she really a good fairy after all?" From time to time radical groups alarmed family and friends by refusing her charms, and arguing that, despite her seeming benevolence, there had to be a better way. And the argument continues 'til this very day.

The Pill Fairy still lives today. No longer dwelling only in caves, or around campfires, she has been promoted to an almost godly rank. Her shrines are found in great cities as well as in backwoods outposts. They are called HOSPITALS. Her attendants receive long years of intensive testing and with initiation are rewarded with a white robe to signify their special function. They are called NURSES and DOCTORS. Their magic is called MEDICINE. And it is awesome, and dearly bought. Doctors and nurses, like the Pill Fairy herself, are powerful and mostly benevolent, laboring long hours to help the suffering masses. Occasionally even they have been known to wonder if there is, perhaps, another way. But then the people still need them so desperately, and reward them so handsomely, that few have the time or motivation to look beyond.

The general attitude of "tell me what to do and I'll do it," or "you do it for me," seems initially easier. We appreciate that the training of the specialist gives him or her a special skill. You would probably never get to wash your dishes if you had to fix your own watch, TV, or sewing machine. Experts are necessary in all aspects of life. But the problem is not that we *have* experts. The problem is that we often *shift all responsibility* to something outside ourselves. When we do this, we don't have to suffer the guilt that might follow upon fail-ure. We remember only too well the terrifying admonition: "You'll have no one to thank but yourself!"

To take charge of your own life and health implies taking calculated risks. It means a recognition that you have choices, and carries with it your willingness to live with the consequences of those choices. For instance—in order to meet a dead-line you may place yourself under prolonged stress, neglect your diet, and forget your exercise. These are your choices. If they are short-term, you will probably bounce back easily. But occasionally, they might result in a cold, or other condition, that sends you to bed. Are you responsible for the cold? Yes, at some level you are. You may have no conscious awareness of it, but you created the condition which weakened your body and made it an environment of "dis-ease." If you are self-responsible, you will accept the cold as an important message from your body, and use it as a chance to rest and rebalance.

Taking responsibility for choices which result in illness does not mean taking on blame. There is a big difference. With blame you berate yourself for not learning a lesson, or burden yourself with guilt which creates more stress. With responsibility, you accept that you engineered your life situation, and that you can change it as well. You open yourself to learn the valuable lessons which the consequences offer.

We resist self-responsibility when we assume we are helpless in the face of a "foreign invader." The belief that germs *cause* disease is still widely accepted. Disease is viewed as that something "out there" which "happens to" us poor, unsuspecting victims. Our primitive ancestors lived in terror of the invasion of evil spirits, and called upon the magical incantations of their shamans to drive them out. Unfortunately, much of medical practice today reflects this same thinking. The forms of exorcism have radically changed, but the attitudes which motivate them are embarrassingly similar.

We are reluctant to take responsibility, or even to assert an opinion, because we have lost touch with our reservoirs of knowledge and intuition, our physical body-signals (both internal and external), and our gut-level, emotional responses. We mistrust ourselves and turn instead to the others who *really* know. The end result is a diminution of personal freedom, a weakened self-concept and a power-robbed existence. Certainly a high price to pay.

To accept responsibility for your health in no way implies that you should never seek the help of a doctor or a healer. To assume this is to misunderstand the concept completely. Your doctor probably has

· · · · · · · · · · · · · *John's Journal* · · · · · · · · · · · · ·

January 1973

I hated medical school. "Memorize this," "Do it this way," "Don't question why they're sick, just diagnose and learn the right drugs to give." I was depressed most of the time. Depression was the way I had learned to handle anger (I found out later on). I dragged my feet and passively resisted and hurt inside a lot.

When I got out of school and would see patients in the clinic at my own pace, I began to see how their lifestyle had been leading up to this symptom or disease they were now presenting to me to fix. Sometimes it looked like the pattern had been going on at least twenty years before any symptom had shown up. I would think to myself:

"Here you are sick and hurting, wanting me to take the responsibility to fix you up. That's not the problem—that's just the tip of the iceberg. The problem is in your lifestyle, yet I can't convince you of that, let alone help you change it. I'm depressed by your family (job, social, etc.) situation too. I guess all I can do is write you this prescription for Valium (or an antihypertensive, pain killer, sedative, or mood elevator). I hate to expose you to the awesome side effects of these chemicals, just to try to sweep something under the carpet for awhile. What you really need to do is some internal vacuum-cleaning but if I sent you to the psychiatrist to help you do it, you'd either be insulted, or s/he would say you're not crazy enough and wouldn't have time to see you. There must be another way. This way simply doesn't work."

I've decided to discontinue doing sick care. It feels like a huge weight lifted from my shoulders. I will focus full time on learning ways to help people see their responsibility for their health and then consciously take it. I will use the Transactional Analysis training I've been getting, the body therapies I've been exposed to, and much more. I will continue to use myself as a laboratory, learning how to express anger more effectively, seeing how to deal with problems more directly. (The sore right foot I developed during my 4th year in medical school was nearly crippling me as I began my residency. It seemed to be my body's way of resisting walking, to avoid stepping into more of this stuff which didn't feel good. It cleared up when I began enjoying my work.)

This script that the only way to be OK is to follow in Dad's footsteps and be a family doctor has run out. I can make my own script and be what and who I want to be.

· ·

How I Learned To Be Sick

As children, we all receive messages about illness and health from many different sources—our parents, relatives, friends, teachers, movies, books, T.V. . . . Often, these communications are so strong that we adopt them and carry them with us for years. This exercise will refresh your memory about how you *learned* to be sick.

Directions: List the names of persons you knew as a child, or cite experiences you had as a child, and then go on to explain what messages you received from them.

I learned to be sick from:

Person/Experience	*Explanation*	*Messages*
Mom	She took lots of aspirins everyday to cope with her arthritis	Messages I remember hearing/ getting about illness/health: example: "All the women in our family have arthritis." "Tall people always have low-back pain."

valuable experience which you have not had, and can be a fine resource. But you need to assert your rights as a consumer in the medical economy, to ask questions, to seek other opinions, and to accept that you know yourself better than anyone else does.

And finally there is just good common sense. Call it awareness, call it care—it is about self-responsibility. It shows itself in the use of safety about ourselves, our homes, our automobiles, our children and loved ones, our environment. Sometimes, it is as simple as wearing a seat belt, or removing poisons to a place that children can't reach. Sometimes it is more involved—a plan of escape in case of fire in your home.

Moving one step beyond personal/familial issues, we come face to face with our responsibility for the neighborhood, the city or town, the county, the state in which we live. One vote does make a difference! And many votes can make a bigger difference. As we assume more consciousness and accountability in our own lives, the more we will see and enjoy our interdependence with one another. A beginning may be as simple as getting to know who our neighbors are, which easily extends to work-

. . . . *Exercise* . . . .

Bodily Symptoms— Trackdown on Deeper Meanings:

Introduction: Illness, pain and accidents are often signs of deeper, sometimes hidden, needs that are going unmet. This trackdown method is one way of helping you to identify some of the these needs.

Trackdown Steps	Regina's Example (tension headache)	Your Example (Symptom: _____)
1. It feels like:	a knife over my right eye	
2. It happens when:	I've been pushing myself hard for several days	
3. It prevents:	reading, feeling excited about life	
4. It encourages:	more sleep, less work, admitting my weaknesses	
5. It provides the reward:	attention and help from Jere	
6. It may indicate the deeper need for:	Jere's acceptance of me	
7. A more direct way to meet this need might be:	expressing this to him; scheduling more special time with him	

. . . .

ing together in protecting our shared, local environment from overdevelopment and pollution.

The awareness that Spaceship Earth is a finite vessel should strengthen our willingness to conserve resources and energy by recycling glass, aluminum, etc., insulating our homes, and buying products which are not wastefully packaged or unnecessarily disposable. Once we begin to view our daily decisions in the light of our awakening responsibility, we learn that nearly every individual choice we make is a choice for the rest of humanity as well.

Self-Responsibility = Self-Trust

You don't trust what you don't know! It is paradoxical that a culture like ours which promotes an almost pornographic obsession with the appearance of the physical body could encourage a pervasive ignorance and mistrust of it. Sex education, or the lack of it, provides an excellent case in point. This subject is still discretionary within most school districts in the U.S. today, despite increases in both teenage pregnancies and the incidence of venereal disease. Need

more examples? Ask a number of people where the pancreas is. You may find yourself directed to a local restaurant down the block.

What can you say about a population that may know more about the structure and the function of the automobile than it does about the workings of the human body?

It's hard to love when you feel guilt and fear! For all of our scientific sophistication, the sad fact is that many of us sense that our bodies are somehow inferior to our minds. Some parts of the body are felt to be shameful. Some of its processes considered "dirty."

Exercise

Remembering a Childhood Illness

Your past experiences are shaping your present reality, whether you are aware of them or not. Recalling a childhood illness and reflecting upon it may help you better understand yourself and how you interpret illness/wellness today.

Write about an illness experience you remember having as a child. Describe it in as much detail as possible—unpleasant symptoms, your sickroom, any medicines, how long it lasted, how your parents responded, the "goodies" it provided, etc.

As you read over your description, look for carry-overs to your present situations.

Where's the Pancreas?

Match the letter to the number. (Not all are shown.)

_____ 1 Pancreas
_____ 2 Pituitary
_____ 3 Thymus
_____ 4 Ovaries
_____ 5 Spleen
_____ 6 Thyroid
_____ 7 Adrenals
_____ 8 Stomach
_____ 9 Pineal
_____ 10 Testes
_____ 11 Parathyroid

Answers

1 g	5 none	
2 a	6 c	
3 e	7 f	
4 h	8 none	
5 none	9 b	
6 c	10 i	
7 f	11 d	

Young children know nothing of shame and fear. But once learned, these beliefs and feelings will surface throughout life. It takes some active involvement to overcome these influences, to re-establish a trust, a love, a sense of reverence for the body. It really is pretty remarkable.

Twenty-four hours a day throughout your entire life you make use of your body's built-in feedback system. Too hot—take off your coat. Too cold—put on a sweater. Hungry—eat. Thirsty—drink. Headache—take an aspirin.

These are the easy ones. There are many more, however, which are suppressed or disregarded because you have more important things to do. You are neither ready nor willing to do anything about them. Tired muscles, sore throat, congested head? Swallow a cold capsule and keep on pushing! That knot in your stomach as you walk into the office each morning? Have another cup of coffee and start working! Light up a cigarette and begin coughing? Decide to quit as soon as this project is over! The list of examples goes on. This most

sensitive machine is constantly trying to tell you something. It will do its best to keep a molehill from developing into a mountain, but most of us simply will not listen to its messages. We are only too quick to anesthetize pain and alleviate symptoms, forgetting that these are only warning signals, not the real problem. If we are to be well, we need to start listening to every cell in the body, then provide it the best conditions possible so that it can continue healing itself. And that is something the body knows how to do. All the medical tech-

. . . . *Exercise* . . . .

A Conversation With a Body Part or Symptom

The body/mind is very wise. It knows a lot more than we give it credit for. The purpose of this exercise is to access some of this hidden wisdom by "speaking" with a body part or symptom. Use this technique when you are sick to learn ways of supporting your own healing, and use it more often to simply get to know yourself better and have a good time.

A. Getting prepared:

   1. Take pen and paper. Use your personal journal if you wish.

   2. Move to a quiet place where you will be uninterrupted for at least 20 minutes.

   3. Close your eyes and rest for 3 – 5 minutes, breathing deeply. Then open your eyes and go on.

B. Setting the stage:

   1. Think of your symptom or body part as if it were a "person" with its own separate history. Recall this history, and write it down if you care to. For instance:

   When was this symptom/part "born"?
   How and where did it grow?
   What have been the high and low points in its life?
   When does it come to visit or remind you of its presence?

   2. Rest with eyes closed for a few minutes.

C. The Conversation:

   1. Now, imagine the symptom/part sitting in a chair across the room from you.

   2. Give it a name.

   3. **WRITE**, as fast as you can, without editing and without rereading, **A CONVERSATION** between yourself and the symptom or body part. For example:

   Regina: Headache, I hate you.
   Headache: You hate me? I think you hate yourself!
   Regina: . . .

   Continue writing until you are complete. Expect nothing. When finished, reread what you've written.

D. The Wrap-up:
   Record your reactions and insights from this entire process. What has this experience taught you?

   Try this same procedure, with the same symptom or body part, on several different occasions. Compare, contrast, learn from the results.

. . . .

nology at our disposal does not really "cure" anything. *Only the body heals itself.*

What all of this has been leading up to is a definition of one of the general principles governing the approach to wellness taken in this book. It is sometimes called body trust, sometimes simply self-trust. Turn around ignorance, shame, fear, neglect, and the tendency to praise or blame something out there for what's happening in here, and you have its components.

Self-trust means learning about how your body works, and at the same time loving and respecting it for the magnificent and powerful creation it is. It means attuning to the signs and signals, both internal and external. It includes listening to yourself to discover what you want to change. Most importantly, body trust/self-trust involves a new way of thinking based on the knowledge that the only true healer is the one inside the skin, and the realization that patience and compassion are the key words in the process.

Love and Compassion

If you were going to climb a mountain you would make a number of necessary preparations. An important one might be to consult with those who have taken the trip already. Then you would carefully pack the minimal amount of essential gear, checking and double-checking to make sure everything was in good working order. Only then would you set out on your adventure.

The journey toward higher levels of wellness poses a similar challenge, and requires similar

Self-Acceptance—from Regina

When we were writing the first edition of this book, John and I both had difficulty with the fact that I was a cigarette smoker, and our book was about wellness. What would people think? Should we tell them? In working out this problem, we realized that it was more important to accept each other as we were than to try to fit other people's expectations. His acceptance of me, and my willingness to go outside when having a cigarette, led to his writing a little piece like this about the process. He also shared some of *his* "vices."

We have each received more comments about those three paragraphs than about almost any other part of the book. Smokers were relieved. Nonsmokers were touched. The whole process of dealing, personally and together, with our inconsistencies has inspired patience and compassion for ourselves and for others.

Come to think of it, I've learned a lot about patience and self-acceptance in the past four years, and all of it motivated by seeming crises. In 1981, while traveling in India, I contracted hepatitis and spent eight weeks sick and alone in a foreign country. Here was an opportunity to face my deepest fears of death and abandonment. Which I did. Then, in the winter of 1982, I fell on the ski slopes and broke my left leg in three places. Four months of greatly restricted mobility were the result. The "monsters" met this time were dependency and self-recrimination. Will the lessons never end? Not as long as I'm alive, I suppose.

I consider myself a "well being" and yet I've probably been laid up more than most people I know. But then, my definition of wellness has more to do with learning and loving than it does with sickness and health.

preparation. The equipment is less tangible, so it may be easy to neglect what is most essential. In remembering knowledge, self-trust, and perseverance, you might forget love and compassion. Yet these form the knapsack that carries all your other resources.

Compassion is an attribute of love. It means an empathic consciousness of weakness or distress, together with the desire to alleviate it. Any attempt at change which

lacks it is doomed from the start. It is just that important! Let's examine it in detail as it applies to the subject of health and "wholeness."

From our earliest years we have been rewarded for being strong, for achieving. We got "stroked" (touched, acknowledged, rewarded) for being what others defined as OK. As a result we often assumed that our self-worth depended upon "doing the right thing." Needing these strokes to

·Exercise·

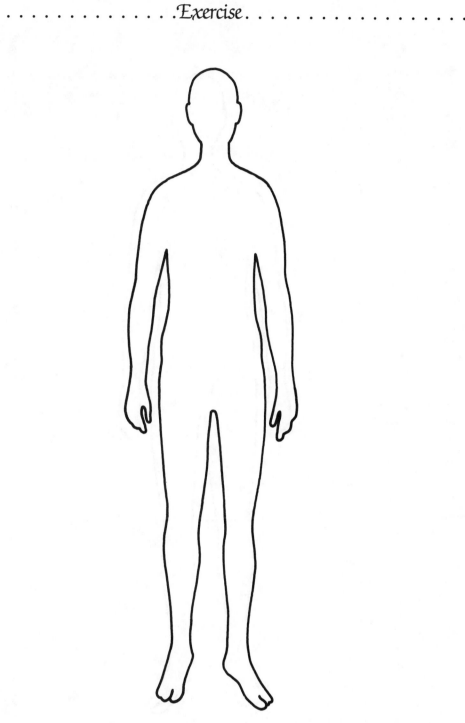

Here I Am #1

Imagine that the outline above represents your body as you are right now. Color it, choosing colors to signify how you feel about all the different parts of yourself. Write on it, or around it, commenting on each part of you, head to toe, inside and out. For example: short, curly hair—looks good on me; I don't like my legs—too skinny; a sense of darkness around my head—too many headaches; strong arms—I'm proud of them . . . Also note how you feel about your body/ your self in general. Include those comments/statements here too.

Here I Am #2

Now imagine that this outline represents your Ideal Body. Color it. Write all over or around it, commenting on yourself as you would like to be. For example: 20/20 vision—no more glasses; 143 pounds—just right; lungs clear—asthma gone.

    Compare your two pictures. You may find that you are unduly critical of yourself. Some things simply cannot be changed—accept them. Be aware of how you are influenced by media images of what health and beauty look like. Don't be fooled. Focus on loving yourself as you are, and with this foundation, inspiring yourself to change what you can.

live, we set about trying to accumulate them, only to be disappointed and frustrated when our best attempts sometimes failed. We were often weak, unprepared, and misinformed, and we accepted that this meant that we were "not OK." An interesting paradox then emerged. Some of us learned that by getting hurt through accident or illness we got stroked even more. Perhaps we were soothed with candy and ice cream, or permitted to stay home from school while Mother brought hot soup and the TV set to our bedside. And so the pattern was reinforced. If we couldn't get sufficient attention with our achievements, we could get it by our sicknesses. The seeds planted in our childhood continued to grow as we moved through adolescence and into adulthood. They are with us today and will be as we advance to old age.

The comedian on a popular late-night talk show remarks about his eighty-two-year-old mother: "She loves her new therapy. The doctor is all the time touching her, touching her!" We laugh, knowingly, because most of us recognize how readily people use suffering to get the strokes they haven't gotten through other means.

You can accept this insight and resign yourself to it as "the way things are." You can criticize the hypochondriacs of the world, of your own household, and resolve to steel yourself to their needs. Or you can examine your own life to see why this tendency shows itself, and resolve to do something about it. What would it be like to arrive at a place where you could ask for the strokes you need, *when* you need them? Suppose you start viewing

your own illness as a need for strokes in some broader context of your life? Imagine the many lessons you would learn, and the growth you could achieve, if you used the experience of disease as an opportunity to reevaluate your lifestyle and environment. What answers might surface if you posed yourself the question "Why do I need this problem at this time?" Could you possibly let go enough to enjoy the rest which an illness may afford? Are you willing to stroke yourself in the midst of your weakness, rather than in spite of it? Can you believe that it is OK to be weak, in need, out-of-balance at times; basically that it is OK to be just as you are—a glorious series of contradictions?

As we've noted before, the process of high-level wellness does not preclude an occasional bout with illness. If we view sickness as an evil to be eliminated under all circumstances and at any cost, we make death the ultimate enemy. This attitude can lead to the support of the quantity of life above its quality. One of the aspects of self-love and self-acceptance is allowing disease to be an instructive and positive life force. The lessons which accompany it are essential to the fully functional human being.

Regina slipped on the ice one cold day and broke her arm. It was right in the middle of a very pressured period of working on this book. The situation forced her to slow down, to rest, to struggle with her general reticence to ask for help from someone else. It became an opportunity rather than a problem.

History is filled with examples of individuals who experienced personal transformations as a result

Basic healthiness describes the quality of natural health or well-being which is fundamental to human beings. This quality of healthiness is *not* dependent on physical well-being for its expression. It is an unconditional state of health which may be *obscured* but *not destroyed* by illness. It is therefore possible to discover well-being in the midst of serious or chronic illness. Although this may seem simple and obvious, it is a major statement that sets our approach (of basic healthiness) apart from the many wellness and preventative health theories so prevalent today.

Lamen Mitchell Levy
Executive Director,
Amara Association of
Health Professionals[6]

of serious disease or crippling handicap. The writings of Helen Keller, or the music of Ray Charles, for instance, have inspired millions of people all over the world. Wellness may be encouraged by a physical handicap as much as by a vigorous exercise program or a pure diet. Of themselves, none of these things automatically leads to wellness. When used as tools for self-exploration, for education, for growth, everything leads to wellness.

Disease is not really the problem. It is more likely the body's attempt to solve the problem—a feedback of sorts that says "something isn't working properly." That "something" is probably lots more than cramped, disfigured fingers, or the headache over the right eye.

. . . . *Exercise* . . . .

To Accept, To Forgive, or To Change?

> God, grant me the serenity
> to accept the things I cannot change,
> The courage to change the things I can,
> And the wisdom to know the difference.

Much valuable life energy is wasted in burdening ourselves with guilt and blame. ("I should have done this . . . I shouldn't have said that. . . .) The objectives of this exercise are to identify the "shoulds" you are shouldering, and then to allow you to choose which are worth keeping, and which you need to accept and forgive.

Part I

A. Reflect upon all the ways in which you are hard on yourself. What do you blame yourself for? What do you feel guilty or "bad" about? What "mistakes" of your recent past still burden you with feelings of inadequacy or regret? Start making a list. Write it below.

The List:

B. Next to each item on your list, record your judgments or interpretations—the internal messages you give yourself about your actions. For example:

The List:	The Messages:
overeating	"I'm undisciplined. I hate myself."
losing my temper with Alaina	"I don't know how to handle children. I should be more patient."

C. Now that you've compiled this list, what do you think or feel about yourself? What have you learned about yourself in doing this?

. . . .

Part II

Using the questions below, test each item listed in the left column above to find out if you really intend to do something about it now.

Test Questions:

1. What is the "problem"?

2. Realistically, can I do anything about this situation now?
   If YES, go on to question #3.
   If NO, move ahead to Part III, and focus on acceptance/forgiveness.

3. Am I willing to face this situation now or soon?

4. What will it take in terms of time, energy, money, etc. to handle this situation?

5. How important is this situation in the context of the rest of my life?

6. Am I willing to **commit** to working on this problem **NOW**?

If your final answer is YES, see the section on Brainstorming in chapter 7 for some ideas on how to begin.

If your final answer is NO, or MAYBE, read Part III and focus on acceptance/forgiveness.

Part III

Acceptance, Forgiveness and Wellness

• The willingness to accept things as they are is the first step towards lasting change. Without the compulsiveness of "have to's," changing can be a joyous adventure.

• Acceptance is often confused with resignation, but the two are not the same. At its best, resignation may be a necessary, preliminary step towards acceptance. Resignation is dry, passive, and lifeless. It is an attitude of defeat. Real acceptance, on the other hand, is a choice, an active and lively process that requires your participation.

• You can't rush acceptance, or forgiveness, or force yourself into them. Any life change (positive or negative) entails some grief, some letting go of what was. And grieving takes time. Acceptance and forgiveness are results of adequate grieving.

• To forgive means to refuse to hold onto the past; to release grievances, recrimination, blame; to reconcile.

• Forgiveness includes the willingness to look below the surface of behaviors or feelings. Here we find the essence of the precious, loving being—which is you. When you connect here, and acknowledge who/what you find . . . forgiveness is so much easier.

• Forgiveness of yourself or others often brings with it a relaxation in the body, and peace of mind. This harmony is the essence of healing, and the heart of wellness.

Like the metaphors of a poem, or the images in a dream, these body-signs can often be interpreted at many levels. The most apparent says, "I've got arthritis," and "Mother had it too." Reflecting deeper, however, you might realize that all your life you've swallowed anger and clenched your fist behind your back. With this awareness, the focus of attention changes radically. Instead of determining how many aspirins you can safely continue to take, you ask what other, more direct ways there are for expressing your feelings. Then, you're ready to hit the road toward high-level wellness, generously reinforced with the compassion and love which will encourage your continuing success.

Being in love is what it's all about! As you fall in love with yourself you just naturally get healthier. All the do's and don't's of health education can only serve to build a house of straw, if love is not the foundation. When you see love in operation in a relationship, you see trust, acceptance of the uniqueness of each person, understanding of differences, and forgiveness of failings. To love yourself is to love your body, your emotions, your intelligence, your spiritual nature. It is to trust, to accept, to understand, and to forgive yourself. The challenge is in remembering that love is all around you, and in opening yourself to receive it. Love is not out there waiting to be found; it is within you wanting to be recognized. The fact is that all things in the universe are connected. All things in the body are connected as well. There is simply no place where the body starts and the mind stops; no place where the universe starts and the individual stops.

Self-Acceptance—from John

As we prepare this second edition of the *Wellness Workbook*, I reflect on how well I've measured up to what I've helped write. If I compare myself to what most people think of as wellness (see No Fascism Please, p. xviii), I'm a poor example. I've had more physical problems in the past four years than ever before in my life. My back chronically aches and periodically leaves me flat on it. Since passing forty, my body's aging has made itself known. I've grown many gray hairs, and lost a lot on top. And all of this I find hard to accept.

Regular exercise has always been a struggle for me. I get no pleasure whatever from doing anything with my muscles. And, I'm at the point of breaking that barrier because my discomfort level is rising fast, along with my cholesterol, which is 230, even though I eat a well-balanced diet. I suspect it's both the lack of exercise and the chronic stress I create that keeps the cholesterol so high. I'm hard on myself. I fear that I'll never get anything done without deadlines, and so I set up ones that I can never quite meet.

Oftentimes I compare myself with some "ideal" and find myself wanting. Despite all I know about self-responsibility and blame being two different things, I still berate myself for not being a "better person."

Then I remember that wellness isn't perfection and that it's OK to be just the way I am. I'm actually learning to love myself (or at least not to punish myself) even when I don't do things "right."

So I hope you do not see this book as prescribing answers or telling you the one true way. Likewise, don't think you need to "have it all together," no matter which paths you take.

I believe we all teach what we most need to learn. As long as this wellness stuff is still big in my life, I might as well enjoy learning it.

Finally, love means taking it easy on yourself. As you begin to realize how many things affect your state of wellness you might at first be overwhelmed, thinking that you have to *do something* about each of them. But the connectedness of all things actually makes this whole business of living wellness a lot easier. As you breathe better, you move better, and digest your food better, and relax more deeply, and develop greater self-awareness, and . . . The associations multiply. When this happens, we appreciate one of the basics of wellness—that it's all one process.

The challenge of living well is the challenge of becoming the most loving, clearest, most aware channel of energy you can possibly be. To do so simply means to become a natural alchemist in the highest sense of the word. It is to become a transmuter of energy. It is to transform yourself.

. . . . *Exercise* . . . .

How to Practice Forgiveness

It's simple. You make the intention to do so; watch as you fall short of your goal time after time, day after day; and then you make the intention again. Be patient. Your *willingness* to forgive yourself and others is a monumental step. Renewed intention slowly and surely takes its effect. You may not *feel* any differently after forgiving yourself/someone. Don't worry. Forgiveness is not a feeling; it's a decision.

Here are a few exercises which focus awareness about forgiveness.

1. The inability to forgive may be indicative of insufficient grieving of a loss. Ask yourself: What have I lost in this situation? Forget about trying to forgive, and concentrate on telling the story of your pain or problem to every willing ear. Find friends who are not afraid of strong emotion, and cry with them. Write letters to yourself, or to others, describing and lamenting your loss. Enlist the help of a support group, or seek professional counseling to work out your grief. And it is work, so don't give up too soon.

2. Review all the things for which you blame yourself. With each one repeat to yourself: "I forgive you for _____, _____. I release you from any guilt or blame, now and forever." This may seem foolish or magical especially if you don't "feel" forgiving. Do it anyway. It's up to you to *create* its reality by directing your intention.

3. Repeat the name of the person you want to forgive (this may include yourself) as you picture him/her in your mind's eye. Begin to see/feel good things, blessings, happening for him. Don't be satisfied with a few good things. Let your imagination have free reign and bless yourself or the other abundantly and outrageously.

4. Lack of forgiveness may be a failure to acknowledge the beauty and strength of who you really are. Focusing on appreciation of these qualities in yourself or others is helpful in practicing forgiveness. Make a list of all the things that are great about you (or the other). Include your talents, accomplishments, sensitivities, caring and generous activities, courage or other virtues—everything you can think of. Don't be satisfied until you have a good, long list. Now post this list where you will see it frequently, and READ IT!

5. Visualize the person you want to forgive surrounded in a warm, golden light. See this light melt her/him, layer by layer, revealing the fears and pain she is hiding within. It also reveals her loving center—the hunger she has for love and peace. Allow yourself to feel her pain, her fear, and her love. Keep this picture in your mind for a few minutes. Allow forgiveness to be there.

Suggested Reading*

American Friends Service Committee. *Taking Charge of Our Lives: Living Responsibly in a Troubled World*. Joan Bodner, ed. San Francisco, CA: Harper and Row, 1984.

Ardell, D. *High Level Wellness: An Alternative to Doctors, Drugs, and Disease*. Berkeley, CA: Ten Speed Press, 1986.

Bricklin, M. *The Practical Encyclopedia of Natural Healing*. Emmaus, PA: Rodale Press, 1983.

Carlson, R. *The End of Medicine*. New York, NY: John Wiley and Sons, 1975.

Cassell, E.J. *The Healer's Art*. Cambridge, MA: The MIT Press, 1976.

Deliman, T., and Smolowe, J. *Holistic Medicine—Harmony of Body, Mind, Spirit*. Reston, VA: Reston Publishing Co., 1982.

Dossey, L. *Space, Time and Medicine*. Boston, MA: Shambhala, 1982.

———. *Beyond Illness—Discovering the Experience of Health*. Boston, MA: Shambhala, 1984.

Dunn, H. *High Level Wellness*. (7th ed.) Arlington, VA: R. W. Beatty, 1972.

Ferguson, T. *Medical Self Care*. New York, NY: Simon and Schuster, 1980. Also a quarterly magazine of the same name and edited by the same author: Box 1000, Point Reyes, CA 94956.

Illich, I. *Medical Nemesis*. New York, NY: Bantam Books, 1976.

*This is only a representative sampling. Many excellent books have been omitted. At the bookstore or library, look over the whole selection and choose according to your judgment.

Jampolsky, G. *Good-Bye to Guilt: Releasing Fear through Forgiveness*. New York, NY: Bantam Books, 1985.

Knowles, J., ed. *Doing Better and Feeling Worse: Health in the U.S.* New York, NY: W.W. Norton, 1977.

Kripalu Center for Yoga and Health. *The Self-Health Guide: A Personal Program for Holistic Living*. Lenox, MA: Kripalu Publications, 1980.

Miller, J. *The Human Body*. New York, NY: Viking Press, 1983.

Moss, R. *How Shall I Live: Transforming Surgery or Any Health Crisis into Greater Awareness*. Berkeley, CA: Celestial Arts, 1985.

Pelletier, K. *Mind as Healer, Mind as Slayer*. New York, NY: Delta Books, 1977.

Reader's Digest Family Safety and First Aid. New York, NY: Berkley Books, 1984.

Rubin, T.I. *Reconciliations: Inner Peace in an Age of Anxiety*. New York, NY: Berkley Books, 1980.

Samuels, M., and Bennett, H. *The Well Body Book*. New York, NY, and Berkeley, CA: Random House/Bookworks, 1973.

Schutz, W. *Profound Simplicity*. San Diego, CA: Learning Concepts, 1979.

Weil, A. *Health and Healing*. Boston, MA: Houghton-Mifflin, 1983.

. . . . *Regina's Journal.* . . . .

I believe that most of my illnesses and accidents have been self-imposed punishments for not being perfect (or "sinless").

One day in a session with a therapist I recalled a time when I was thirteen years old. I remembered lying in bed and giving up in total despair: "God, send me to Hell! I just can't fight sin any more." I was so tired of waging this battle within myself that I was ready to die.

Now I see that from my earliest days I had accepted the idea that the only way to please God, the only way to be truly good, was to be perfect. And I have been beating myself up in an endless variety of ways since then whenever I have fallen short of my own unattainable ideal.

I prayed that God would forgive me, and when things got tough, took my pain as punishment. It was not until years later that I learned a different conclusion, i.e. that **God did not have to forgive me, because God had never condemned me.** I had condemned myself. It followed then, that if I was to heal, and grow, and experience wholeness again, I had to forgive **myself.**

When I understood this—I cried.

. . . .

Notes

1. National Health Expenditures, *Statistical Abstract of the United States 1985*, U.S. Dept. of Commerce, Bureau of the Census.

2. "Examination of the Pharmaceutical Industry," Hearings Before the Subcommittee on Labor and Public Welfare. U.S. Senate 93rd Congress, 1st and 2nd sessions on S.3441 and S.966. Dec. 18–19, 1973, Part I. See pages 188–89, 233–34.

3. For an interesting treatment of how statistics on life expectancy can be misleading see:

Kuntzleman, C. *The Exerciser's Handbook*. New York, NY: David McKay Co., 1978, pp. 92–94.

4. Kuntzleman, C., pp.92–93.

5. Lerner, M. "When, Where and Why People Die," in *Death: Current Perspectives*. Shneidman, E., ed. Palo Alto, CA: Mayfield Publishing Co., 1977, p. 153.

6. Reprinted with permission from: *Vajradhatu Sun*, June/July 1985, p. 18.

Amara is an association of Eastern and Western health professionals founded by Chogyam Trungpa Rimpoche to explore the relationship between body and mind. Its main focus is "basic healthiness" as it affects our appreciation of health and treatment of illness. For further information write: Amara Association of Health Professionals, 1345 Spruce St., Suite A, Boulder, CO 80302.

Two

Wellness and Breathing

THE HUMAN BODY is remarkably adaptive and resilient. Human beings can survive for many weeks without food, for several days without water. But without air, life ceases in only a matter of minutes. The fact is that every cell in the organism requires a continuous charge of oxygen in order to carry out its assigned function.

. . . .

Air is the first food of the newborn.

—EDWARD ROSENFELD

. . . .

The job of breathing is to supply this energy to the bloodstream, but since it has been happening automatically for every moment of your life, you've probably given very little attention to it. Yet without it, everything stops. So this is where we will begin our investigation of wellness.

When the air is clear, your lungs strong, your body relaxed,

Breathing is synonymous with living. It is our most basic energy-transforming process. In the Wellness Energy System, oxygen is the first energy input. All the cells of our body depend upon oxygen for the production of the high-energy chemical bonds necessary to maintain life.

and your mind at peace, you experience total well-being. Unfortunately, this ideal is seldom realized. In the language of the Wellness Energy System, the *input* source, the air, may be polluted in some way. Or perhaps there just isn't enough

of it available. High altitude climbers must carry their own oxygen, or risk light-headedness and even death around 24,000 feet. Being in an overcrowded room without proper ventilation will have a similar effect. The *channel* (which is you) may have breakages (poorly functioning organs, illness, accident), or be blocked by foreign objects, by the restriction of muscles created from emotions such as fear, anger, and grief, by tight clothing, or by chronically poor

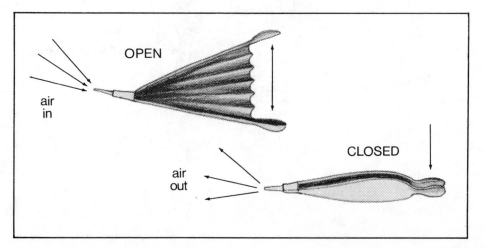

posture. It may also be contaminated by the poisons of nicotine and tar accumulated in lung tissues.

The resulting *output*—your general metabolism, and your ability to work, play, and communicate with others—will depend upon these factors *and* upon how effectively the energy has been used.

The Process of Breathing

Breathing may be likened to the functioning of the old-fashioned blacksmith's bellows. Lift up the handles, opening the bellows, and air is sucked in. Press down, flatten the bellows, and the air rushes out.

. . . .

Adult human beings breathe an average of 16,000 quarts of air each day.

. . . .

The components of the process here are those of volume and pressure. As the volume of the bellows increases, the internal pressure decreases, creating a vacuum-effect which draws in the outside air. When the bellows collapse, the volume decreases, and the increasing internal pressure forces the air back out again.

The bellows at work within your body are a number of fascinating muscles. The most active of these is the diaphragm—a dome-shaped muscle located at the base of the rib cage and above the stomach. It contracts during inhalation and pulls down on the bottom of the chest, increasing the volume inside the chest cavity. At the same time, the chest capacity can be further increased by elevating the ribs slightly and moving them outward and upward. When all is working smoothly what results is maximum volume and minimal pressure. Air is drawn in—you are "inspiring." Relax these muscles and the elastic property of the lungs causes them to contract. The diaphragm is pulled back up, ribs move back in and down, the pressure builds, and the air is exhaled. The diagram (left) will further clarify it.

The oxygen taken into the lungs contains the life force—"prana" the Hindus call it. The red corpuscles of the blood moving through the lungs pick oxygen up and proceed to carry it throughout the body, charging every muscle, bone, nerve, and organ with its necessary fuel. Quite an impressive process, especially when you consider that it has been going on day and night from your first moment in the world. Fortunately, it happens without need for your conscious direction.

Breathing, you understand, is not something you DO. Rather, it is something which you ALLOW. Left alone, the body will do what it needs to do, and most efficiently at that. So then why devote a chapter of a book to it?

The answer is that we *don't* allow our breathing to happen smoothly and naturally. We continuously do things which restrict it. Changing this around is going to mean that we pay some attention to it for a while. Rather than add-

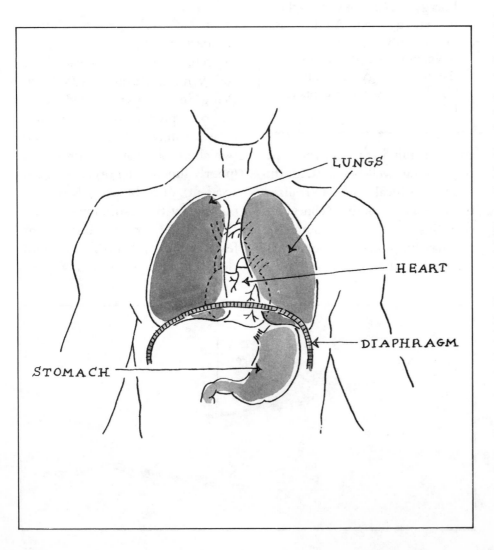

LUNGS

HEART

DIAPHRAGM

STOMACH

. . . . *Exercise* . . . .

Experiencing a Full Breath

Introduction: While it is not possible or necessary to fully expand the lungs with every breath, it is vital in heightening awareness to experience how a really complete breath feels. Used periodically, this exercise utilizes the lungs to capacity and extracts great amounts of "life force" from the air.

Directions: Try this exercise sitting, standing, and lying down.

1. Exhale deeply, contracting the belly.

2. Inhale slowly as you expand the abdomen.

3. Continue inhaling as you expand the chest.

4. Continue inhaling as you raise the shoulders up toward your ears.

5. Hold for a few comfortable seconds.

6. Exhale in reverse pattern, slowly. Release shoulders, relax chest, contract the belly.

7. Repeat.

This exercise will require gentle practice in order that inhalation and exhalation be smooth and balanced. Beginners should only do it 2 or 3 times continuously.

. . . .

ing something new, most of our work will be centered around removing the obstacles, the conditions, which are blocking our breathing and consequently depriving us of a full life.

Problems in the System

Disease and Damage

Recent testing conducted by the U.S. Environmental Protection Agency verifies that breathing polluted air causes not only coughing, chest tightness, and eye irritation, but actually impairs lung functioning and weakens the ability of white blood cells to fight infection.[1] Thus affected, the respiratory system may become the weak link in the body's chain, and therefore a receptive environment for diseases such as influenza, bronchitis, TB, and other types of pneumonia.

The condition known as emphysema, which is principally linked to smoking, occurs when, through repeated abuse, the lung tissues lose their elasticity. The lungs are no longer able to expel air on their own, so breathing becomes more difficult and even impossible. Since we generally use less than half our lung capacity in usual breathing, a heavy smoker may only become aware of lung damage when s/he exercises. The slow, subtle progression of this disease makes it more serious because it may not be detected until it is too late. Emphysema is a major cause of death in the U.S.

Asthma is another condition which affects the ability to breathe. It is a reaction triggered by allergenic substances as well as by threatening emotional situations. Anita recalls that during the summer of her tenth year she traveled across the country with her parents in a small trailer. She awoke one night to hear her parents making love. Her father's groans frightened her. Her mother sounded hurt. Fearful that they would discover her listening, she stiffened her body and tried not to breathe. The following day she suffered the first of many attacks of asthma.

The realization of the connection between emotions and asthma strengthens our premise that disease is more than damage or infection. It is a state of mind.

. . . . *Regina's Journal*. . . . .

Dec. 18, 1979

A Reaction to Grief

The news of Sheila's death came by phone early this morning from Frank's sister in New York. I took the call.

My body immediately shocked. A feeling of breathlessness—all morning long I am gasping for air. The sensation in my body is hard to describe—something like cotton candy in the veins. I am simultaneously enervated and numbed. The reality does not penetrate. Jere is breathless as well. He allows a few tears to flow and then becomes silent. We hold each other for a long time, unable to speak.

. . . .

Tension

Fear, grief, anger, and even exhilaration are emotional states which produce physical changes in the body. These changes increase the overall body tension, and restrict breathing. Any excess tension will upset the balance, and interfere with normal breathing.

Marjorie experienced an asthmatic attack when she noticed the flowers on her doctor's desk. She panicked. Her mind issued a "red alert" to her body, and sweating and gasping for air was her response. The flowers, she later learned, were artificial. But the pain she felt was real. Whether the danger is real or imaginary makes little difference. Fear will create tension, and tension will affect the ability to breathe. What we perceive, believe, trust, and fear in our minds will spill over into the body and manifest in some way. There is simply no place where the mind stops and the body starts and vice versa.

Recall a recent fearful event in your own life and reflect how your breathing was affected by it. Perhaps you have had a near accident in your car. No impact or injury, but upsetting none the less. The scenario may look something like this: You narrowly miss hitting a child who has run into the street. A few moments pass and you pull over to the side of the road . . . because something has knocked the wind out of you. That something is fear. You take some slow, deep breaths, and pinch yourself in relief that you are still in one piece. Your fast-beating heart begins to slow to its normal rhythm, and you proceed on your way. Retelling the incident, or waking from a dream about it, you experience the same breathlessness which accompanied the event itself. Once again, you pause to get your breath to complete your story, or to fall back to sleep again.

The inability to breathe fully is also one of the most common reactions to grief. People experiencing great sadness at the loss of a loved one often describe feeling as if steel bands were binding the chest. The heart has been wounded or broken in the figurative sense, but the physiological reaction is literal. The muscles associated with respiration tighten in an attempt to protect this vulnerable region from further injury. Shallow breathing serves the self-protective function of cutting off feeling, and this is often temporarily necessary. Holding, stroking, and massaging the grieving person give the feeling of security again. This contact and the acceptance it symbolizes can encourage the crying and deep sighing necessary in working through a loss experience. Releasing grief breaks the vise-like grip around the rib cage and allows breathing to happen normally again.

Holding in emotions such as fear, grief, or anger restricts breathing; the conscious use of breath can be an invaluable tool in learning to express emotions appropriately.

Posture and Clothing

Physical posture is one of the main factors in restricting breath. Years of presenting ourselves to the world with "chest out and stomach in" can create poor breathing habits. These take their toll in a whole range of imbalanced conditions from hemorrhoids to headaches. Is it any wonder? How can the diaphragm possibly do its job of expanding if the abdominal muscles refuse to move? The body will compensate by breathing from the upper chest, but the result is only a half-breath. Our furniture, our cars, and our clothing serve to further aggravate the situation. Observe the cramped school desks that we sat in for so many hours a day over twelve or more years of our lives, desks that forced us to double over at the waist, to strain the neck, and to keep our legs tightly crossed and out of the way.

Cars, too, are rarely designed to allow for the relaxed posture so vital for natural breathing. Cramped legs, lower back pain, tense arms and shoulders are common, even on short trips. Truck drivers and others who frequently drive long distances often suffer more serious problems.

Clothing design may discourage freedom of movement and restrict breathing. Our culture prizes the flat belly and continues to invent torturous means of assuring it. Figure controlling panty-hose, all-day girdles, and tight-fitting jeans are big business, and therefore not easily dismissed. If you note the gently rounded belly of the relaxed child, or the pictures of the "uncivilized natives" in *National Geographic Magazine*, you see what a natural posture would look like. As you tighten the abdomen to flatten the belly you prohibit free-flowing breathing. You may also tighten the genitals and anus in the same motion. Doing this blocks the flow of sexual energy as well.

The diaphragm connects the upper half of the body with the lower half. Above the diaphragm is the domain of the intellect, the rational mind; below it, the emotional realm, the "gut," the pleasure centers and reproductive organs. Breathing then becomes the harmonizing force, the integrating process which unites and balances us, head with heart with belly.

A Metaphor for Life

. . . .

The gift of giving inspiration to others is the gift of life.
—KAREN GIARDINO

. . . .

The way you breathe is the way you live your life. Actually, the

---

Ways of Breathing, Ways of Being

- "The more I smoke, the shallower I breathe. The more I smoke, the less I feel." —J.F.

- "I go to the mountains because breathing the air there makes me more creative." —K.M.

- "I don't want any more conflict in my life. I walk on egg-shells. I never think about breathing." —J.P.

- "When I'm happy I remember to breathe." —D.W.

- "When I heard the news, I couldn't breathe." —S.R.

- "I love to breathe." —R.S.

---

words for "spirit," meaning life force or the power of God, and "breath," are the same in many languages. For example, in Sanskrit it is called *prana*; in Hebrew *ruach*; in Greek *pneuma*; in Latin *spiritus*. In English, to inhale is to inspire—which is to take in the spirit. To exhale is to expire—to release the spirit. To conspire literally means to breathe together. All of life can be observed as a taking in and giving out, of movement and rest, of controlling and letting go.

Experienced body therapists report dramatic changes in people who start to practice full breathing. Breathing heightens awareness and encourages the release of long-held tensions. Tears, deep sighs, and the recollection of old and painful memories commonly accompany deep massage or manipulation of the muscles involved in respiration.[2]

A psychologist friend told about a game he used to play as a child. He had practiced the ability to control his respiration so completely that he used to challenge his brother to detect any movement which would indicate breathing. He was trying to make himself invisible—to insulate himself from hurtful emotional situations. As an adult, this self-protective approach had become a source of great sadness, of joylessness. Now that he has become aware of what he has been doing, he checks frequently to find out if he is breathing fully, and uses daily exercise to encourage richer breathing. He claims that his whole life is richer as a result.

How do you breathe? How would you describe your general approach to living? You are invited to explore the possible connections.

Breathing for Awareness

. . . .

With awareness comes movement.

—JOEL KRAMER

. . . .

Your breath is a built-in alarm clock which rings on the average of ten to sixteen times every minute, reminding you that you're alive, right now! But like so many habitual cues in your environment, you can easily become so accustomed to it that you don't hear it any more. Ruminating about the past and attempting to anticipate the future, you neglect the RIGHT NOW which is slipping away before you can stop to enjoy it.

Failing to live in the present can be a source of great sadness and dissatisfaction about life. A well-to-do psychiatrist was once asked

Life means rhythm!—With its first breath the new-born baby enters into the rhythm of life; with its inhalation and exhalation, it begins to experience the flow of life in its alternating positive and negative phases, pulsating within it like an alternating current. Life is thus an uninterrupted chain of rhythmic breaths, in and out, until with his last breath man "expires," i.e. "breathes out" and closes the final link in the chain.[3]

—SELVARAJAN
YESUDIN AND
ELIZABETH HAICH

the secret of his success. His patients praised his methods, and his waiting room was always filled with people. "It's easy," he remarked. "I simply tell them to do one thing at a time, and to do it as if it were all they ever had to do in the world." That's part of what is meant by awareness.

Helen recalls little of her wedding ceremony which took place on a hillside in Massachusetts less than five years ago. She was so preoccupied with remembering what she needed to say, and so anxious that everything go smoothly that she missed the magic happening all around her. Learning to be more fully present in the here and now is another aspect of awareness.

The use of the breath can help you in achieving an expanded sense of awareness in your everyday life. You start the practice of cueing in to the process of breathing in all different circumstances (waiting for the bus, watching the sunset). The

inhalation reminds you to open yourself as fully as possible to what is happening NOW.

What is my body doing? Where are my thoughts taking me? Who is this person I'm talking with? What does this food feel like in my mouth? Why is my shoulder feeling so tight? The exhalation allows you to let go of worrying about the past and the future. The inhalation opens you again.

In its purest form, this awareness is the unverbalized appreciation of the way things are—the experience of just "being with" the flower, the other person, the movement of your body as you dance. This is the stuff of which awestruck moments, the "peak experiences," are made. Coming back

from such a high, a normally grey world is seen in technicolor, and words fail in communicating what has occurred.

Normally, we do not so much look at things as overlook them.

—ALAN WATTS

It is easy to misinterpret awareness training as a methodology for neglecting rational planning and goal-directed behavior. "Don't think about the future, man, just be here now!" Nothing could be further from the truth of what real awareness is about. Instead of living only *for* the moment, awareness encourages living fully *in* the moment. And this moment may be

---

I'd Pick More Daisies

If I had my life to live over, I'd try to make more mistakes next time. I would relax. I would limber up. I would be sillier than I have been this trip. I know of very few things I would take seriously. I would be crazier. I would be less hygienic. I would take more chances. I would take more trips. I would climb more mountains, swim more rivers and watch more sunsets . . . I would eat more ice cream and less beans. I would have more actual troubles and fewer imaginary ones. You see, I am one of those people who lives prophylactically and sanely and sensibly, hour after hour, day after day. Oh, I have had my moments and, if I had it to do over again, I'd have

more of them. In fact, I'd try to have nothing else. Just moments, one after another, instead of living so many years ahead each day. I have been one of those people who never go anywhere without a thermometer, a hot water bottle, a gargle, a raincoat and a parachute. If I had it to do over again, I would go places and do things and travel lighter than I have.

If I had my life to live over, I would start barefooted earlier in the spring and stay that way later in the fall. I would play hooky more. I wouldn't make such good grades except by accident. I would ride on more merry-go-rounds. I'd pick more daisies.

Nadine Stair, 87
Louisville, KY

. . . . *Exercise* . . . .

"I Am Relaxed"—A Simple Form of Meditation and Relaxation

1. Sit comfortably and quietly.

2. Tell yourself that you are going to use the next 5, 10, or 20 minutes to rebalance, to heal, to relax yourself.

3. Surrender the weight of your body, allowing the chair, or floor, to support you.

4. Close your eyes, gently cutting out visual stimulation and distraction.

5. As you inhale, repeat to yourself: "I AM . . ."

6. As you exhale say ". . . RELAXED."

7. Continue to breath normally not trying to change it in any way. Just watch it happening and continue to repeat: "I AM" with inhalation; "RELAXED" with exhalation.

8. As your mind begins to wander, gently bring it back to the awareness of your breath and your statement "I AM RELAXED."

    Be compassionate and loving with your "leaping frog" mind which wants to be anywhere but here.

9. Continue doing this for as long a time as you have established.

10. To conclude, discontinue the phrase and slowly stretch your hands and feet, your arms and legs, your whole body.

11. Open your eyes a sliver at a time—like the sun coming up in the morning.

12. Continue on your way.

. . . .

devoted to designing a new strategy for environmental protection, planning for your retirement, or studying for tomorrow's biology exam. The point is that you choose consciously to address yourself to each issue. You immerse yourself in the task at hand with energy and concentration. You attune yourself to all the input—at the rational, emotive, physical, and even psychic levels. You do it with passion—*knowing* that you are doing it!

Try the simple experiment of eating a piece of fruit with awareness. You take the first bite. The coldness excites your mouth. You start chewing, experiencing the exquisite flavor, the sweet juice. Before you can swallow, you realize that you've checked the time, picked up a magazine, looked out the window, decided to make an apple pie for dessert, and wondered if you need to go to the drycleaners this afternoon. Not such a simple task, this eating with awareness. As you begin to practice it you are often overwhelmed with how unconscious so much of your life has become. This is when compassion needs to step in. Then you can relax into the experience, and laugh at how much learning you have to do, without judging yourself harshly for not yet being there.

Using breath-attunement on a regular basis will aid you in maximizing the body's built-in feedback system—those constant messages it offers you are its attempt to regain balance. Responding to them will create that state of relaxed awareness which it most wants to have.

Breathing and Relaxing

"I knew I was back in the driver's seat in my life," reported the prominent college professor, "when I smiled at the elevator in my office building." He went on to tell the story about this slow, unreliable elevator which had become such a great source of tension and frustration to him over the years. Day after day he waited for it, pacing anxiously, checking his watch, cursing it. One day, he became involved in a research experiment on the campus, and learned a simple technique of relaxation. This involved a short, daily practice of rhythmic breathing and the repetition of a meaningless word—a "mantra." The discipline was enjoyable, and the study intriguing, so he kept it up. The morning that he found himself smiling at the elevator, he woke up to a whole new appreciation for life. He credited the change to the relaxation practice, and has stayed with it since.

Stories of this nature are becoming commonplace in the literature about relaxation and consciousness development. Nearly all of the relaxation techniques support the use of breath control or awareness. No longer the sole privilege of religious adepts, these practices are being encouraged, and adopted, by educational and industrial groups because they show results. In Denver, Colorado, educational consultants train classroom teachers in relaxation methods which serve to both reduce stress and encourage creativity in children.[4] Biofeedback training, which relies heavily on slower, deeper breathing, is receiving wide acceptance throughout the medical

Biofeedback

Biofeedback is the process of becoming aware of physiological events we normally are not aware of, with the intent of ultimately gaining voluntary control of such events. Basic examples of biofeedback include weighing yourself, taking your pulse when exercising and taking your temperature when you are sick. Biofeedback, an acronym for biological feedback, revolutionizes the area of physical and mental health by providing a means for receiving feedback on areas previously labeled involuntary: the brain, the heart, the circulatory system.

Using sophisticated instrumentation, an individual can learn to reestablish mind-body connections and regulate muscle tension, brain waves, skin temperature, skin resistance, and other physiological processes. The implications in preventive medicine and health maintenance are tremendous. Deviations from the body's homeostatic state can be prevented or overcome by consciously reestablishing homeostasis. Clinical applications of biofeedback include stress management, migraine headache, tension headache, anxiety neurosis, neuromuscular rehabilitation, hypertension, Raynaud's disease, and gastrointestinal disorders.

The principal instruments used in biofeedback training are:

1. Electromyogram (EMG): the feedback of bioelectric information from muscles. Audio-visual information provides the user with information on levels of muscle tension.

2. Electroencephalogram (EEG): the feedback of bioelectric information from the brain. Audio-visual information provides the user with knowledge of changes in brain wave states: theta (creativity, meditation), alpha (relaxation, internal orientation, meditation), beta (cognitive activity, external orientation).

3. Thermal trainer: the feedback of changes in skin temperature, which is a function of blood flow.

4. Electrodermal response (EDR): the feedback of changes in skin resistance, which is a function of skin perspiration.

Source: Aims Biofeedback Institute, Aims Community College, Greeley, Colorado.

community.[5] Large companies are incorporating workshops in stress-management and meditation for their employees because they find it beneficial.[6] Many of these stress-reducing techniques include using breathing for relaxing.

As a society we are constantly exposed to anxiety-producing circumstances which cause excess tension. Driving your car or bicycle to work, the pressures of job production, deadlines, term papers, the noise of technology, the music

······· Exercise ·······

Breathing for Balance

Introduction: As you breathe, the air traveling through the nasal passages will stimulate the sensory nerve linings here and consequently affect the nerve origins in the brain. Involving both nostrils more fully will assist your body in its great balancing act. Use this exercise to increase awareness of imbalanced breathing as well as to relax and energize your whole system.

Directions:

1. Begin by exhaling completely using both nostrils.

2. Press your thumb or forefinger against the right nostril, closing it completely, and then inhale slowly and easily through the left one alone.

3. Hold the inhaled breath for a few comfortable seconds and then exhale through the right nostril, while keeping the left one closed. Hold while comfortable.

4. Now inhale through the right nostril, hold, and then exhale through the left nostril, while you keep the right one closed. Hold. Inhale left . . .

5. Continue for 5 to 8 cycles. Then stop. Allow breathing through both nostrils.

Goal: Short daily practice periods will enable you to make your breathing smooth and balanced.

on the radio—all of these can set us on edge so easily that we tend to lose touch with what life would be like without them.

If you have recently found yourself in a situation in which you were threatened—a near accident, the start of an important examination—you may recall that breathing came with some difficulty. Anger, fear, sedentary work, and the pace of fast-food restaurants, to name a few, may cause a dramatic change in your breathing. Slowing down, attuning to the breath, taking a few deep inhalations and exhalations will assist you in releasing the unnecessary distress which so easily builds up.

The link between states of tension/relaxation and the rate and depth of breathing is clear. Endangered from without or from disturbing thoughts within, the body reacts to protect itself. The instinctive response has been called the "fight or flight" mechanism. Described by Dr. Hans Selye, perhaps the world's leading authority on the subject of stress, it involves a whole range of automatic reactions.[7] These serve to energize the body to do battle or to run away, whichever seems right at the moment. The physical changes include a surge of adrenalin which raises blood pressure, and increases heart rate, blood flow to muscles, general metabolism, and the rate of breathing.

There are other measurable changes that characterize the "fight or flight" response. Hand and foot temperatures below 70°F/21°C in a room temperature environment, are commonly found among very tense individuals. (And despite the old saying, cold hands have nothing to do with warm hearts.) Palms and fingers may become moist with small amounts of perspiration released by the adrenalin discharge. Such clammy hands are another signal that chronic tension exists. Similarly, there is an increase in muscle tension throughout the entire body which may show up as morning stiffness or excessive facial wrinkles. These wrinkles are caused by the constant stretching and bunching up of skin due to overactivity of the underlying musculature. If you notice any of these symptoms with regularity, you can be sure your body is aroused unnecessarily.

As an occasional and temporary condition it serves the whole organism well, but when this "alarm" state characterizes your

. . . . *Exercise* . . . .

Cleaning House . . . Waking Up . . . Calming Down . . .

There are numerous occasions when you feel cloudy and tired due to the atmosphere in a smoke-filled room, accumulated carbon dioxide stored during sleep, or tense, sit-down work. These exercises can be used to help you to clear out your head, and wake up your body, as well as to calm down by releasing tension.

Exercise 1: Stand up. Bend from the waist; relax the knees and muscles around anus and genitals. Place your hands on your upper thighs.

> Inhale deeply through the nose.
> Exhale forcefully through the mouth.
> Push all the air out of the lungs.
> Repeat.

Exercise 2: Stand up. Raise arms above your head. Begin to jump up and down rhythmically as if you were jumping rope.

> As you jump up, you inhale quickly.
> As you land the air is expelled from the mouth with the sound of "hu."
> Continue for about 30 seconds in the beginning.
> Stop. Allow your breath to come naturally.

Exercise 3: Stand up. Inhale through the mouth as you raise your arms above your head. Pretend that you are trying to grasp the stars. Get up on your tiptoes. Reach even higher, inhaling all the way. Release. Go limp. Exhale vigorously. Bend from the waist and let head and arms dangle like a rag doll. Stop. Breathe normally.

---

general approach to living, you sap huge energy reserves which are needed for other purposes. Sooner or later the results will show up in some destructive way both in the body as well as in the spirit. As Selye says, ". . . stress plays some role in the development of every disease."[8] The constructive, conscious use of the breath can break this pattern of tension as a way of life.

While we're on the subject of tension here, let's remember that it's not all bad. It is, in fact, a necessary component of most life situations. Death is the only stress-free condition. A tension-less state—the limp handshake—is far from

desirable. But equally discomforting is the tight, rigid grasp. What we're looking for is a balance between these extremes—the firm, yet relaxed handshake, the supportive, yet gentle embrace. This happy combination is seen in the performance of the dancer, the movements of the accomplished skier, and heard in the music of the masterful pianist.

The problem is that most of the time we fall far short of this state of relaxed-tension. We use excessive amounts of energy in striving for perfect form. The result is often loss of balance, early fatigue, and accidents. Many of us live an "uptight" existence absorbed in and

surrounded by anxiety-producing situations. We end up with headaches and ulcers. Releasing this vise-grip approach to life can begin with paying conscious attention to breathing. Try out some of the exercises and cueing methods suggested in this chapter, and you may be pleasantly surprised by the results in joy and health which they can promote.

Breathing for Work and Play

Some excellent examples of the positive and therapeutic uses of rhythmic breathing and breath awareness come from such diverse

Remembering to Breathe—Allowing Natural Breathing

As you go through a day, there are many occasions during which you block breathing by your posture or level of tension. Use this exercise to remind yourself to check your breathing and to remove factors which may be restricting your natural breathing.

Purchase a supply of self-adhesive, colored dots at a stationery store. Go through your house, your office, your car, your wallet, your purse, and place these dots in prime locations. Each time you see one, use it as a cue to remind yourself to allow breathing.

AND/OR

Make signs such as BREATHE or WAKE-UP or REMEMBER and put them around where you are sure to be surprised by them regularly. When you notice them, attune to your breathing, or lack of it. Allow it.

P.S. When people ask about the dots on the signs, use this as an opportunity to breathe again, and to spread the good word!

activities as childbirth and sports. More women today are choosing natural or drugless childbirth—a variety of techniques for using deep breathing to decrease overall anxiety and pain, as well as for assisting the normal bodily processes involved in birthing a child. The father, or another supportive person, serves as the "coach" to encourage the woman to regulate her breathing as the infant moves down the birth canal.[9]

In sports, controlled breathing in swimming is absolutely essential in maintaining a steady, smooth movement through the water. Observe weight-lifters going through their paces and you will see the results of much practice in the coordination of breath and movement. In dancing, skiing, yoga, and running, breath control plays an important part.

Whether or not you participate in such recreational activities you can profit from breath awareness as you work. Pause for a moment and check out your posture as you read this book. Does it enhance your natural breathing, or restrict you to shallow, constrained intake of air? Those of us who work at sedentary occupations suffer a whole range of health problems including low back pain, headache, hemorrhoids, stomach and intestinal maladies, congested sinuses and other respiratory complications. Sitting for hours at a stretch, hunched over, neck strained, legs cramped, can certainly discourage the easy flow of oxygen into the lungs. The result is a partial blockage in energy flow. The consequence is that we tire easily, start to feel foggy, and may soon lose interest in the task at hand. Time out for a coffee break, when what we really need is more oxygen!

Examine the position of your desk, or work table, the structure of the chair you use, and the posture you most frequently assume. Evaluate how these are affecting your ability to breathe fully. And while you're doing this don't forget to check out the clothing you're wearing, too. Tight waistbands and collars are prime offenders in promoting poor breathing habits.

A friend recently replaced the THINK and PLAN AHEAD signs on his desk with new ones that read AWARENESS and BREATHE. He claims that it has made a tremendous difference in his level of enjoyment, and his productivity.

Breathing for Healing

Left alone, the body knows best how to heal itself. The technical word for this is homeostasis, the natural tendency to reestablish balance. With illness, energy is blocked—the balance is upset. The state of "dis-ease" is the result. Breathing is a primary method for correcting this disharmony.

. . . . *Exercise* . . . .

Breathing with Every Cell—For Healing

Part 1:

Sit in a comfortable position with arms and legs uncrossed.

Surrender the weight of your body, allowing the chair or floor to support you.

Softly close your eyes.

Bring your attention to your nose and imagine what air looks like as it enters here. Follow its path down into your lungs, observe it swirling around, and see it moving back up and out. As it leaves tell yourself that it is carrying away tension, pain, and disease.

Do this for about 1 to 2 minutes.

Part 2:

Bring awareness to the center of your belly. Imagine a tiny opening here through which you are breathing.

Visualize the oxygen coming in, swirling around in the abdomen, lower back, anal and genital regions, and then flowing out.

Tell yourself that it carries away tension and pain as it leaves.

Continue breathing from here for another 1 to 2 minutes.

Part 3:

Focus now at a point in the center of your chest, close to your heart.

Visualize a tiny door opening here.

As you inhale, you draw air into your chest and upper body, into your heart as well.

Watch it swirling around, and carrying away tension as it departs.

Do this for 1 to 2 minutes.

Part 4:

The point of breathing now moves to the center of your forehead.

Breathe from here, releasing tightness in all muscles of your face, and clearing out the cobwebs in your brain. Again for 1 to 2 minutes.

Part 5:

Repeat this same process in other areas, especially those which are diseased or in pain.

Breathe from the palms of your hands, the tips of your big toes, the undersides of your knees, the base of your spine, etc.

Now breathe with every cell of your body.

To Conclude:

Complete your directed imagery. Breathe naturally. Begin to stretch. Slowly open your eyes.

. . . .

Breathing deeply and rhythmically will assist your body in healing itself. As we mentioned in discussing the process of respiration, oxygen is needed by every cell, every muscle, bone, and organ. When part of you is ailing, the whole organism is thrown out of balance. Vigilant red corpuscles in the blood rush to the aid of the injured or diseased member. Since it is the oxygen you inspire which provides the energy to the cells, it naturally follows that these cells need to be charged to their fullest potential in order for healing to occur.

It has long been known that pain is intensified by the anxiety which accompanies a threatening situation. Fear causes the body to tense itself, a spontaneous reaction to the need to fight or run away. So what we have is a two-stage process—fear giving rise to tension; tension increasing pain. Using the breath to limit tension will help to quiet both the fear and the pain. The intuitive wisdom used by parents of young children provides us with an excellent example. The child who has been crying and gasping for breath is cautioned to "calm down" and "take a deep breath." Mother knows that the child's pain is worsened by the scare and the sight of blood. Panic reactions generally involve this same gasping or fast, shallow breathing pattern. Bringing it to the attention of the injured party can immediately change the level of anxiety. In order to use this in a crisis situation for yourself, it helps to be attuned to it on a regular basis.

What is true for the relief of physical pain is also applicable to mental and emotional pain as well. Sadness, depression, and boredom

Jim's Story

Shortly after my thirtieth birthday, I developed asthma for the first time in my life. Over a four-month period the asthma attacks increased in frequency and severity. I incurred asthma while exercising outside, when briefly exposed to cat fur, and fairly often at bedtime. At the peak of my debilitation, I couldn't even throw a Frisbee for ten minutes without gasping for breath. Many times I became very angry with myself or panicked in my plight, which only served to exacerbate my breathing.

In desperation, I visited a pulmonary specialist who treated me very clinically and expressed doubt that I could do anything (e.g., breathing exercises and dietary change) short of taking cortisone to relieve my condition. No way was I going to subject myself to the long list of side effects accompanying cortisone ingestion. Enraged and resolute, I began an holistic campaign to eliminate my asthma. I developed a routine of special breathing and "lung-energizing exercises," minimized my intake of dairy products and bread, received weekly therapeutic massages, and did a lot of emotional and intuitive work.

My combined efforts enabled me to alleviate my asthma, but not to eliminate it. The turning point came during a complex visualization experience, when I vividly realized that asthma was like a coat I'd have to wear until I traded it in for a deep commitment to love and express myself powerfully. My intention came gushing forth, and in a matter of weeks, my story seemingly had a Hollywood ending.

That was nearly a decade ago. Since then, I've had no asthma from exercise, but frequent, though much milder, asthmatic reactions to cats. Also, each year I have had a few onslaughts of asthma, sometimes up to twenty hours in duration. Each of these attacks began during or shortly after highly intense emotional situations. However, I have had numerous overwhelming experiences without any asthmatic backlash. Well, throughout my thirties, I have remained convinced that self-responsibility is the foundation of empowerment. Yet I no longer think life involves a neatly packaged series of cause-effect events. These years I take in lots of fresh air while riding on the wings of mystery and innocence.

can frequently be turned around by a change in breathing. So, as you reach for the aspirins, the antacid tablets, or the telephone to call your doctor, let that serve as a reminder to you to breathe as well. And remember, breathing well is letting go of the restrictions to the natural process.

The Person Breathes/
The Planet Breathes

• • • • • • •

No one knows the exact extent of death caused by workplace exposures to the thousands of toxic substances in common industrial use today. But we do know the toll is in the thousands—perhaps more than a hundred thousand per year becoming ill.

—EULA BINGAM
FORMER U.S. ASSISTANT
SECRETARY OF LABOR, OCCUPATIONAL
SAFETY AND HEALTH

• • • • • • •

It's not easy to be a healthy fish in a polluted lake. It's hard to remain a healthy person while breathing polluted air. The reality is that air pollution in the United States has reached crisis proportions.

The whole planet is breathing—lakes, forests, mountains, fields. Its needs are identical with those of human beings—a clear and ready input source, and an unrestricted channel. And the sad fact is that the planet is gasping. Where will it turn for help in releasing its tensions? Where can it go for some fresh air?

Since all things are connected, all beings breathing the same air, then self-responsibility means social responsibility. We are all dependent upon one another. We all need to examine many of the details of our lifestyle with this realization in mind. With respect to the environmental crisis created by air pollution we must weigh our decisions about the size of the car we drive, and how much we drive it.

We need to look at the type and quantity of the fuel we use in heating our homes. We can involve ourselves in local, neighborhood efforts for improving the environment in which we live, as well as voice our support for political candidates who represent a consciousness about pollution-control issues.

Keeping yourself balanced will keep you focused upon your own real needs, and those of the planet on which you live. Despair, panic, and compulsiveness in approaching any problem only serve to intensify it, and often divert you from the real issues.

Remember the basic principles of wellness—trust, compassion, self-responsibility, and the positive value of "illness." Rightly used, these can bring about health for you, and for the entire planet as well.

Citizen Suits

Citizens long have had the right to file suit under nuisance laws for damage to health and property caused by pollution. Under the Clean Air Act of 1970 (PL-91-604), and the Federal Water Pollution Control Act of 1972, citizens can now take direct action to enforce compliance with Federal air and water pollution requirements.

Both laws empower citizens to take court action against anyone violating those laws. And citizens can also file suit against EPA itself if it fails to perform any mandatory duty required by the two laws.

Rules governing citizen suits under the Clean Air Act are available in the Federal Register, Dec. 9, 1971.

Air Pollution and Your Health

The gist of the scientific studies and the clinical evidence can be summed up briefly. Air pollution is related to human sickness and sometimes to premature death: People of both sexes and all ages can be affected, but the danger is greatest for the very old and the very young and people already sick with certain chronic ailments.

Air pollution probably causes and certainly aggravates:

• Diseases of the respiratory (breathing) system: nose, sinuses, throat, bronchial tubes, and lungs. All these organs have direct contact with breathed-in air:

• Diseases of the heart and blood vessels. Pollutants can pass through the lung membranes into the blood.

• Cancer, especially of the lungs. Airborne cancer-causing agents can enter the body through the skin as well as the lungs and be carried by the blood to any organ.

• Skin diseases, allergies, eye irritation.

Source: U.S. Environmental Protection Agency, March 1979.

How's The Air Out There?

(PSI) Pollutant Standards Index Value	PSI Descriptor	General Health Effects	Cautionary Statements
500 400 300	hazardous	Premature death of ill and elderly. Healthy people will experience adverse symptoms that affect their normal activity.	All persons should remain indoors, keeping windows and doors closed. All persons should minimize physical exertion and avoid traffic.
200	very unhealthful	Premature onset of certain diseases in addition to significant aggravation of symptoms and decreased exercise tolerance in healthy persons.	Elderly and persons with existing diseases should stay indoors and avoid physical exertion. General population should avoid outdoor activity.
100	unhealthful	Significant aggravation of symptoms and decreased exercise tolerance in persons with heart or lung disease with widespread symptoms in the healthy population.	Elderly and persons with existing heart or lung diseases should stay indoors and reduce physical activity.
50	moderate	Mild aggravation of symptoms in susceptible persons, with irritation symptoms in the healthy population.	Persons with existing heart or respiratory ailments should reduce physical exertion and outdoor activity.
0	good		

Source: U.S. Environmental Protection Agency, Washington DC 20460.

Suggested Reading*

Acharya, P. *Breath, Sleep, The Heart, and Life*. Clearlake, CA: The Dawn Horse Press, 1975.

Ballentine, R., Rama, S. and Hymes, A. *Science of Breath*. Honesdale, PA: The Himalayan Institute, 1976.

Benson, H. *The Relaxation Response*. New York, NY: Avon Books, 1975.

Davis, M. The Relaxation and Stress Reduction Workbook. San Francisco, CA: New Harbinger Publishers, 1980.

Hittleman, R. Yoga: *28 Day Exercise Plan*. New York, NY: Bantam Books, 1973.

Nakamura, T. *Oriental Breathing Therapy*. Tokyo: Japan Publications, 1981.

Ramacharaka, Y. *Science of Breath*. Des Plaines, IL: The Yogi Publication Society, 1905.

Rosenberg, J. *Total Orgasm*. New York, NY and Berkeley, CA: Random House/Bookworks, 1973.

Rozman, D. *Meditating with Children*. Boulder Creek, CA: University of the Trees Press, 1975.

Selye, H. *Stress Without Distress*. New York, NY: J. B. Lippincott Co., 1974.

Shealy, N. *90 Days to Self-Health*. New York, NY: Bantam Books, 1976.

Smith, P. *Total Breathing*. New York, NY: McGraw-Hill, 1980.

*For a catalog of excellent tapes to breathe and relax with, write: Source Cassette Learning Systems, Box W, Stanford, CA 94305. Also see Appendix A at the back of this book.

Notes

1. Research conducted by EPA at the Clinical Laboratory for Evaluation and Assessment of Noxious Substances, University of North Carolina, Chapel Hill. See: Perham, C. "A Matter of Life and Breath," *EPA Journal*, October, 1978.

2. For more information about therapies which deal with breathing, muscle tension, and emotional release see:

*This is only a representative sampling. Many excellent books have been omitted. At the bookstore or library, look over the whole selection and choose according to your own judgment.

Johnson, D. *The Protean Body—A Rolfer's View of Human Flexibility*. New York, NY: Harper Colophon Books, 1977.

Lowen, A. *Bioenergetics*. New York, NY: Coward, McCann & Geoghegan, 1975.

Dychtwald, K. *Bodymind*. New York, NY: Pantheon Books, 1977.

Barlow, W. *The Alexander Technique*. New York, NY. Knopf, 1974.

Orr, L,. and Ray, S. *Rebirthing in the New Age*. Berkeley, CA: Celestial Arts, 1977.

Janov, A. *Primal Man: The New Consciousness*. New York, NY: Crowell, 1976.

3. Yesudin, S., and Haich, E. *Yoga and Health*. New York, NY: Harper and Brothers, 1953.

4. For more information contact: Marty Belknap, Salina Star Route/Gold Hill, Boulder, CO 80302.

5. According to the directory of the Biofeedback Society of America (4301 Owens, Denver, CO), some of the hospitals and medical centers using biofeedback are:

Stanford University Medical Center, Palo Alto, CA

Mayo Clinic, Rochester, MN

Menninger Foundation, Topeka, KS

Institute of Living, Hartford, CT

Langley Porter Psychiatric Institute, San Francisco, CA

Cleveland Clinic, Cleveland, OH

Memorial Hospital, St. Joseph, MO

The Family Center, Department of Psychiatry, Georgetown University School of Medicine, Washington, DC

6. "Phone Company Workers Offered Meditation for Stress," *Brain-Mind Bulletin*. Vol. 5, No. 4, pp. 1, 3. Copies of the study may be obtained from Carrington, Psychology Dept., Princeton University, Princeton, NJ 08540.

7. Selye, H. *Stress Without Distress*, Philadelphia, PA, and New York, NY: J.B. Lippincott Co., 1974.

8. Selye, p. 47.

9. For more information on childbirth methods that recommend breathing exercises see:

Ewy, Donna and Rodger. *Preparation for Childbirth: A Lamaze Guide*. Boulder, CO: Pruett Publishing Co. (3rd ed.), 1982.

Kitzinger, Sheila. *The Complete Book of Pregnancy and Childbirth*. New York, NY: Alfred A. Knopf, 1985.

McCutcheon-Rosegg, Susan, with Peter Rosegg. *Natural Childbirth the Bradley Way*. New York, NY: E.P. Dutton, Inc., 1984.

Peterson, Gayle. *Birthing Normally: A Personal Growth Approach to Childbirth*. Berkeley, CA: Mindbody Press, 1984.

Three

Wellness and Sensing

> Sensory information (light, heat, touch, sound, odor, taste, movement, etc.) is the second form of energy input in the Wellness Energy System. Vast amounts of energy are received from our environment and channeled by our five physical senses, and possibly through other less well understood senses. These energies are necessary for our protection and survival, and serve as our most basic form of communication.

I T IS THROUGH the senses—seeing, touching, smelling, hearing, tasting—that we come to know and enjoy the world. Our ability to work, to feel pleasure, to communicate with others, and to impact the world is directly related to our efficient use of sensory energy. In the context of wellness this means eliminating the abuse of our senses, appreciating them, and using them more creatively.

. . . .

These are our first real experiences of life—floating in a warm liquid, curling inside a total embrace, swaying to the undulations of the moving body, and hearing the beat of the pulsing heart.

—DESMOND MORRIS

. . . .

Everywhere there is sad evidence that many of us have "lost our senses." You probably know people who burn their skin, allow it to blister and peel, and then go back for more in an attempt to look "healthy" and "sexy" in their summer clothes. The noise of dishwashers, air conditioners, power tools, trucks, and loud music invades everywhere, making us irritable, angry, listless, or unable to sleep. Loud sounds from machinery and traffic can actually damage our delicate hearing mechanisms and cause headaches and hearing loss. When it comes to tasting, lots of us tax our digestive systems constantly with food that is too hot and beverages that are too cold,

ending up with burnt tongues and stomach pains. We move apathetically through an environment filled with chemical pollutants, and hope that we're not absorbing too much nuclear radiation from the power plant upwind. The more we abuse our senses with these types of overstimulation, the more we dull ourselves to their subtle warning signals—the body's cries for help, for balance.

The flip-side of this sorry state of affairs is the withdrawal from sensory stimulation. Our fears cause us to freeze up when we are being touched. With depression and boredom we turn inward and often neglect the necessity for sunlight and fresh air. With grief we numb ourselves to the outside world as we attempt to cope with a loss. Studies with young mammals clearly indicate that early deprivation results in lowered activity, improper physical development, and many failures in sexual functioning.[1]

Your senses are marvelous in-

41

struments which require vigilance to keep them in tip-top operating condition. Becoming skilled technicians in their care and creative use is one of the foundations for wellness. This chapter is your owner's manual for the senses. It will deal with touch and temperature, sight, sound, and smell. (Taste is covered in the next chapter.) This chapter is about coming to your senses.

The Sense of Touch

As the largest organ of the body, the skin comprises almost one-fifth of the total body weight and engages a major percentage of the operation of the brain. The skin is constantly growing and changing in sensitivity as it performs its many functions: protection, sensation, regulation of temperature, excretion, respiration, and the metabolism and storage of fat.

Touch is the earliest sense to develop in the newborn. As the infant takes its first breath, it reaches out to learn what this new world is all about. Sensory receptors located in the skin start picking up enormous quantities of information and sending them to the brain. Pressure, temperature, pain—each stimulation carries a message about the environment. Each one adds another dimension to the infant's accumulating experience.

The Need for Touch

There is a biological need for touch, an actual skin hunger, which can be met only in contact with another human being. When touching is denied, or severely restricted, infants die. Children, abandoned at birth and transferred

to foundling homes, died by the thousands during the 19th century. They literally wasted away, despite the fact that they were fed, kept clean, and protected from danger. The condition, known as marasmus (from the Greek, meaning "wasting away"), claimed the lives of nearly 100% of the infants under the age of one in U.S. foundling hospitals as late as 1920.[2] What these children lacked was physical contact. Other infants, raised in their own homes, were cradled and fed at their mothers' breasts. These foundlings weren't. When this connection between life and touch was realized, doctors and nurses in many institutions cooperated in a plan to supply "mothering" for these children. It consisted of holding, stroking, speaking to the infant, and allowing significant periods of cuddling the child, especially at mealtimes. The results were dramatic and immediate. Infant mortality rates dropped within one year of adopting these touching procedures.

. . . . . .

Reach out . . . reach out and touch someone.

—BELL TELEPHONE AD

. . . . . .

Despite the lessons we have learned about the necessity for touch, many child-rearing practices endure today which discourage it. So-called experts have encouraged mothers to feed children only on schedule, discouraged breast-feeding, and convinced us that independence was to be learned by exiling the little person to an oversized crib in a separate room of the house. In many cultures it is common practice for par-

ents and children to share the same bed, yet in our society this is often considered unnatural. Tanya's friends were recently shocked to learn that she slept with her son until he was four.

The lack of sufficient touch has far-reaching effects on our development, and shows itself in problematic ways when we reach maturity. Some people devise destructive means of compensation to satisfy the hunger for touch. These include:

- overeating—which serves to gratify oral needs by stimulating the lips and mouth to fill us up with more of what we really don't need, to deaden the pain of emotional isolation

- destructive habits—smoking, nail biting, pulling out hair, rubbing the skin excessively, and even self-mutilation

- compulsive sex, physical violence and aggressiveness, rape and other forms of sexual abuse

The biggest problem that touch deprivation creates, however, is a sense of alienation from ourselves and isolation from others. We see this manifested as:

- boredom and lack of energy for life in general—the experience of being out-of-touch, or disconnected from the world

- sexual dysfunction—an unresponsiveness to the special electricity of the touch of another human body; overanxiousness which can encourage both premature ejaculation and overall bodily tension; and fear of one's own body

- unsatisfying relationships and the unwillingness to attend to the needs of the other; self-preoccupation; excessive shyness; the fear of reaching out; and the fear of sustained intimacy.

The need for psychological touch—acknowledgment, love, praise—is as great as that for physical touch. As a primary input in the Wellness Energy System it will be dealt with as "strokes" in chapter 6.

Why We Don't Touch

By now you should have a good idea of how important touch is for human growth and development, and how grave the consequences may be when it is lacking. The question now becomes—"Why don't we do more of it?" There are at least five possible answers.

First: Not everyone knows how essential it is. Here, as in so many areas of life, we are often sadly lacking in information about what it takes to promote personal wellness. In an attempt to counter this ignorance one group has printed a bumper-sticker which reads: "Have You Hugged Your Kid Today?" An holistic health network in Denver distributes buttons which say: "I Need a Hug," and the Council of Nurse Healers recommends a minimum of four hugs a day.

Second: Much of our reluctance to touch and be touched stems from fear of our bodies, a fear we learned as children. To touch yourself and gain pleasure is still considered sinful by many segments of society. Infants who masturbate frequently get their hands slapped. Many of us were told that mastur-

· · · · · · · · · · · · · *Regina's Journal* · · · · · · · · · · · · ·

Rosemary's Teaching

Rosemary was a student of mine for several courses, a remarkably talented woman—a counselor, a fine cook, and a weaver. Rosemary was born with a degenerative spinal condition which left her body twisted and hampered normal development.

One day in class we were working at the front of the room. One at a time, the students left their seats and came forward to take part. Rosemary remained at her place. When I asked her, "Shall I bring the equipment down to you, or clear some space so that you can get your wheelchair up to the front? Or," I hesitated, not sure that I really wanted to make the offer, "shall I carry you?"

"I want you to carry me," she replied immediately. And so I did.

My reaction startled me. I was really afraid to touch her. Her body was no larger than that of a five-year-old child. I love to pick up children. But here was an adult. Here was a twisted body. Old voices filled my head. For one split second I was repulsed as if I might catch something. Catch her paralysis, her deformity? No, catch my own. . . . What was happening was that I was touching deep within myself—to the hidden, ugly places, which I don't usually let people see. I was reminded of my own weakness, my vulnerability, my mortality. Tears streamed down my cheeks. Rosemary was crying too. I looked up and saw the entire class, as one pair of eyes, connected with us. Many others were crying too.

"I asked you to carry me," Rosemary reported, "because I needed to be touched."

As we left class that day, everybody touched. Hugs went all around—to me, to Rosemary. Men hugged men. Women hugged women. We had all learned an invaluable lesson.

· ·

bation was disgusting behavior. Messages like this communicate negativity about the body, and create distrust of it.

Third: Societal attitudes frequently connect touch with sexual advances, and label as improper any public displays of affection. These attitudes show up in numerous ways:

- a woman who breast-feeds her child outside the home receives disapproving looks

- a preschool teacher tells her class that while it's permissible for girls, boys are not supposed to kiss each other

- two friends who recently met in the local bank after many years apart were asked to leave when their embracing extended beyond forty-five seconds in duration.

Fear of the body in general and sexuality in particular are deeply

I Am Touched—Remembrances of Growing Up

We learn to touch by being touched. Some of us were raised in homes where physical contact was commonplace. Others rarely received touching of any kind. A few remember only the hurtful incidents—the spankings. What do you recall about your early life relative to touching?

Settle back into a relaxed position. Put your feet up. Close your eyes. Take yourself back in time, as far as you can go. Don't feel that you have to progress logically or chronologically. Simply let your imagination suggest to you incidents which relate to your experiences of touching. Let them stay as long as they wish. Let them go when they are ready, especially if they are unhappy memories. Record your recollections.

In writing, here or in your journal, ask yourself:

What does this mean to me today? Does it help to explain some things for me? Does it highlight areas which I would like to change?

. . . .

A Self Massage—The Head

You can use these suggestions to design your own method of self-massage. Remove glasses or contact lenses. Let your body tell you what needs attention, what feels good.

Begin by rubbing your hands together to warm them and generate energy in them.

Place the palms of your hands on your face. Hold them there for a few seconds. When they are ready, let them move as they wish over the whole surface of your face. Movements may include circular motion with fingertips, pulling the skin in different directions, kneading, slapping, following the contours of the face with finger-pressure.

Move your fingertips up onto your skull, run them through your hair. Try tapping vigorously with fingertips, scratching with fingernails, grasping hair by the roots and firmly moving the skin of the scalp in different directions. Smoothly and gently move hands over hair, ears, face, neck. Talk to yourself as you do it. Tell yourself positive and loving things. Enjoy. Allow yourself to be creative.

Use fingertips to massage your gums by feeling them through the cheeks. This is a rare treat. Some people love it.

Follow by giving yourself a "facial" treatment. Open pores with hot towels placed over the face. Cleanse thoroughly with warm water and pure soap. Rinse with warm water until all soap is gone. Splash with cold water. Moisturize your face with natural oil—sesame, avocado, wheat germ, almond. Love yourself.

embedded in the consciousness of the culture.

Fourth: We refrain from touching and allowing touch because we are depressed, anxious, withdrawn, living chiefly in our heads, or just simply unaware that we may be needing it.

Finally: It is risky to touch. To be "touching" or "touchable" is to be vulnerable. If you reach out to another person you might be rejected, and this would hurt. If you allow yourself to be touched by another, your defenses are down and you might be hurt as well. Consequently, many of us have learned that it is easier to simply "keep our hands to ourselves."

When people lose touch with their inside world, when they fail to be sufficiently touched in a positive way by the world outside, they slowly die—sometimes physically, but more often socially, sexually, emotionally and spiritually. We need to touch and be touched in order to learn, to communicate, to experience pleasure, to be healthy and to grow. As you appreciate your needs for and fears of touch, you lay the groundwork for more creative ways to touch your world.

Creative Uses of Touch

Communication

Our everyday language is filled with references to the sense of touch. Besides the act of physical stimulation of the skin, we use the word "touch" to mean communication at a deep level—"Your words touched me"; correspondence or contact at a casual level— "do keep in touch"; and the experience of just about every emotion—"how touching."

The sense of touch communicates without the need for words. Gently stroking a child will induce sleep, quiet rage, and soothe pain. Physical contact informs the other of our presence, our caring, our support. We hold the person who is grieving. We touch to say "Hello," "Goodbye," and "It's OK." A pat on the back signals approval, a slap on the hand says the opposite. And we rely upon the chemistry of touch in our sexual interactions.

Limiting ourselves to verbal expression cuts us off from the full range of communication. Since

. . . . *Exercise* . . . .

Creative Massage

Here are some creative ways to use massage. Add your own experiments to the list.

Roll a tennis ball under your hand as you apply pressure. Roll it over your feet, your partner's back, any muscular part of the body. It provides an interesting and stimulating sensation.

Remove shoes and socks. Sit down and roll the bottom of your foot over a golf ball; or fill a basin with marbles and rub your feet over them.

Dry brush massage, or massage with a loofa sponge, is popular at health spas in Europe. Make sure the bristles of the brush are not too firm. Experiment until you find one that stimulates, but doesn't hurt. Use circular motions. Start with the soles of your feet and work up. Avoid the face.

Try a texture rub. See how various parts of your body respond to different textures. Take a piece of fur, a silk scarf, a flannel shirt, a terry cloth towel, a bunch of fluffy cotton, etc., and gently massage yourself. Try this with a partner.

Additional massaging effects can include warm scented oils, warm mud, a vibrator, a wooden roller. What are your suggestions? Be creative.

touching means closeness, it can help to bridge the distances which separate us from one another. Thus connected, you can communicate better. As you approach the other with your defenses down, and your hand extended in a gesture of acceptance, you stand a better chance of reaching a mutual understanding.

In sex, touching becomes a special form of communication. Among the most frequent complaints voiced by women about sex is that their male partners do not use enough stroking and caressing prior to, during, and after intercourse.[3] What these women are really asking for is the communication of presence, of acceptance, of tenderness, throughout. Sex therapists who work with couples encourage them to explore meaningful and pleasurable ways to touch each other, besides strictly genital involvement.[4] Experiment-

ing with touch in sex sensitizes you to an awareness of the non-verbal messages which the body is expressing and opens up new options for intimacy.

Massage

We are fortunate to be living at a time when touch is being liberated. While walk-in massage parlors may still remain suspect, the growing popularity of books on massage and new schools for the training of massage therapists indicates an increasing acceptance of this practice.[5]

Massage is nonfattening, and, if you do it yourself, it's free! Some of its uses include:

- relief of pain and tension

- the improvement of muscle tone

- the maintenance of a healthy complexion

- release of emotional blockages caused by trauma and repression

- the increase of blood flow and electrical energy to "wake up" dead parts of the body

- foreplay for sexual intercourse, or sensual arousal, and

- general balancing of right and left, upper and lower parts of the body.

And it's so simple to do. You put your hands on, and start moving them. Lotions, varied techniques, and training can certainly enhance the experience, but they can also lead you to believe that you need them to do it right. This is just not true. The only rule that applies is to listen to the feedback from your own body, or ask your partner if s/he likes what you are doing. If it feels good—do it. The more you can quiet the chatter and judgment in your mind, and allow your hands to move intuitively, the more creative, relaxed, and enjoyable the results will be.

Give yourself permission to receive and administer pleasure, if for no other reason than that it is a proven method of increasing overall health.

Clothing

Anthropologists report that people who wear little or no clothing show much greater skin sensitivity than do people who are usually clothed.[6] Observations of infants verify this. Babies who are almost always covered are less active and less sensitive than those who are generally lightly clothed or naked.[7] There is little chance that nudity will ever become the social norm, but we can still learn how to *use* our clothing rather than be used by it.

The skin must be allowed to breathe if it is to remain healthy. Numerous skin disorders are the results of irritation and improper ventilation caused by clothing. Popular synthetics, such as nylon, dacron, and polyester are made of smooth fibers that can be very tightly woven. These fabrics are often favored because they resist wrinkling. They are unfavorable because they don't "breathe." Nylon pantyhose, for instance, were discovered to promote vaginal infections in women because they trapped heat and moisture, making an ideal environment for infection. Fortunately, cotton panels which breathe are becoming commonplace in women's underwear. Our bodies invisibly eliminate a substantial portion of waste products from the skin, and unless these can pass out via the open weaves of cotton and wool we will need to use more chemical deodorants to keep us all smelling as fresh as daisies.

People who wear skin-tight plastic pants may cause a sensation at a party, but do so at considerable cost to their skin. (For ages, religious ascetics have used coarse fabrics and even hair shirts as a method of penance and self-discipline for the subduing of the flesh.) If you have to wear tight, coarse materials in uniforms or suits because of your work, you can minimize their numbing effects by wearing soft undergarments next to your skin and by changing into something more comfortable as soon as you return home.

As you look over your wardrobe today take note:

- How many of your clothes are constructed of natural fabrics?

- How many contain synthetics?

- Ask yourself what differences in mood and behavior various textures produce in your body?

- Are most of your clothes really comfortable—soothing to the skin, loose enough to provide for freedom of movement, enhancing of sensual pleasure?

- And finally, does your clothing really reflect you—your moods, your personality, your ideals of how you want to be?

Go without clothing whenever appropriate in order to air your skin. This will enhance its sensitivity and promote its health. Even Eskimos who live in snow huts sleep in the nude under thick furs. We can all profit from their example.

Water

Getting some of your needs for touch met may be as simple as filling your bathtub. Certainly a much livelier alternative than drowning your sorrows in beer, dulling them through drugs, or passing them on to your doctor.

Being in water is a healthy experience. Water will stimulate every cell of the skin as it relaxes tightened muscles and promotes healing. It wakes you up, and calms you down, and washes away the problems of the day along with the dirt.

Shower massagers are becoming very popular. More people every day are enrolling in health spas, swimming year-round, and building whirlpool baths and hot tubs in their own homes. It has always been difficult to get children out of the water—and now the same is true for adults.

The Japanese have championed communal bathing for centuries. An entire family shares the intimacy and pleasure of being naked together, as each fulfills the basic needs for personal cleanliness and relaxation. Our reticence to accept such a practice in the West reflects our fear of the physical body and its functioning.

There is more to bathing than promoting cleanliness. Water has always been a religious symbol because of its connection to purification, refreshment, and regeneration. We all come from the water—evolving from the creatures of the sea, bathing in the uterus of the mother. Water, like air, has the capacity to touch us all over, in every crack and crevice of the body. Immersing yourself in it is one of the greatest and simplest pleasures known to human beings. The security of being surrounded in it can be a great source of healing. And the possibilities for its creative use are limitless. Here are some of them:

Drinking it—Water is an important source of minerals and serves to wash out the system. Drink lots of it.

Showering—Alternate hot and cold showers—it's great for circulation. Feel more alert and energetic. Play with a shower massager. Shower with a friend.

Bathing—Fill the tub with hot water, and a mild bubble bath. Light a few candles and some incense. Put on your favorite music, or take in a good book. A glass of wine or favorite fruit juice or tea makes a loving accompaniment.

Soaking in a hot tub—If you don't have a friend who has one, inquire at local gyms or health spas. Whirlpool jets soothe and untangle tired muscles.

Sweating in a sauna or steam bath—Follow this exposure to heat with a short, stimulating, cold shower.

Having a water fight—Establish a few ground rules. Fill everything in sight—water guns, plastic bags, cups, buckets, hoses. Avoid glass bottles! Have fun.

Swimming—Even if you don't know how, just get in there and splash out your frustrations with the problems in your life. Guaranteed to make you feel better. Float—head back, belly up, lower back arched—surrender to the healing touch of the water.

Floating—Check out places in your area where you can rent the use of a sound-proof, light-proof, isolation tank in which you safely float on your back for an hour or more. It is an experience not to be forgotten.

Soaking your feet—Fill a basin with hot water and mild soap or baking soda. Experience your whole body relaxing as your feet do. Finish off by drying them with a coarse towel. Then give yourself a foot massage.

Applying hot compresses —Buy some fresh ginger root at your local supermarket. Grate it and wrap it in a cheese cloth. Place it in a large pot of water. Heat the water, but do not let it boil. Soak a towel in the water, remove it and let it cool until it is comfortable to handle, and then wring it out. Apply the towel to any ailing body part. Leave on until the heat is exhausted. Then do it again.

Visiting a hot springs—If you don't live near any natural hot springs, or mineral springs, check into them on your next vacation. Often they are not well advertised. Ask local residents. The curative powers of these waters have been praised for ages.

Making medicine—Some very famous American Indian healers have used water to cure lots of ailments.[8] As the saying goes: "It wouldn't hurt!" Try it yourself. Fill a glass or bottle with water and place it on a window-sill of your house where it will receive the first rays of the rising sun. Before you retire for bed, sit with the water, telling it what you need for your increased health and well-being. In the morning, drink the whole glass. Believe it!

Baptize yourself—This is one of the most beautiful and effective ways of loving yourself. Compose a ceremony in which you use water to symbolically cleanse your body (or the body of a loved one), and your mind and soul from illness, darkness, "sin," and painful memories. Make it a beautiful occasion. Take a new or additional name to signify your new life. Be at peace.

Healing

Prophets and teachers in most of the world's great religions have been credited with the power to heal through touch. In our own time, reports of modes of healing which involve the "laying on of hands" are many.

• At McGill University in To-ronto, Dr. Bernard Grad demonstrated that wounded mice who were touched by a "healer" healed significantly faster than those who were untouched, or those touched by his lab assistant.[9]

• Jere Pramuk (Regina's husband) was relieved of chronic back pain for three months after a charismatic Christian "healer" imposed hands and prayed with him.

• Dolores Kreiger, R.N., Ph.D., a professor at New York University School of Nursing, conducts classes in healing touch for nurses to use in encouraging the healing process in their patients.

• Affectionate touch, whenever appropriate, in communicating with dying people and grieving family members, is recognized as an effective therapeutic measure. The dying experience extreme loneliness as they leave everything they have known and loved. Reassuring touch can reconnect them with the family, the community of support. Healing of this type is a healing of the spirit.

It is not the skin alone which is touched—it is a whole person. Touching brings with it a stimulation of the capillaries and increased blood flow to the area, a sharing of body heat, and a relaxation of muscular tension. Each of these factors will encourage the normal healing process. But more important, perhaps, is the way touching comforts a troubled mind, provides security for a lonely and scared victim, and communicates caring person-to-person. You probably know that pain is increased by anxiety, and that emotional imbalance feeds physical disease. Touch serves to ground a patient in the realization that s/he is not alone. That assurance brings healing. For ages, parents have used hugs and kisses to heal their children's hurts. Putting an arm around an asthma-sufferer at the onset of an attack will frequently stop it.

. . . .

Now when the sun was setting, all they that had any sick with diverse diseases brought them unto him; and he laid his hand on every one of them, and healed them.

—LUKE 4:40

. . . .

When you are hurt, your hands will automatically move to the area of pain. Part of this is for protection. The other part is that we connect our hands with some ability to relieve or remove pain. A man will grasp his sprained ankle. The child curls up in a fetal position, hands covering her aching belly. A woman with a headache will frequently rub or hold her head. Watch a person with a severe toothache. You will almost always see a hand tightly pressed against the cheek and jaw. We attempt to heal ourselves through touch without much awareness. To use it more consciously can be a very powerful method of relaxation and pain reduction.

Therapeutic procedures such as acupressure, which use touch for rebalancing and healing, are growing in number and popularity. Some are based on ancient Chinese medicine and the belief that a universal energy, "chi" or "ki," circulates throughout the body. This

. . . . *Exercise* . . . .

A Sensuous Foot Massage

Gather what you need—a large basin, your favorite scented soap, a bottle of scented oil or lotion, a loofa or a soft brush, a fluffy, soft towel, and a comfortable chair or pillow.

Create a relaxing atmosphere—play your favorite music, burn some delicious incense, brew a cup of soothing tea, be in touch with your breath, breathe deeply, close your eyes, visualize healing colors, be centered . . . be refreshed.

Fill your basin with comfortably warm water and add your soap, sit comfortably, and immerse your feet in the water, let your feet soak, and the water relax you and your feet.

Enjoy your tea, savor the incense, flow with the music, be calm, be centered . . . let your body's energy flourish.

Talk to your feet, communicate with them, thank them for supporting and transporting you during the day.

With your loofa or brush, *slowly cleanse* away the soil and old skin, let it tickle you and clean your feet. Laugh and enjoy your feet.

Dry your feet with your towel, as caringly as you would a tender babe. Sit on your pillow or chair in a comfortable position, stroke your feet . . . let them grow warm.

Pour lotion or oil into the palm of your hand. Let the oil or lotion grow warm, with love and healing energy. Let your eyes close, and send energy to your hands . . . offer your hands and your lotion or oil to your feet. Let this be a gift of renewal.

Caress, rub, massage, stroke and explore your feet, learn the contours of your heels and the texture of your toes, give your feet pleasure with every caring, gentle motion. . . . Take all the tension, tightness, soreness and stress from your feet with every loving touch; and be aware that you are relaxing.

Be in touch with your feet, nurture them when they speak to you through pain or uncomfortableness. Close your eyes, and feel your feet; come to know and cherish your feet as an old, dear friend, or a tender lover.

This exercise was a gift of love from Gregg Pickernell, Greeley, Colorado

. . . .

energy, it is believed, can become blocked at any point, creating an imbalance in the system. Using massage and pressure at specified points may release the blockage.[10]

Much of this can be done by yourself with the guidance of a clear book and a little practice. Imagine being able to relieve a headache by pinching the skin below your nose and above your upper lip, or by pressing at a point on your hand between your thumb and forefinger! Strange as this may sound, these techniques sometimes work faster for many people than the leading brand of aspirin.

One of the most ancient of arts—the rubbing of tired feet—has recently been systematized into a science. Called Zone Therapy or Foot Reflexology, it correlates points on your feet with every part of your body—organs, glands, spinal column.[11] Working on the feet is then comparable to massaging the entire body. Energy blocks broken up in the foot mean a recharging of the corresponding segment of the body. (Or so its proponents believe.) Many of these claims have yet to be clinically verified, but the values of foot massage as a simple, loving, and healing tool remain undisputed by anyone who has ever received one.

Nurturing yourself through touch is a way of accepting and loving yourself—a form of preventive medicine, easy to do and immediately rewarding. Using touch with others is a primary way of opening communication and establishing intimacy with them. And intimacy is healing.

Touching the Earth Touching the Sky

We ought to touch the earth and sky with the same respect, balance, and moderation with which we touch ourselves and others.

Dave, who lives in a mountain community in Colorado, speaks of "living lightly on the planet." The images this evokes are beautiful ones—dancers tip-toeing across fields and floating through forests, graciously thanking the other beings in the environment for the beauty, shelter, and energy they provide.

People who live lightly consciously evaluate their behaviors with regard to how they may enhance or disrupt the natural balance of all things. They are aware that exhaust gases from cars and industrial pollutants are painting a brown haze across the horizon; and fluorocarbons are destroying the planet's ozone layer, exposing us to harmful radiation. They realize that unrestricted urban sprawl is wantonly eliminating our green space;

weed and insect killers are poisoning our soil, and consequently our food. Greed and waste are the characteristics of a population which has lost touch with itself.

Take some time to reflect about your own lifestyle and the ways in which you touch the earth, the waters. Your wellness, our wellness, and that of our children depend upon it.

Temperature

Of all the forms of energy we can sense, the most fundamental is thermal energy. Given this basic source of energy, our bodies are able to function and sense a myriad of other stimuli: electromagnetic radiation (particularly visible light), vibration of air which we experience as sound, physical contact which we experience as touch, and chemical stimuli which we experience as taste and smell.

The human body maintains a very narrow temperature range, averaging 98.6°F/37°C, and generally, is equipped to handle temperature fluctuations in wonderfully adaptive ways. Our senses are geared to detect a lack of thermal energy or a surplus of it. If it is cold, the blood vessels constrict. We breathe more and circulation in the extremities slows down to conserve heat energy in the central portions of the body. If it is warm, we breathe less. As we metabolize the food we eat, and when we exercise, we create large amounts of internal heat. This is used to maintain our temperature, with any excess being released to the environment.

The need for heat has been a major factor in the development of

civilization. Our clothing, the structure of our homes, the socialization process—all are affected by the presence or absence of external heat. This is probably why most great innovations have been developed in the temperate zones of the world, necessity being the mother of invention. The need to develop energy sources to bring the sun indoors has led to the creation of our transportation systems and the revolution to heat-powered machinery.

Heat Distribution and Health

The way your body generates and uses heat reflects your overall well-being. More heat is generated in the trunk of the body and distributed to the limbs and head through the flow of blood. Hands and feet, ears and scalp act like radiators. When you are hot they help dissipate heat; when you are cold the blood vessels in these parts constrict and send heat back to the center of the body. This happens not only in response to the temperature around you, but in emergency and chronic stress conditions as well. Faced with a life-threatening crisis, this diversion effect is helpful in providing a maximum amount of energy to the heart, lungs, brain, and muscles. Over a longer period, if stress becomes chronic, this adaptation can be more harmful than helpful. It leads to a retention of energy, and is manifested by cold hands and feet. An extreme example is seen in the disorder known as Raynaud's disease where hands become painfully cold. Many people have a less serious form of this condition, without even being aware of it. The first manifestation of the con-

. . . . *Exercise*. . . . .

Warm Hands/Good Health

By relaxing and focusing on warming your hands you can raise your hand temperature as much as 20° F in 5 minutes. The result of hand warming is usually a deep state of relaxation, or one of the altered states of consciousness experienced in meditation. It is an effective stress reducer, and can be used in the control of migraine headaches. It helps the body to carry out its self-repair.

Sit in a relaxed position. Place your hands on your lap, palms facing up, fingers easy.

Begin to say slowly to yourself: "My hands are getting warmer."

Repeat this many times.

Combine the repetition of the words with a mental picture which suggests warm hands. For instance, see your hands being bathed in warm water, imagine that you are holding your hands up to the sun, visualize someone rubbing your hands to encourage circulation, see rivers of warm energy flowing from the trunk of your body into your hands. In your mind's eye surround your hands with a glowing yellow light. Feel them getting gradually warmer.

. . . .

dition is consistently cold hands, even when the temperature outside is above 70°F. Later complications include migraine headaches, blood sugar problems such as hypoglycemia or diabetes, menstrual problems, and depression.

If you have this tendency, you can learn to consciously make your hands warmer. Some of the methods for doing this are visualization processes and temperature biofeedback. You can monitor your hand temperature by touching your lips, a stable reference point, to note if your hands are warm or cold. Soaking in a hot tub, or taking a sauna, produce relaxation in a similar way by encouraging blood to flow to the periphery of the body. When this happens, your tissues expand with more blood and you experience pleasure.

Wellness and Weather

Despite our technological sophistication we are still subject to the powers of wind and rain and sun. Being well includes a rekindled respect for the natural rhythms of things—and an attempt to harmonize ourselves to the changes, both internal and external, which weather brings. Today it is almost possible to ignore the weather as we move from heated or cooled homes to heated or cooled automobiles to heated or cooled offices or schools or department stores or supermarkets and back again.

These luxuries have brought with them negative effects on life and health. Summer colds are frequently the result of air-conditioning which creates January in June and upsets the body's equilibrium in the process. As we move in and out of these super-cool environments we repeatedly chill and dry the mucous membranes of nose and throat. The glands must work overtime, often to the point of exhaustion, pumping extra fluids and then slowing down dramatically. The lungs are shocked by differences in temperature of sometimes twenty or thirty degrees as we leave an air-conditioned car or building to walk across the street. Humidity fluctuations may be even greater. In this tenuous state, the body is ripe for the hosting of some confused virus. It's the summer cold!

Winter brings its own unique stresses for the body in question. Many of us in North America suffer colds and other more serious respiratory problems during the winter. One woman we know waits every October in fearful anticipation of her annual case of strep throat. The dryness which central heating produces in the air plays havoc with the whole respiratory tract. The extremes experienced in moving from the over-heated home into the stabbing cold create similar imbalancing effects.

Because the need to generate and conserve heat is increased in cold climates, the heart, especially, works harder at this time. Heart failure and other coronary fatalities occur more frequently in winter than at any other time of year. The same individual who rakes leaves or exercises vigorously without difficulty in the gentle autumn weather may suffer a heart attack in shovelling snow from the front walk in near freezing temperatures.

While the solution for some may be a move to a more moderate climate, most of us will reject that option. If body trust, self-responsibility, and moderation are your governing principles, you can celebrate the changing seasons in good health. Here are some simple suggestions:

Moderation

1. In warm weather keep air-conditioning no more than 10°F cooler than outside air.

2. Keep humidity generally between 40 and 50%.

3. Acclimatize yourself with outdoor exercise as soon as the seasons start to change.

4. In cold weather keep the temperature in your home about 65°F/18°C.

5. Loose clothing over tight will form a natural air insulation and keep you warm.

6. Resist all temptations to "suffer" the cold—quit working if you start sweating.

7. Check your pulse occasionally—if too fast, rest from your work or exercise. (See p. 100.)

Self-Responsibility. Make your needs for comfort and health known to those who control the thermostats. If they refuse to cooperate then take your business elsewhere.

Body Trust. As the seasons change your body will slowly adapt to them. Learning to respect your internal rhythm during seasonal transitions is an important aspect of wellness. Don't be too hard on yourself. Work during hours which support your personal efficiency rhythm. Rest or "goof off"

when work-energy wanes. Nourish yourself throughout the seasons but most especially during the transitional times.[12]

The Sense of Sight

. . . .

If the doors of perception were cleansed, man would see things as they are, infinite.
—WILLIAM BLAKE

. . . .

Adults receive the majority of sensory stimulation through their eyes. The ability to learn, to navigate, and to communicate depend upon visual input. So strong is the connection between seeing and knowing that the words have become synonymous in our language. Like Doubting Thomas in the Gospels, we have to *see* in order to *believe*. Or, like the man from Missouri, we have to be shown.

Few people in our overstressed culture escape problems associated with sight. Can you name ten friends who do not use glasses or contact lenses? Can you name five? Some degree of near-sightedness, far-sightedness, or other refractive error is experienced by the vast majority of people in industrialized countries of the world.[13] If we are to experience greater wellness, we need to address the real reasons behind this epidemic of poor eyesight. We need to heal our eyes, since it is with them that we feed our souls.

Stress and Sight

Like breathing, seeing is not something you need to do, rather it is something which you allow. Most people, however, do not appreciate

. . . . *Exercise* . . . .

Relaxing the Eyes

Resting

To relax your eyes is to relax your whole body. Since so much of our sensory input is visual, temporarily closing off this channel will almost immediately cause the rest of the body to slow down. Brain wave patterns change to a lower frequency as soon as the eyes are closed. Resting your eyes is an important way of reestablishing balance throughout the system and reducing unnecessary strain.

Palming

This is a technique developed by Bates for relieving eye strain.

Sit or lie down and take a few moments to breathe deeply.

Now gently close your eyes.

Place the palms of your hands over your eyes, with your fingers crossing over your forehead.

Use memory and imagination to realize a perfect field of black. See it so *black* that you cannot recall anything *blacker.*

Do not *try* to produce any experience. Simply *allow* the blackness to happen.

Continue for 2 to 3 minutes, breathing easily.

Remove your hands from your eyes, and open them slowly.

Do this several times a day, or whenever you need to relax.

. . . .

that seeing is essentially a passive process. They strain to count the stars in the sky, to read the tiny print of newspapers, and to keep awake while studying organic chemistry long into the night. The conditions of civilized life place our minds and bodies under continual tension which blocks our ability to let seeing take place naturally.

The idea that poor eyesight is primarily a result of stress was pioneered by ophthalmologist William Bates, M.D. The solution to our vision problems, according to Bates, is not to stop reading, or looking at the stars, or studying for an exam, but rather to relax the mental strain which supports the imperfect functioning of the eye in both near work and distant vision. Aldous Huxley was one of the many who succeeded in doing this. Relaxation is the key.

Poor vision, like so many other dis-eased conditions, is not something which invades, or happens to us. Rather it is something which we encourage by our lifestyle. The traditional treatment has been to prescribe glasses. While they serve to correct an imbalance, they also keep the condition in a relatively static state—something like using a crutch to compensate for a broken leg.

Bates himself was rejected by his colleagues who preferred to think of refractive errors as static problems unrelated to lifestyle or habit, and to treat them only with lenses. The approach to treating them with stress reduction exercises is slow and time-consuming. But the long range effects of improved functioning are causing more people to take them seriously.[14]

Light and the Body

As light enters the eyes, it passes along neurochemical channels to the pineal and pituitary glands, the master controllers of the endocrine system. Any change in endocrine balance will cause major alterations in body chemistry and physiology, and will affect both health and behavior.

Experimentation with animals

is showing us the relationship between hormone secretion in the body and the presence or absence of light. A Wisconsin research team found that they could increase both weight and milk yield in cattle by 10% to 15% simply by increasing the numbers of hours of light the animals received. The normal nine to twelve hours of light exposure was raised to sixteen hours per day. No additional consumption of food was necessary to accomplish these gains. The entire effect seems to be the result of the manipulation of the light.[15]

Industrialized egg farming has relied on the same techniques for years. Confined to their cages inside large, light-controlled buildings, the chickens readjusted to a rhythm motivated by the increased light. The result was increased production of eggs (although quality may be adversely affected).

Sunlight reaching our skin should be our primary source of vitamin D.[16] This vitamin is essential for the development of tissues, bones, and teeth, as well as for regulating the level of calcium in the blood. Inadequate amounts of vitamin D lead to rickets, a disease resulting from the body's failure to assimilate calcium and phosphorus and characterized by softened and deformed bones. It is seen dramatically in neglected and confined children who have been kept in dark rooms for many years. Their bodies are underdeveloped.

Too much sunlight creates other problems. Ultraviolet radiation from the sun, while beneficial in small quantities, can be hazardous or even fatal in large doses. The cultural message that a deep, dark tan makes you more socially acceptable is a dangerous one. Many

---

How To Get More Full-Spectrum Light

For specially shielded light fixtures, designed to house a separate UV tube in addition to standard tubes, contact:

Environmental Systems
1140 Dillerville Rd.
Lancaster, PA 17601

For those who wear spectacles, UV transparent plastic stock which your optician can grind to your prescription can be obtained from:

Younger Optics
3788 S. Broadway Pl.
Los Angeles, CA 90007

The hardened coating used to scratch-protect plastic lenses blocks UV and should not be ordered.

For soft contacts that pass near-UV: Bausch and Lomb Sof-Lens

Hard contact lenses can be obtained from:

Wesley-Jessen Co.
400 W. Superior St.
Chicago, IL 60610

For current information on Dr. Ott's work and publications, send a stamped self-addressed envelope to:

8118 Sanderling Rd.
Sarasota, FL 34242

---

people disregard the body's warning signals in an attempt to be beautiful. Overexposure to sunlight will encourage rough, blotchy, dry, wrinkled and sagging

---

skin, and even the development of cancer. The short-wave, ultraviolet light generated by sunlamps can be equally dangerous.

We have seen how light affects milk production in cattle, egg-laying in chickens, physical development in children, and the health of the skin. What about fertility in the human female? Light surely plays some part in the regulation of the menstrual cycle, which generally occurs every twenty-eight days—the same time it takes the moon to complete its phases. Perhaps there is more than folklore and superstition involved in the ancient practice of dancing in the moonlight! More conscious birth-control methods, which seek to eliminate the use of drugs or mechanical devices, are being developed as we learn more about these connections. Light is touching and changing us in many subtle ways. The more we learn, the more we realize how interdependent all things are.

Natural Light. One area of investigation that has been receiving wider attention in the last few years concerns the harmful effects of certain types of lighting, particularly that created by fluorescent lamps. Work in this field has been pioneered and carried out almost exclusively by John N. Ott, Sc.D. (Honorary), of Sarasota, Florida. During the 1940s, while perfecting the process of time-lapse photography, Ott discovered that plant growth was significantly altered in greenhouse conditions. Sunlight passing through glass was being filtered, eliminating the near-ultraviolet (UV) portion of the light spectrum. The plants suffered from this deprivation. He found a similar problem in the animal kingdom. A group of minks was not breeding properly. Raised in a basement where they received only artificial light, the animals' normal patterns were seriously affected by a lack of near-UV light.[17]

The National Cancer Institute found that ordinary fluorescent lights were causing mutations in the chromosomes of hamsters, and could possibly stimulate cancer. Mayron and Kaplan found, in 1976, that fluorescent illumination was killing both bacteria and human cells. They also observed serious inhibition to the growth of bean sprouts which were germinated under such lights.[18] Ott further reported that the brightness, the buzzing, and the flickering of fluorescents contribute to irritability, inattention, and impulsive behavior. Perhaps, the hyperactive behavior of some children reflects this form of input which they have received in school, exposed to these lights for long periods of time over many years.

Ott's recommendations are offered here for your consideration. He suggests that you get outside for a good part of every day, and make use of natural lighting whenever possible. At the same time, you should protect your skin from too much short-wave ultraviolet radiation by protective clothing, or the use of sun-screening lotions. Incandescent indoor lighting should be used in preference to fluorescent, unless these latter are special fixtures with near-UV bulbs, and are specially shielded to prevent the escape of harmful radiation. Those who wear corrective lenses should choose a special type of plastic lens which allows the full spectrum of light to pass. Because the glass in the windows of your

Seeing with the Imagination

The extreme reliance on the visual sense which is so encouraged by television can cause us to neglect the development of our own creative sense of "inner seeing"— the imagination. When everything is shown to us as someone else envisioned it we may fail to stimulate our internal visualizing mechanism. What suffers is our creativity.

An experienced art teacher lamented the sorry consequences of this situation. Her children wanted to see what they "should" draw. They wanted a model from her before they could begin to express themselves. One of her approaches was to play music and recorded fairy tales for her students. She then asked them to draw the pictures that they had constructed in their imaginations. Her advice to their parents was to tell their children stories without showing them illustrations in books, and to balance visual stimulation with increasing amounts of auditory and tactile input. The reinstitution of radio as a dramatic medium, rather than simply for music and news, would undoubtedly be beneficial for all of us.

The subject of "inner seeing," sometimes called mental visualization, will be discussed in depth in chapter 7, Thinking.

home blocks the near-UV, you might want to install plexiglass in some windows, since this does not have the UV inhibitor added to it. If you get enough near-UV, your eyes will be better able to adapt to bright light, and you may not need to wear sunglasses.

Ott has also pioneered the study of the harmful effects of X-rays given off by color television sets. His work has resulted in improvement in the design of color picture tubes. Most recently, he has turned his attention to the video display terminals of computers, thought by many to pose a major health risk.

For millions of years, life on planet Earth has been bathed in a sea of radiation from our sun. Like plants in greenhouses, or minks in basements, humans, too, are bound to experience some detrimental effects from living most of their lives within walls. When we fail to get a healthy dose of natural light on our bodies every day, we cut ourselves off from a very important source of input energy.

Beyond the Neutral Point

Sight is more than a useful way to keep from stepping into holes. If our needs for safety and survival are provided for by care and attention, we can nourish a sense of joyfulness and wonder by using light and sight to feed our souls, and heal our bodies. The aesthetic senses of the human being are high up on the scale of needs.

Light and color have been used in therapy for a long time. In fact, Pythagoras used color for healing. Color therapy is based on the concept that selected colors beamed at the body will change its rate of vibration and so stimulate new life and new energy in diseased parts.

The public at large is beginning to appreciate the mood-setting qualities of light. Dimmer switches, track lighting, and high intensity lamps—indoor lighting has become a huge, artistic industry in the U.S. Some businesses are utilizing it effectively. Restaurants have always done so. They are often rated relative to how much atmosphere they possess, one of the primary factors being the quality of the lighting.

Examine your home, your office, in this light. What moods are created by the lighting in various rooms? If green plants can't thrive in your room, how do you expect to? Learn some valuable lessons from your green, growing friends. Experiment with lights of different colors, with altering the color scheme of a setting. You will discover that certain colors will have a more relaxing effect on your nervous system. Trust your intuition. Surround yourself, dress yourself, in colors that you really like. You alone are the judge of what feels good to you. Go ahead and do it.

Light in the Environment

Light pollution? Now there's another evil for you to rally against. Anyone who has ever lived in a big city near flashing neon signs knows about it.

Your ability to see the stars is one of your inalienable rights and that right is slowly being taken away. You see the sky clearly in the mountains or out in the country because the amount of outdoor lighting in the vicinity is at a minimum. There are really no more

You used to be able to go up in this valley and see Mt. Baldy fifty miles away. Now you can't even see the stars at night because of the smog.

—A FORTY-EIGHT-
YEAR-OLD NATIVE
OF A LOS ANGELES
SUBURB

stars over the country lane than there are over the city street. But we are seeing fewer and fewer of them.

Outdoor lighting is growing in the U.S. by about 10% every year. Because the technology of lighting is also becoming more sophisticated this means an actual increase in the intensity of actual light produced. Estimates are that by the year 2000 your night sky will be thirty times brighter than it is today, which means that you will see thirty times less than what you see now, unless you decide to do something about it. The technology exists, in fact has been in use in Tucson, Arizona, since 1972, to fit outdoor lights with shields that extend below the horizon, and to equip them with filters that will not interfere with astronomical photography or naked-eye viewing.

Smog and high-rise construction are also blocking out the light and shrinking your horizons. The hundreds of small decisions that precede the creation of these big eyesores are the responsibilities of those of us who know. We see—so we should know! When are we going to really open our eyes?

The Sense of Smell

The sense of smell is probably one of the most neglected forms of energy exchange. Our primitive ancestors, like the animals, depended on their noses to warn them of approaching danger. Yet, most of us in the Western world have not developed our sense of smell to any great degree. It lies dormant. Other than detecting a skunk on a country road, a cloud of fumes from a passing bus, or the odors of rotting garbage, we pay little attention to the constant though subtle input of olfactory information.

The sense of smell is designed to serve both as a source of warning and a source of pleasure. Food is probably the most common and most pleasurable stimulus to the sense of smell. Most of what we commonly assume to be our sense of taste is actually our sense of smell. The four basic taste sensations of sweet, sour, bitter, and salt are combined with the wide range of smells to provide us with the sensations we experience while eating.

The olfactory portion of the brain is closely tied with the limbic system (see chapter 6)—that ancient and primitive part of the brain where emotions are felt. Often strong feelings associated with childhood experiences can be triggered by a whiff of a long forgotten scent. Recall the smell of grandmother's house? Of the incense or candles in church? Of a funeral parlor? A new car? We often respond to smells of food cooking with emotional intensity, and strong memories. Hamburgers on the grill? A slow-cooking soup? The spices in the spaghetti sauce? The cotton-candy at the circus? Sometimes the smell will generate an emotional response even though we are unaware of the specific memories associated with it.

Almost every living thing

emits a scent. Along with water vapor the skin is constantly secreting unnecessary by-products. These odors produce each individual's unique body scent. While these scents change with emotional state, diet, and season, they are a chemical signature. An animal detects its baby from a group of many similar babies based on this.

In some cultures, it is only when two persons are within smelling distance of each other's bodies that they feel themselves to be making meaningful contact. This is an essential part of their social interchange. Sexuality is closely tied to the sense of smell.

In our ultra-hygienic culture such organic body odors are usually abhorred. We go to great lengths to cover them up with artificial scents and deodorants for underarms, genitals, mouth—in the same way that we deodorize the bathroom, kitchen, or trash can. In our obsession to eliminate natural odors we have surrounded ourselves with a host of new unnatural ones.

As we move toward high-level wellness, we often experience our sense of smell becoming more acute. On the unpleasant side, smoke which didn't bother us before becomes offensive. The fumes from a single car passing us on a deserted road smell horrible; imagine what effect the thousands on the freeway must be having on our bodies. We taste the sodium benzoate in bread. We are overpowered by the deodorants in public toilets. When we can detect these warning signals, we can choose to suffer and be discouraged that things are getting worse, or we can choose to minimize the amount of poisons in

our environment, or separate ourselves from them.

On the pleasant side, we can become aware of the unique scent of each of our loved ones and of our own bodies, of the wonderful scents of flowers and trees calling out to us from afar, and the subtle aromas of food. A fuller appreciation of the fragrance of life is one of the benefits of wellness.

The Sense of Hearing

The energy conversion which allows us to hear happens in the inner ear. The cochlea is lined with about 24,000 tiny hair cells of extreme sensitivity. When stimulated with sound, these hairs vibrate, creating impulses which pass along the auditory nerve into the brain, where they are interpreted. "Ah, yes. It's you, mother."

It is through the child's acute hearing that s/he will learn the sounds which make up the language used for communication. Moreover, infants depend upon the soothing sounds of a familiar voice for their security. As adults, we know this and so approach a strange child with gentle talk in order not to frighten.

We need, expect, and appreciate sound. The sound of music, of the rain, of the wind in the trees, of the stars in their travels in the night sky—these are the food of the soul. Just imagine what your world would be like without them.

On the other hand, excessive sound input can cause serious complications, and this is a growing problem in our industrialized world. The insidious background noise in our environment, which many of us have come to take for

granted, has been increasing on the average by about 1 decibel per year.

We have known for a long time that hearing loss is one of the occupational hazards of being around noisy equipment. In reporting on the causes and treatment of deafness one doctor wrote back in 1831:

The blacksmiths' deafness is a consequence of their employment; it creeps on them gradually, in general at about forty or fifty years of age.[23]

These losses are due to prolonged exposure to sound levels of between 90 and 100 decibels, and because they damage the nerve

Noise Around Our Homes

Noise Source	Sound Level for Operator (in dB)
Refrigerator	40
Floor Fan	38 to 70
Clothes Dryer	55
Washing Machine	47 to 78
Dishwasher	54 to 85
Hair Dryer	59 to 80
Vacuum Cleaner	62 to 85
Sewing Machine	64 to 74
Electric Shaver	75
Food Disposal (Grinder)	67 to 93
Electric Lawn Edger	81
Home Shop Tools	85
Gasoline Power Mower	87 to 92
Gasoline Riding Mower	90 to 95
Chain Saw	100
Stereo	Up to 120

Source: EPA

they cannot be mended. Hearing aids are largely ineffective in remedying the condition. Realizing the magnitude of this problem, the U.S. Department of Labor publishes occupational safety and health standards which include guidelines for the levels of noise allowable in industrial and business establishments. The Environmental Protection Agency makes recommendations for acceptable levels of noise in the environment at around 45 to 55 decibels.[24]

Hearing loss is not the only problem associated with noise. Noise increases stress and irritability and may even be a factor in more serious emotional disturbances. People who live near Heathrow Airport in London showed a 31% higher rate of nervous breakdown—than did those in similar economic areas away from the airport. In the community of Inglewood, California, where the noise level of jet aircraft exceeds 90 decibels, University of California at Los Angeles researchers Meecham and Smith found that the mental hospital admission rate was 29% higher than in a comparable, but quieter community.[25]

Awareness and self-responsibility in regard to noise pollution may be as simple as using a set of acoustic earmuffs, or earplugs, to protect yourself when working around loud machinery. Attending certain concerts or parties where loud music is played will require some conscious action on your part. We hear stories of rock musicians who at the age of thirty or forty are suffering from severe hearing loss. The sound levels at discos have been reported to average about 100 decibels. Some are

Jerry's Story

About seven years ago, I was arrested and sentenced to serve forty weekends in a county jail. I found the experience very degrading, especially the strip search, which happened each Friday evening. On the eighth weekend, I started becoming sick within the first hour after I arrived at the jail. I had contracted the London Flu that was going around that year.

As a child, I learned to use illness as a way of eliciting sympathy from my parents and other authority figures. In this way, I got lots of attention, and was able to get out of doing things I did not want to do. One of my favorite ways was to contract a sore throat, which became a head cold and fever, swollen glands, and finally an earache. As a result, I developed a severe hearing loss in my right ear, which stabilized at puberty.

In jail, I suffered the highest fevers I have ever had. I would complain to the jailers, and they would give me some aspirin and tell me to go see a doctor when I got out on Sunday evening. They said there was no doctor available to see me. So, I kept making myself sicker.

When I finally was let out on Sunday evening, I would go home and receive care from a nurse-friend. I got better during the week, but would still feel pretty weak when Friday rolled around again. I had a lot of anxiety about having to return to jail each weekend. One day, I was listening to the noon news on the radio, when my left ear "popped." I couldn't hear anything out of it. I assumed that this was just a temporary situation, and that my hearing would soon return. It didn't. I still have enough hearing left in my right ear to profit from a hearing aid. My left ear does not have enough hearing left for me to even use an aid.

In retrospect, I realize now that I did not just lose my hearing. I turned it off. My subconscious mind was trying to do whatever was necessary to get me out of an intolerable situation. Past experience had taught me that making myself sick was the way to accomplish this. So when one method didn't work, I would just try another. I also know that since I turned my hearing off, I am also capable of turning it back on. Obviously, there is still a "payoff" for me to continue the status quo.

even blasting away at up to 140! The longer you stay in these environments, the more accustomed your ears, your whole nervous system, will become to the sounds. It may no longer bother you. But what you are doing is drugging yourself with a form of sensory overload. It will therefore take greater amounts of input to stimulate you, at the same time that you lose an appreciation of the subtleties.

Hearing loss is not always physically caused. Some losses result from the desire to avoid hearing something, or the wish for distance in a relationship. Sometimes the event which triggers it occurs long before the actual hearing loss is detected. Our associate, Jerry, remembers deciding when he was a teenager to turn off his hearing. The decision was certainly related to his later problems. (See Jerry's Story.)

Care and consciousness; moderation and body trust; self-responsibility and love—these need to be the guiding principles in exercising respect for this magnificent sense.

Creative Sound and Silence

Just as sound can cause illness and injury and set you on edge, so it can be one of the easiest ways to relax you, supply you with new energy, and even transport you into other states of consciousness. Listening to the movement of air through your nostrils, the music of a beautiful symphony, the sounds of a chime—these can be great aids to awareness and balance. For centuries, people have used music and singing as a part of ritual celebration.

. . . .

Without music life would be a mistake.

—NIETZSCHE

. . . .

Chanting—intoning the same note—serves to tune the chanters

Sound Levels and Human Response

Common Sounds	Noise Level (dB)	Effect
Carrier deck jet operation Air raid siren	140	Painfully loud
	130	
Jet takeoff (200 feet) Thunderclap Discotheque Auto horn (3 feet)	120	Maximum vocal effort
Pile drivers	110	
Garbage truck	100	
Heavy truck (50 feet) City traffic	90	Very annoying Hearing damage (8 hours)
Alarm clock (2 feet) Hair dryer	80	Annoying
Noisy restaurant Freeway traffic Man's voice (3 feet)	70	Telephone use difficult
Air conditioning unit (20 feet)	60	Intrusive
Light auto traffic (100 feet)	50	Quiet
Living room Bedroom Quiet office	40	
Library Soft whisper (15 feet)	30	Very quiet
Broadcasting studio	20	
	10	Just audible
	0	Hearing begins

This decibel (dB) table compares some common sounds and shows how they rank in potential harm to hearing. Note that 90 dB is the point at which noise begins to harm hearing. To the ear, each 10 dB increase seems twice as loud.

Source: U.S. Environmental Protection Agency, Washington, DC 20460

into the same vibration. Songs generate energy for patriotism, for propaganda, for religious devotion. A rhythm and a frequency set the nervous system, the brain, the whole body in motion. In Appendix A you will find a detailed list of musical recordings and chants which you may want to investigate.

The sounds of the environment around you can serve as constant reminders to you to breathe, to cue into what your body is doing, to refocus your attention to the task at hand, to repeat a positive and loving prayer to yourself. Here are

......

When real silence is dared, we can come very close to ourselves and to the deep center of the world.

—JAMES CARROLL

......

some ways to use sound:

Outside

- Close your eyes and stand very still. Listen carefully. What is the furthest sound you can hear? Concentrate on that one. Hear it with the "ear" of every cell of your body.

- Stand very close to a tree or bush. Listen only for the sound of the wind playing with the leaves or branches. Experience yourself as the tree. Listen for what the wind does to your body.

- Locate a source of running water—a river, a stream, a waterfall. Close your eyes and allow the sound of moving water to fill you. Try to attend to nothing else. Hear the water with your whole body. Imagine that it is running through you—the channel. Allow it to cleanse and refresh you. Become a part of the water.

Indoors

- Most large buildings have an air-conditioning system or heating system which makes a continual background noise. Close your eyes and listen for this sound. Identify it with the sound of the wind, or another soothing sound. Use it to relax yourself.

- At home use the sounds of your oil-burner or the whirr of your refrigerator motor to do

Some Helpful Hints for a Quieter Home

- Use carpeting to absorb noise, especially in areas where there is a lot of foot traffic.

- Hang heavy drapes over windows closest to outside noise sources.

- Put rubber or plastic treads on uncarpeted stairs. (They're safer too.)

- Use upholstered rather than hard-surfaced furniture to deaden noise.

- Install sound-absorbing ceiling tile in the kitchen. Wooden cabinets will vibrate less than metal ones.

- Use a foam pad under blenders and mixers.

- Use insulation and vibration mounts when installing dishwashers.

- Compare, if possible, the noise outputs of different makes of an appliance before making your selection.

- Install washing machines in the same room with heating and cooling equipment, preferably in an enclosed space away from bedrooms.

- If you use a power mower, operate it at reasonable hours. The slower the engine setting, the quieter it will operate.

- When listening to a stereo, keep the volume down.

- Place window air conditioners where their hum can help mask objectionable noises. However try to avoid locating them facing your neighbor's bedrooms.

- Use caution in buying children's toys that can make intensive or explosive sounds. Some can cause permanent ear injury.

Source: EPA

the same thing. Remember, if you can't get away from these sounds, you might as well make friends with them and use them to your advantage.

Many of us experience great uneasiness when confronted with a lack of auditory input, because silence may force us to think, to feel, to touch deep parts of ourselves. Learning to be comfortable with silence is learning to be comfortable alone with yourself. It is one of the healthiest habits one can cultivate. Religious teachers speak of the necessity of silence for encountering the voice of God. In the silence of the mind, the heart speaks.

Watch yourself as you go through the course of a day, or several days:

- When and for how long did you experience silence accidentally, deliberately?

- How did you feel about these occasions? What, if anything, did it do for you?

- Would you like to cultivate a more loving relationship with silence? With yourself?

. . . .

Conclusion

The poets among us have written about the marvels of our bodily senses in language which reflects the wisdom and power which they afford. We know of no better way to summarize our considerations of wellness and senses than to share the inspiration of e e cummings who wrote:

> I thank You God for most this amazing
> day: for the leaping greenly spirits of trees
> and a blue true dream of sky; and for everything
> which is natural which is infinite which is yes
>
> (i who have died am alive again today,
> and this is the sun's birthday; this is the birth
> day of life and of love and wings: and of the gay
> great happening illimitably earth)
>
> how should tasting touching hearing seeing
> breathing any—lifted from the no
> of all nothing—human merely being
> doubt unimaginable You?
>
> (now the ears of my ears awake and
> now the eyes of my eyes are opened)

Used with permission

. . . .

Suggested Reading*

Downing, G. *The Massage Book.* New York, NY, and Berkeley, CA: Random House/ Bookworks, 1972.

Gunther, B. *Sense Relaxation: Below Your Mind.* New York, NY: Collier Books, 1968.

Halpern, S., and Savary, L. *Sound Health—The Music and Sounds That Make Us Whole.* San Francisco, CA: Harper and Row, 1985.

*This is only a representative sampling. Many excellent books have been omitted. At the bookstore or library, look over the whole selection and choose according to your judgment.

Kime, Z. *Sunlight.* Penryn, CA: World Health Publications, 1980.

Krieger, D. *The Therapeutic Touch: How to Use Your Hands to Help or Heal.* Englewood Cliffs, NJ: Prentice-Hall, 1979.

Montague, A. *Touching: The Human Significance of the Skin.* New York, NY: Columbia University Press, 1971, pp. 31–37.

Ott, J. *Health and Light.* New York, NY: Cornerstone, 1976.

———. *Light, Radiation and You.* Greenwich, CT: Devin-Adair, 1985.

Rosen, S. *Weathering: How the Atmosphere Conditions Your Body, Your Mind, Your Moods—And Your Health.* New York, NY: M. Evans and Co., 1979.

Selver, C. and Brooks, C. *Sensory Awareness: The Study of Living as Experience.* New York, NY, and Esalen, CA: Viking Press/ Esalen Books, 1974.

Tappan, F.M. *Healing Massage Techniques: A Study of Eastern and Western Methods.* Reston, VA: Reston Publishing Co., Inc., 1980.

Notes

1. Montague, A. *Touching. The Human Significance of the Skin.* New York, NY: Columbia University Press, 1971, pp. 31–37.

2. Montague, pp. 82–84.

3. Hite, S. *The Hite Report: A Nationwide Study of Female Sexuality.* New York, NY: Dell Publishing Co., Inc., 1976.

For a discussion of males' needs for touch see: Zilbergeld, B. *Male Sexuality.* New York, NY: Bantam Books, 1980.

4. Exercises for getting in touch with the skin, called "sensate focus," are recommended and explained in: *S.A.R. [Sexual Attitudes Restructuring] Guide,* published by National Sex Forum, 1523 Franklin St., San Francisco, CA 94109.

5. For list of schools write: Robert K. King, National Education Director, American Massage and Therapy Association, 1329 W. Pratt Blvd., Chicago IL 60626. Include self-addressed stamped envelope.

6. Montague, pp. 147–48.

7. Montague, p. 144.

8. Boyd, D. *Rolling Thunder.* New York, NY: Random House, 1974, pp. 10, 11.

9. Bernard Grad's studies are discussed in:

Bowles, N., and Hynds, F. *PSI Search.* San Francisco, CA: Harper and Row, 1978, pp. 53, 128.

Mishlove, J. *Roots of Consciousness.* New York, NY, and Berkeley, CA: Random House/Bookworks, 1975, pp. 141–42.

10. These techniques include acupuncture, acupressure, do-in, shiatsu, and others. See:

Carter, M. *Body Reflexology: Healing at Your Fingertips.* West Nyack, NY: Parker Publishing Co., 1983.

Namikashi, T. *The Complete Book of Shiatsu Therapy.* Tokyo: Japan Publications, 1981.

Teeguarden, I.M. *Acupressure Way of Health: Jin Shin Do*. Tokyo: Japan Publications, 1978.

Tohei, K. *Book of Ki: Coordinating Mind and Body in Daily Life*. Tokyo: Japan Publications, 1976.

11. For more about foot reflexology consult:

Carter, M. *Helping Yourself with Foot Reflexology*. West Nyack, NY: Parker Publishing Co., 1969.

Ingham, E. *Stories the Feet Can Tell Thru Reflexology: Stories the Feet Have Told Thru Reflexology*. St. Petersburg, FL: Ingham Publishing, Inc., 1984.

Kunz, K., and Kunz, B. *Hand and Foot Reflexology—A Self-Help Guide*. Englewood Cliffs, NJ: Prentice-Hall, 1984.

12. Palmer, B. *Body Weather*. New York, NY: Harcourt Brace Jovanovich, 1976.

13. Bates, W., M.D. *Better Eyesight Without Glasses*. New York, NY: Pyramid Books, eighth printing, 1975, p. 9.

14. Additional books on vision improvement:

Corbett, Margaret D. *Help Yourself to Better Sight*. Hollywood, CA: Wilshire Book Co., 1975.

Huxley, Aldous. *The Art of Seeing*. Seattle, WA: Montana Books, 1975.

Jackson, Jim. *Seeing Yourself See*. Brooklyn, NY: Saturday Review Press and Dutton, 1975.

15. "Supplemental Lighting Stimulates Growth and Lactation in Cattle," *Science*, Vol. 99 (February 24, 1978), pp. 911–12.

16. In actuality, so few of us get enough regular sunlight that a primary source now is milk irradiated with ultraviolet light, "enriching" it with vitamin D. (See chapter 4.)

17. Ott, J. *Health and Light*. New York, NY: Cornerstone, 1976. See also: Ott, J. *Light, Radiation and You*. Greenwich, CT: Devin-Adair, 1985.

18. For a general overview of research in this field see: "Fluorescent Lamps," *Consumers Research Magazine*. 62 (August 1979), pp. 27–294.

19. We recently learned that the full spectrum fluorescent tubes, such as Vita-Lite, mentioned in the first edition of this book, have a major shortcoming. The phosphors which emit the near-UV portion of the spectrum wear out after about one-third of the life of the tube. Since you cannot see the near-UV, you can't tell when you stop getting it from these bulbs. In addition, the plastic light diffusers of most fixtures also block the near-UV generated by these bulbs.

20. Recently, some controversy has arisen about the damaging effects of near-UV. Experimental studies attempting to show that near-UV is harmful do not adequately simulate the conditions of real life. These studies involve massive doses administered to animals over short periods of time. Despite the shortcomings of these studies, we do not dismiss them completely. Rather, we recommend that people who have been deficient in their intake of near-UV and suddenly expose themselves to sunlight at high altitudes or low latitudes should take special precautions.

21. Clark L. *Color Healing*. Old Greenwich, CT: Devin-Adair Co., 1972.

22. "Enemy Light," *Astronomy*. Vol. 7 (August 1979), pp. 63–64.

23. Fosbroke, J. "Practical Observations of the Pathology and Treatment of Deafness." *The Lancet*, Vol. I, No. II (1830–31), pp. 645–48.

24. E.P.A., Office of Noise Abatement and Control, Washington, DC 20460.

25. Reported in: "Noise to Drive You Crazy," *Psychology Today*, Vol. II (June 1977), p. 33.

Wellness and Eating

IN FEBRUARY OF 1977, a select committee of the U.S. Senate, under the chairmanship of Senator George McGovern, published a report entitled *Dietary Goals for the United States*. Its purpose, Senator McGovern stated, was "to point out that eating patterns of this century represent as critical a public health concern as any now before us."[1] Now, nearly a decade later, the findings of this committee remain relevant not only in the U.S., but in other highly developed countries as well. They serve as a powerful indictment of a lifestyle that glorifies immediate satisfaction and neglects the long-term consequences of actions.

The major concerns expressed in this study are that many U.S. citizens are malnourished, and/or overweight, and/or dying in increasing numbers from conditions linked with dietary patterns, particularly heart disease, cancer, and stroke. The "minor" concerns, we would add, are that few of us really

> Our third energy input is food. Eating (including digestion and assimilation) is the process whereby molecules are extracted from food, combusted with the oxygen supplied by breathing, and transformed into electrochemical and heat energy. These newly acquired molecules are also used in the production of raw materials needed for building and repairing body parts.

experience happiness, peace of mind, and good health. We suffer:

- tooth decay
- indigestion
- constipation
- allergies
- headaches
- hyperactivity
- lethargy
- skin disorders
- poor nails and hair

and the list goes on and on. And each of these conditions is connected with what we eat, as well as how and why we eat it.

The basic problem is that our diets and eating habits are imbalanced because we lack information about nutrition, we are stressed, we have learned to use food to relieve emotional and physical pain—because we have lost touch with ourselves.

. . . .

As a nation we have come to believe that medicine and medical technology can solve our major health problems. The role of such important factors as diet in cancer and heart disease has long been obscured by the emphasis on the conquest of these diseases through the miracles of modern medicine. Treatment, not prevention, has been the order of the day.

—DR. PHILIP LEE
PROFESSOR OF SOCIAL MEDICINE
UNIVERSITY OF CALIFORNIA
FROM *DIETARY GOALS FOR THE UNITED STATES*

. . . .

Exercise

I Already Know What I Need to Know

Think back to the meals and snacks you've eaten in the past few days, and list the foods below. When you're done, you may want to star those foods you think you should eat more of, or add foods to that list. You can also add a third category—foods you consciously avoided eating because you knew they would not be good for you.

Good Foods I Ate

Poor Foods I Ate

Besides what we eat or don't eat in the way of nutrients, many of us are addicted to various drugs: caffeine, alcohol, nicotine, and a wide variety of pharmaceuticals.

The situation is a vicious circle in which each imbalanced factor leads to another and then turns back to reinforce itself. The more stressed you are, the more you may tend to eat in an attempt to relieve your pain. The more you eat, the more pain you may create through increased weight or compounded guilt. The more pain you create, the more you may want to eat to relieve it. Round and round you go. It makes no difference at what point on the circle you jump in. Anywhere you turn, you lose. Winning requires breaking this cycle—moving into another circle altogether.

In this chapter we will present

some basic data about nutrition, examine the reasons behind our imbalanced use of food, and highlight ways of growing in awareness and love through our diet and eating habits. These suggestions will help us define a whole new circle.

The Food Story— Back to Basics

All foods are made of one or more of six essential nutrients—so called because they are necessary to sustain life in the body. These nutrients are:

- PROTEINS
- CARBOHYDRATES
- FATS
- VITAMINS
- MINERALS
- WATER

Nutrition is the study of how to provide these six nutrients in the right amount for good health. Changing these nutrients into smaller, simpler substances for ready use within the body is the process of digestion. Its main activity is breaking down:

- carbohydrates into simple sugars (glucose)
- proteins into amino acids and
- fats into fatty acids and glycerol.

Proteins, carbohydrates, and fats are the only three nutrients that contain heat-producing energy. They are the fuels which the body burns in order to provide it with the heat energy it needs. The amount of heat generated when food is oxidized is measured in cal-

ories, a unit of heat which represents the quantity necessary to raise a kilogram (roughly one quart) of water, 1°C. Each of these three nutrients burns at a different rate—some providing instant, but short-lived "flames," others burning slowly and efficiently for the warmth needed on a cold winter's night. Fats contain about 225 calories per ounce and are the slowest burning fuel. They are the coal. Proteins contain about 115 calories per ounce, and burn almost twice as fast as fats. They are the hardwood. Carbohydrates contain 115 calories or less per ounce, and burn quickly. They are the soft wood and kindling.

Protein

The word protein comes from the Greek *proteios,* meaning primary. Your body is composed chiefly of proteins (18% to 20% by weight),

---

The need for protein

- Only proteins contain nitrogen, sulphur and phosphorous which are essential to life.

- Protein is needed to build skin, hair and nails, muscles and bone.

- Enzymes and hemoglobin are protein.

- Protein synthesis forms antibodies to fight infection.

- Proteins are needed to keep the blood "neutral"— neither too acid, nor too alkaline; and to regulate the balance of water in the body.[2]

---

and consequently needs to be supplied with them in order to build new cells, replacing those which are constantly dying. Energy-wise, they are slow to digest and thus may be likened to efficient hardwoods which create a slow-burning but steady fire. Every naturally occurring food contains some protein—so the sources are indeed abundant.

. . . .

Never eat more than you can lift.

—MISS PIGGY

. . . .

Twenty-two different amino acids are needed to build all the proteins needed by humans. Fourteen of these can be manufactured within the body. The other eight cannot be easily synthesized by the body, and must be supplied with regularity, and in certain proportions. A food source in which all eight are present in the right amounts is a *complete protein.* Some foods, like grains and vegetables, are incomplete proteins. When eaten in the right combinations, however, they become complete protein foods—rice with beans, or a cheese sandwich on whole wheat bread, for example.

Proteins are like words, and the amino acids which comprise them are like letters. When a protein is digested, it is taken apart and the "letters" made available to spell whatever new words the body needs. In order to spell all the words necessary, a good supply of all the "letters" of the alphabet is imperative. Before you start worrying, however, realize that your cultural heritage and your body's own wisdom have oriented you toward a diet already replete with complete proteins: meat, fish, eggs, milk, soybeans, nuts, and many other foods.

Carbohydrates

Carbohydrates are the most common source of food energy. Our grandparents lived quite well on diets which were high in unrefined or natural carbohydrates—vegetables, fruits, and whole grains. These foods supplied starches, natural sugars, vitamins, minerals, and adequate fiber to keep everything in good working order. So why do carbohydrates have such a bad name today?

The question has many sides to it, and lack of understanding is rampant—the old "potatoes are fattening" myth, for example. The most important point to remember about carbohydrates is that there is a significant biochemical difference between unrefined carbohydrates (like potatoes, for instance) and refined carbohydrates, such as bleached flour, white rice, and sugar.

Refined carbohydrates, like kindling in the fireplace, provide a burst of flame which is soon gone. They are immediately absorbed into the bloodstream, creating the short-lived "quick pick up" that you experience after eating a chocolate bar or drinking a soda-pop. What the advertisers neglect to tell you, however, is that refined carbohydrates provide just as quick a letdown. Read what William Duffy, the author of *Sugar Blues*, has to say on the subject:

The sugar pushers have been harping on the energy building power of sucrose for years because it contains nothing else. All other foods contain energy plus. All foods contain some nutrients in the way of proteins, carbohydrates, vitamins or minerals—or all of these. Sucrose contains calories—period. The "quick" energy claim the sugar pushers talk about which drives reluctant doughboys over the top and drives children up the wall, is based on the fact that refined sucrose is not digested in the mouth or the stomach but passes directly to the lower intestines and thence to the bloodstream. The extra speed with which sucrose enters the bloodstream does more harm than good.[3]

And today we find sugar in just about all processed foods—cold cereals, pies, and snack foods, as well as in canned vegetables, fruits, and meats, and in many prepared baby foods.

Unrefined, natural carbohydrates (vegetables, fruits, whole grains, potatoes) burn like soft woods in your fireplace. In addi-

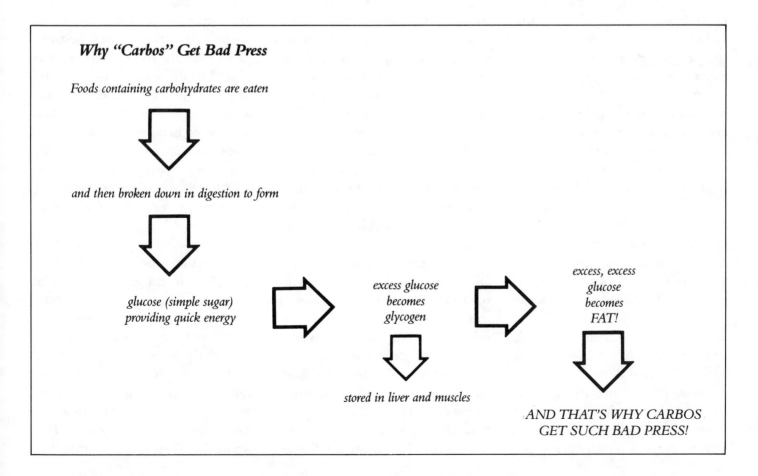

Why "Carbos" Get Bad Press

Foods containing carbohydrates are eaten

and then broken down in digestion to form

glucose (simple sugar) providing quick energy

excess glucose becomes glycogen

stored in liver and muscles

excess, excess glucose becomes FAT!

AND THAT'S WHY CARBOS GET SUCH BAD PRESS!

tion to being rich sources of vitamins and minerals, these foods provide a steady burning fire which will last many hours.

In a well-balanced diet, it is generally believed, more than 50% of the foods should be in the form of complex carbohydrates. Don't panic! But do examine your diet. Whole grain cereals for breakfast, lots of salads, fresh or lightly cooked vegetables and fruits, whole grain breads, rice and other grains, beans, nuts, and seeds — these foods will adequately supply this need and set you squarely on the road to a more healthful and satisfying life.

Fats

Few people would deny that fat is a big problem in our society. It is also big business! How easily our television-motivated culture is bandwagoned into eating "Big Jacks," and french fries, and then shamed into joining a health club, eating diet-bread, or buying a figure-control girdle. Is it any wonder our lives are not happier and our bodies healthier?

Let's clear up one common misconception—there is fat, and then there are *fats*. The latter need not be singled out as the cause of the former. You can *be fat* as a result of eating excessive amounts of protein or carbohydrates too. The fats we're talking about here are an essential ingredient in a well-balanced diet. Oils, which are fats, supply us with vitamins A and E, and aid in the production of healthy hair and skin.

Fats, in the fireplace analogy, burn like coal, the hardest and slowest burning fossil fuel. They contain twice as much energy per

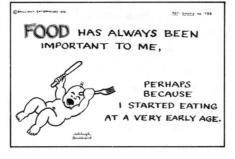

gram as the other fuels—proteins and carbohydrates. With significant exercise, which requires a large turnover of energy, our bodies can use fats to great advantage. Eskimos consume large quantities of fat with no ill effects. Without activity, however, we would do well to remember the old adage, "A moment on the lips and forever on the hips," and limit our intake of foods which are high in fat.

Vitamins and Minerals

Our concern about vitamins and minerals is relatively recent in human history, and new discoveries are being made all the time. As we continue to alter our natural environment and increase the stress of day-to-day living, we will need to change both the quantity and quality of our food consumption in order to maintain any semblance of balance. This must bring with it additional attention to the vitamins and minerals which our bodies must have.

You need vitamins and minerals so that your body can properly regulate its metabolic processes. In and of themselves, vitamins and minerals are not sources of energy, but they do determine and direct the ways in which ingested foods are assimilated and distributed. Minerals also provide building materials for teeth and bones.

Because each of us is different,

it is impossible to set absolute standards for all. The chart which follows this section lists the essential vitamins and minerals, and tells what they are needed for and where to find them. It is important to remember, however, that the minimum daily requirements and recommended doses are merely averages.

What supplements should you take? One look at vitamin/mineral advertising is enough to make ostriches of us all. Good luck in sorting it out. It is beyond the scope of this book to give that kind of advice. What we do support is that you trust your intuitions about products and the people selling them. In the long run, believing that you are doing the right thing is probably more important than what you actually do.

An important factor in getting vitamins from your vegetables is the method you choose to prepare them. The heat of boiling destroys most vitamins and the rest are dissolved in the water, which is usually just thrown away. Eating your vegetables raw would assure that you got maximum value from them. But since most of us still like our string beans cooked, we suggest lightly steaming or stir-frying to preserve as many essential vitamins as possible.

It is possible to get too much of a good thing. Salt (sodium chloride), for instance, is an essential mineral. It occurs naturally in vegetables, grains, and meats—in nearly all the foods we eat. Because of its flavor-enhancing qualities, and because we have dulled our taste buds through misuse, we have been adding salt to our foods in ever-increasing quantities. This abuse has been found to cause an

"Eat Everything on Your Plate" and Other Lines Your Parents Fed You

Recall some childhood experiences involving food and eating. What messages did you receive from family and friends? Were there rules or rituals that had to be followed, for instance? What problems, if any, did they cause you then? How do you relate to them now?

Messages/Models	Reaction/Consequence	
	Then	*Now*
Example: We always ate dinner at 6 p.m.	I often forced myself to eat.	I sometimes feel guilty preparing dinner at 9 p.m.

Water

increase in blood pressure and hypertension in some people, and is thought to encourage heart disease and migraine headache in others.

The need for water in the human body is absolutely critical. The human body is 90% water, the brain is 75% water, total body weight is 70% water. We rely upon water for digestion, cooling the body, elimination and, of course, for the circulation of nutrients to every cell in the body. Failure to replenish the supply will mean death. Your need for water is clear!

The exact amounts of water required daily will vary depending upon the foods you eat, the temperature and humidity of the air, the amount of exercise you do, and your individual rate of metabolism. (Some of us just sweat more than others!) Fortunately, supplying this element is not a problem. We get water by drinking liquids, and by eating solid foods (some of which, like carrots, lettuce, tomatoes, and watermelons, are more than 90% water). We also get some from body cells as a by-product of metabolism. Water quality is another problem, which we will address later.

Well, this concludes your course in the basics of nutrition. The next one, also a required course, is an examination of the reasons—both attitudinal and behavioral—for our imbalanced approach to eating.

Translated, that simply means:

WHY WE DON'T EAT RIGHT!

The "Why" Behind the Problems

Food as Security

Ashleigh Brilliant, in the cartoon on p. 68, gives some good insight into the first problem we will address—associations. We learned about food long before we ever started feeding ourselves. In fact, our concern with food began even before we were born. So let's go back to the beginning—to that tiny mass of protoplasm within the uterus, sustained by the nutrients

Vitamins and Minerals

This chart[5, 6, 7, 8] lists the essential vitamins and minerals, where they are found in high concentration, the process for which they are necessary, and the recommended daily allowances (RDA) for adults. Since the need for vitamins and minerals varies tremendously from individual to individual and from day to day, these figures are only approximations and statistical averages. An RDA for one person may be too much or too little for another.

Minerals

Mineral	*Processes*	*Sources*	*RDA*
Calcium	bones & teeth; coagulation of blood; vitamin metabolism; heart & nerves; enzyme stimulation; acid/alkaline balance; skin tone	cheese; milk products; green vegetables; oranges	1 g.
Phosphorus	necessary complement to calcium; all cells; bones & teeth; hair, skin, nails; enzyme stimulation	cheese; wheat germ; bran; beans & nuts; grains; tuna	1 g.
Magnesium	use of fat; nervous system; stimulation of enzymes; structure of bones; lung tissues	wheat germ; almonds; tomato; spinach, lettuce, cabbage; bran	400 mg.
Iron	blood cells; hemoglobin; 02 transmission; tissue respiration; liver	liver meats; eggs; dried apricots; blackstrap molasses; beans; grains; nuts; bran	18 mg.
Copper	conversion of iron into hemoglobin; tissue respiration; red blood cells	leeks; garlic; parsley; radishes; broccoli	2.0 mg.
Zinc	normal growth; tissue respiration; healing; sexual development; circulation; preventing high blood pressure	wheat germ; oysters; liver; oatmeal, sunflower & pumpkin seeds; brewer's yeast; eggs	15 mg.
Iodine	size & activity of thyroid gland; prevention of goiter; oxidation of fats & protein; circulation	iodized or sea salt; all sea plants; seafood; spinach	150 mcg.
Potassium	elasticity of muscle tissues; cell activity; counteracts constipation; purification of blood in kidneys	tomatoes; kale; lettuce; celery; cabbage	Not Known
Manganese	nervous system; red blood cells; tissue respiration	vegetable foods which contain Iron	Not Known

Vitamins

Vitamins	Processes	Sources	RDA*
Vitamin A	growth, esp. of skin, hair, nails, teeth; resistance to infection; maintenance of glandular activity; healthy condition of mucous linings & membranes	liver; parsley, spinach, other green vegs.; carrots; sweet potatoes; fish liver oils	5000 IU
Vitamin C	growth, esp. teeth; protects vascular system; defense against bacterial toxins; glandular activity; appetite; tissue respiration	brussels sprouts; citrus fruits; green vegetables; all fruits & vegs.	60 mg.
Vitamin E	skin; sexual glands & reproductive system; circulation; keeps red blood cells from being destroyed	sunflower seed oil; wheat germ; wheat germ oil; cottonseed oil; corn oil; peanut oil; green vegs.; whole grains; milk, eggs	30 IU
Vitamin D	bones, teeth, tissue; regulation of blood calcium	sunshine; egg yolk; butter & dairy products; tuna; salmon	400 IU
Vitamin B1 (Thiamine)	normal red blood count; growth; appetite; digestion & assimilation; protein, carbo. & fat metabolism; nervous system; vitality; muscle tone	wheat germ; soybeans; brewer's yeast; nuts; beans; grains	1.5 mg.
Vitamin B2 (Riboflavin)	healthy eyes; nerve tissues; cell respiration; control of infection; breakdown of fatty acids	liver; brewer's yeast; dried milk; beans; wheat germ; green vegs.; grains; fruits	1.7 mg.
Vitamin B6 (Pyridoxine)	protection from infection; protein & fat metabolism; nervous system & brain, enzyme system	brewer's yeast; wheat germ, bran; bananas; avocados; pecans; green leafy vegs.	2 mg.
Vitamin B9 (Folic Acid)	red blood cells; RNA & DNA; healing; prev. of infection; protein metabolism	liver; oysters; sunflower seeds; cheese; eggs	6 mcg.
Vitamin B12 (Cobalamin)	production & regeneration of blood cells; prevention of anemia; enzymatic process	dark green leafy vegs.; brewer's yeast; nuts	0.4 mg.

*Recommended Daily Allowance

in the mother's blood, awaiting its entry into the big world outside.

Until its birth, the fetus is warm, secure, and totally dependent for all its needs, which nature so generously fills. This is not to say, however, that it is *completely* safe. Mother's diet and mental state are subtly exerting their influence upon the unborn child. The mother's food needs to be rich in the vitamins and minerals essential to growth, and unadulterated by harmful substances and contaminants which may retard the normal development of the vulnerable fetus.[9]

Once it arrives on the scene at birth, the child spends the first months of life in two basic activities—sleeping and eating. The quality of its food is of great importance, not only in keeping it alive and well now, but in setting the stage for later eating habits. Equally important is the way food is supplied. Traumatic or unsatisfying feeding experiences may color the infant's view of the world and have far-reaching effects upon its physical and mental health.

We know that breast-fed babies evidence strong advantages over bottle-fed infants. Breast-fed children have significantly fewer respiratory infections, conditions such as asthma and hayfever, gastrointestinal problems, and skin disorders such as eczema.[10] A Chicago study of 383 children found that breast-fed children were both physically and mentally superior to those who were bottle-fed.[11] The link here may be due as much to stimulation involved in breast-feeding, as to the nutritional value of mother's milk. More than milk is needed to satisfy "hunger."

As we learned in the last chap-

Whether or not children eat proper foods, eat regularly, eat carefully, and eat politely has an effect on their health and their personalities.

—NATIONAL
EDUCATION
ASSOCIATION, 1940

ter, the intimate association between being fed and being cared for is realized very early in life. Need-satisfaction and food are joined so strongly that the union endures throughout our development and into adulthood. And so, at age eighteen, or thirty-two, or fifty-five, sitting in your chair reading this book, you are a complex network of needs and assets. Your hunger may be for security, for companionship, or for self-worth, but the easiest and quickest source of satisfaction will probably be food.

Food as a Pain Reliever

Many of us have learned to use food to alleviate physical pain. Recall for a moment a typical scene. Jenny is riding her tricycle on the sidewalk, the wheel hits a bump and she topples to the ground, crying. Dad rushes from the house, gathers her up in his arms, kissing her baby tears and consoling, "There, there now, don't cry, you're all right. Come inside and I'll give you a piece of candy." For a long time big people have been trying to convince children that vaccinations, vitamins, spinach, liver, and lots of other things will not hurt or taste bad, provided that they are quickly accompanied by a lollipop or chocolate bar. "Be

brave now, don't cry, and Mommy will give you a treat." (Or is it a trick?) We have been programmed from our earliest years to use food to deal with pain.

While some adults who experience migraine headaches lose their appetites during an attack, Regina found that she actually ate more. "Eating may have been simply a good distraction," she explained, "but I really felt an alleviation of pain when I was eating." In fact, there seems to be a physiological basis to this. Current studies indicate that addiction to food is linked with the release of a brain substance called beta-endorphin. This endorphin is governed by the pituitary gland and serves as a natural opiate which may temporarily relieve pain and stress, creating a biologically comforting effect.[12]

Food as Emotional Insulation

A crossword puzzle enthusiast was recently overheard to remark: "One of these days I'm going to quit doing puzzles and start filling in the other empty spaces in my life!" This insightful comment applies well in our consideration of the use of food to handle emotional pain. Food fills up the empty spaces in the body, but not those in the mind and soul. Learning to tell the difference between "mouth hunger" and "stomach hunger" is important if you have a weight problem.

Eating out of boredom, a form of emotional pain, is one of the chief reasons for compulsive eating and poor nutrition. The work ethic and need for achievement which characterize life in contemporary America can lead you to the conclusion that you must be "doing something" to keep busy or to be of value to yourself and society. When the motivation for work or involvement wanes, due to physical exhaustion, an emotional setback, or an inability to find meaning in life, a sense of guilt for not being productive is commonly experienced. Many people attempt to resolve this condition by moving to the kitchen to "rattle the pots and pans," or to the fast-food establishment down the street to have something, anything, to do.

Time and again in the classes and workshops we have conducted we hear stories like this:

"My problems with overeating started when my last child went off to school."

"I'm eating a lot of junk food lately, but I'm under a lot of emotional stress. Since I lost my job, I'm bored."

Deborah, who conducts weight-awareness seminars for women, has some interesting insights on boredom and eating. She has found that many people eat to gain weight so that they will have something tangible to work at, i.e., trying to *lose* weight. No one makes this a conscious plan—but the pattern is common enough that she believes it is a real one. She personalizes it this way: "If I wasn't on a diet, what else would I have to do?" or "If I ever reached my ideal weight and found that I still wasn't happy—what would I do then?"

Weight and Withholding

The ballasting and insulating qualities of fat in protecting us from unpleasant feelings of inner conflict can be seen from another vantage point. Chronic "nice guys" who don't let their negative thoughts or feelings find conscious expressions often "swallow" these sources of conflict, thinking it gets rid of them. I believe we can probably solve any weight problems we may perceive by behaving in a manner that reflects respect for ourselves, rather than letting people take advantage of us. I don't mean we have to tell everyone every negative judgment we experience, but that we just acknowledge to ourselves that we have them and that they can't hurt us unless we take them seriously.

People with weight problems have reported that by beginning to express verbally all those things they thought they couldn't say, their pounds begin disappearing.

—J.W.T.

Many people use food as emotional insulation to protect themselves from further hurt, or as a drug to dull the pain of a meaningless existence, a broken marriage, or the death of a loved one. When the federal government started giving tax breaks for insulating homes to conserve energy, it made environmentalists very happy. Many chronically overweight people have been giving themselves a "feeling" break for a long time as they pile on layer after layer of fat in an attempt to insulate their hearts, and guts, and sexual organs from emotional energy loss. But the break is only temporary and eventually leads to something worse. The real needs aren't being addressed. Cindy's story illustrates this.

Cindy gave birth to a beautiful eight-pound boy only to learn that the child was deaf. Distraught with grief, she began to eat excessively and consequently to gain weight. Fifteen years and an extra eighty pounds or so later, she realized that she hadn't cried since "I can't remember when," her desire for sex had long since died, and her world was shaded in tints of grey. Cindy's body had become her refuge. She had attempted to shield herself from being disappointed and hurt again, but she was far from happy. It had been an unsuccessful and costly strategy which produced new and different problems and had really not alleviated the pain.

It isn't hard to understand the lessons in Cindy's case. At some time in our lives most of us have used food to mask or alleviate pain, or as an unconscious means of punishment and self-destruction. Or we may have denied ourselves food, and so diverted our attention to a new pain.

It is only in the last few years that conditions such as anorexia and bulimia have been brought into public awareness. Alarming numbers of young people, especially women, are seriously jeopardizing their health by using food

On Bulimia

I was bulimic for fourteen years. Today I am free of this destructive binge-purge cycle, and have been for the past three-and-a-half years. My recovery began when I made a commitment to myself—to do whatever it took to stop this obsession that kept me hating myself and feeling powerless.

In 1981, treatment centers for this eating disorder were unknown to me, so it was a lot harder to get help than it is today. I created a support system by deciding to write my master's thesis on the recovery from bulimia. I interviewed therapists and recovering bulimics. Talking to women who were farther along the path of recovery inspired me to keep going even when I felt scared and hopeless. One person in particular, I'll never forget—a woman who had hidden her binge-purge behavior from her husband and children for twenty-five years. She shared so openly, as did many others, and helped me to open to the strong part in me that knew I could and would overcome this destructive behavior.

Here are the major steps I took:

• I became ruthlessly honest with myself and everyone in my life. Basically, I stopped hiding my behavior and my feelings.

• I learned to ask for what I really wanted, and to say "No" to what I didn't—In my relationships, and all other areas of my life.

• I realized that food and weight issues were not really about food and weight, so I attended groups and workshops to work through the underlying emotional issues—like low self-esteem, perfectionism, and a need to be in control.

• I GAVE UP THE NEED TO BE THIN, AND DECIDED I'D RATHER BE HAPPY. (Paradoxically, after a temporary weight gain, I lost weight and have maintained it with ease.)

• I stopped looking for an external authority to tell me how to live my life (i.e., what I should eat, what I should weigh, how I should act or feel) and began to look inside and trust that

I had those answers for myself.

• I stopped beating up on myself when I had made a mistake. Instead, I used my energy to learn about myself, rather than feeling wrong or guilty about my mistakes.

• I STOPPED BEING A VICTIM, BLAMING CIRCUMSTANCES AND PEOPLE IN MY LIFE, AND TOOK RESPONSIBILITY FOR MYSELF AND MY BULIMIA. Once I accepted that I had chosen to be bulimic, I freed myself to choose otherwise.

My life isn't problem-free now by any means. But, knowing that I conquered bulimia gives me courage to face any problems in my life.

If you are currently struggling to overcome any eating disorder you need to know that RECOVERY IS POSSIBLE! Today, most hospitals have special programs for dealing with your particular needs, and there are therapists who are trained to work with you. Please don't be ashamed to seek help. I did it. You can too.

—Jo Sherrill

in self-destructive ways (i.e., by gorging on food, then vomiting or taking laxatives) or by denying food to themselves altogether. For some it is a misguided attempt to gain control over their lives. For others, it is an obsession with weight gain, which is considered the greatest of all evils. In nearly all cases, low self-esteem is strongly evident. The table becomes the battleground, and food, whether it is the enemy or the only trusted ally, is the one thing that matters. Needless to say, when this kind of emotional war is being waged, considerations such as nutrition, or real nourishment, are rarely found.

Still another type of eating disorder is evidenced by "nutrition addicts" who devote the greater part of their day's work to worrying about and planning the balancing of their foods. They can be found wandering the aisles of the health food stores, diligently studying vitamin bottles, and hurrying home to administer to themselves some new intestinal cleanser. They are obsessed with "toxins" and fascinated by the consistency of their feces. This excessive concern may be temporarily necessary during certain critical periods, especially in treating serious illness, but as a way of life, it more likely indicates another obsession with food that fills time, and may serve to discourage the cultivation of relationships with others and the creation of more dynamic and rewarding forms of self-expression.

Eating and Stress

In a remarkable series of books describing his training by the Yacqui sorcerer Don Juan, Carlos Castaneda describes the characteristics of the warrior, the person of power. Far from being a creature of habit, at the mercy of societal convenience, the warrior is attuned to both intuition and the body's natural rhythms. Consequently s/he will sleep when tired, rise when rested, and eat when hungry. Certainly not dramatic prescriptions, but difficult for most of us to follow nonetheless.

How many of us generally eat because the noon-whistle has sounded or the six o'clock news is over, paying little attention to whether we are hungry or not? The whole scene is strongly reminiscent of Pavlov's dogs who were conditioned to salivate at the sound of a bell.

The demands of a job, a school schedule, or raising children frequently necessitate altering our mealtimes accordingly. Thus we compound the problem by eating too quickly. Have you ever seen a

. . . .

People learn the patterns of their diet not only from the family and its sociocultural background, but from what is available in the marketplace and what is promoted both formally through advertising and informally through general availability in schools, restaurants, supermarkets, workplaces, airports, and so forth. . . . Nutrition and health education are offered at the same time as barrages of commercials for soft drinks, sugary snacks, high-fat foods, cigarettes and alcohol.

—DR. BEVERLY WINIKOFF IN
*DIETARY GOALS FOR
THE UNITED STATES*

. . . .

pie-eating contest? Definitely not an aesthetic experience! While most of us will probably never qualify for the national teams, the speed with which we empty our plates or finish off our lunches might indicate that we are in training for a fast-eating competition.

When you eat rapidly so as not to miss your plane, your history class, or your favorite TV program, you put yourself under time pressure which creates stress throughout your body. The body, in its natural wisdom, will generate a variety of hormonal secretions, as well as increase both heart rate and respiration, to attempt to cope with the situation. Eating in this condition will result in any number of sorry effects, including acid indigestion. The remedy for this, offered by high-pressure advertising, is to consume a candy or liquid preparation that "reduces excess stomach acid." So relieved, you can

continue the practice that got you into trouble in the first place. The "American way" really does support a "pill for every ill."

Speed-eating further subjects us to the risk of choking on our food since we don't take the time to chew it properly. Death from choking is the fourth highest cause of accidental death in the U.S.[13]

Regina grew up in a large family and remembers well the humorous Grace-Before-Meals in which she prayed:

Father, Son and Holy Ghost

The one who eats fastest

Gets the most.

While we are on the subject of childhood memories, picture for a moment the family gathered around the dinner table. The TV shows and romantic novels suggest that they are discussing what the children learned in school today, the literary merits of a current bestseller, or plans for the summer vacation. More realistically, they may spend mealtimes watching high-speed car chases on the television, arguing over whose turn it is to do the dishes, or worrying about whether the money will hold out long enough to get the car repaired or the phone bill paid. Sound familiar? It certainly doesn't make for relaxed, aware eating.

Since mealtimes provide some of the rare occasions for getting together with loved ones, and can be tax write-offs for business, they are often used as opportunities to discuss "big deals" or to deal with problems. Handling hassles "over lunch" is an effective way to increase stress and give yourself an upset stomach.

Where you eat can also contribute to stress. The availability of "fast food" has made it possible to buy and consume a meal without ever leaving your car. Simply driving your car through the city, or on freeways, in so many places in the U.S. today can be a very taxing experience. Eating your meals while doing so rings the bell at the top of the stress scale. The foods served at these establishments are usually highly refined, filled with sugar and chemical preservatives, and loaded with unnecessary fat, which makes it even worse.

We Forget Our Uniqueness

We have relinquished awareness and self-responsibility in our eating habits as we have in so many other areas of our lives. Few people are in touch with themselves and knowledgeable enough about their own metabolism to design their own nutritional programs. We therefore follow patterns we learned as children, or the recommendations of "experts," or the lead assumed by the advertising media.

Watch people eat and observe their bodies and you soon realize that what works for one may be the downfall of the other. One friend consumes huge quantities, has tremendous energy, rarely gets sick, and never gains weight. Another generally eats sparingly and yet constantly battles the scale. A chronically overweight woman complains that she merely has to drive past a bakery shop and she puts on a few extra pounds! The truth is that there are tremendous differences in the biochemical needs of any two individuals. Biochemist Roger J. Williams remarks: "If normal facial features varied as

much as gastric juices do, some of our noses would be about the size of navy beans while others would be the size of twenty-pound watermelons."[14]

We are all subject to periodic fluctuations as well. The change from summer to winter, falling in love, preparing for a crucial exam, the death of a dear one—each of these factors will alter the body's chemistry and motivate a change in eating habits. Yet these factors are rarely appreciated and honored. Our diets are imbalanced because we often don't know what we really need. The paradox is that few of us would approach the servicing of our automobiles with as little care and attention as we give to our bodies.

The Problems With What We Eat

We Eat "Junk" and Highly Processed Food

Between-meal-snacks have become a great American pastime indicative not only of our addictions to sweets and "junk food," but also of our lack of attention to when our bodies really need to eat. You may be interested to learn that in 1976 the average U.S. citizen consumed 125 pounds of fat, 100 pounds of sugar, and 295 cans of soda pop. Soft drinks are now second on the list of most consumed beverages, replacing milk, while coffee is still number one.[15]

The McGovern committee report revealed that refined carbohydrates such as white flour products, instant potatoes or rice, pastries, heavily sweetened foods, sodas, candy and alcohol (which behaves

---

"What Color Do You Want?"—Behavior, Dyes and Junk-Food

Toronto, Canada:
Researchers from the Hospital for Sick Children, and the University of Toronto report a study which links food dye consumption and impaired learning performance in hyperactive children.
Science (207) March 28, 1980, pp. 1485–86.

In Oakland California:
Bernard Weiss, University of Rochester, N.Y., School of Medicine and Dentistry, accumulated data suggesting that modest amounts of synthetic colors ingested by children provoked disturbed behavior.
Science (207) March 28, 1980, pp. 1487–88.

University of Maryland:
Zoologists find that Red Dye 3 (used in food) increases release of a brain chemical, acetylcholine.
Science (207) March 28, 1980, pp. 1489–90.

---

like a refined carbohydrate) have become staples for many. They have replaced our consumption of complex carbohydrates—fruit, vegetables, and grain products—which in the early 1900s comprised 40% of the typical diet. Today only a little more than 20% of our calories comes from these sources.[16]

The movement to highly refined and processed foods is a consequence of growing affluence and the accompanying desire for convenience. These foods are typically high in chemical additives, preservatives and sugar—all of which are linked with hyperactivity in children.[17, 18]

The average adult in the U.S. eats approximately ten pounds of these chemicals each year. Currently more than 1300 of these substances are approved by the FDA for use as colors, flavors, preservatives, and thickeners. Some have been rigorously tested, others less so. Almost daily, the observant reader can find reference to studies linking one or another of these additives with cancer of some sort. It is a pretty tricky business.

As long as we demand a vending machine diet of pink cupcakes with yellow cream filling there will be little chance of curtailing the use of these substances in our food. Necessity is one thing, as in the use of small amounts of nitrates to control bacterial growth in meat. But commercial gimmickry is another. Stroll down the breakfast cereal aisle of your local food store and observe that you can now feed yourself and your children pink, orange, and purple puffs which taste like chocolate bars, blueberry muffins, or strawberry shortcake.

If we lived more in harmony with the earth and sea, the probability is that the foods we'd eat would supply us with all the vitamins and minerals necessary for good healthy bodies. But since we have robbed our soils of these nutrients, polluted our waters, and overprocessed our food, we find we must supplement our diets in other ways—through "enrichment" or by taking vitamins and minerals in tablet form. Many people prefer to eat polished (white) rice instead of brown rice, and then buy bottles of B vitamins which are made from the parts removed from rice in the processing!

Where Is Fiber Found?

Whole grain cereals are a major source of dietary fiber. Bran has 9% to 12% crude fiber; dry beans, lentils, and soybean have over 4% (equivalent to 1.2% to 1.5% after cooking with added water); roasted nuts have 2.3% to 2.6%; and most fruits and vegetables contain 0.5% to 1%, although there is some loss during processing.

Our present economic system of food production, transportation, and distribution makes ease of shipping and long shelf-life its most important considerations. Since these are often supported in place of quality, the foods we buy commonly lack a proper balance of vitamins and minerals necessary for optimum health. The bran of cereals, for instance, constitutes more than half of their vitamin and mineral value, but in order to make cereals more palatable, food manufacturers remove this part and feed it to livestock. Cereals are then "enriched" by putting back four of the twenty-two nutrients which were removed. The whole situation is ironic in the wasteful pattern it encourages. Moreover, by the time most of these foods reach our plates they are soft and smooth, and almost lacking the fiber which is necessary to keep the intestines adequately stimulated.[20]

They also "gum up" the works, and help create a variety of very serious conditions. Diverticulosis is one of these. It occurs usu-

ally in people over forty, whose "unstimulating" diet has been the pattern of a lifetime. In this condition the colon wall is stretched into blind pockets filled with accumulated fecal matter. Other related problems include constipation, obesity, and even cancer.

We Eat Too Much Fat

The problems created by overreliance on refined carbohydrates are equaled by those that accompany the consumption of too much fat. Since fat is the most concentrated source of food energy, large amounts prove useful to Eskimos who live in a harsh climate, or to people who do continual vigorous work. But most of us carry on such sedentary patterns of living that we have little need for this long-stored energy. Some of us spend our lives moving only from bed to table to car to elevator to car to table to TV to bed. The consumption of a diet which derives 40% of its calories from fat results in a continual struggle to control weight. It's the great "battle of the bulge."

The McGovern committee reported that ordinary obesity in the general population is a strong factor in the excess development of coronary heart disease, and that strong evidence exists linking dietary fat to cancer of the breast and colon.[21]

The related problem is that filling up on empty calories and fats will temporarily satisfy hunger, and eliminate the desire for the other foods which the body really needs. Mother was right when she said that potato chips would spoil your appetite.

Without the activity needed to

work it off, living on lots of fats is like keeping a fire in your fireplace without ever getting a good strong draft and a roaring blaze. The result of this smoldering heap is a lot of ashes and a sooty chimney.

Problems With Protein Foods

As we approach the subject of the potential problems created by meat, and the high consumption of other protein foods, we enter an area of extreme controversy. The beef, egg, and dairy industries (our main suppliers of protein foods) exercise powerful lobbies and advertising programs to keep us eating their products.

While it is true that eggs, milk products, and meat are high in protein, they are also sources of cholesterol, and excessive amounts of cholesterol in the system are linked to heart disease.[22] There is no secret, moreover, that growth-producing hormones, chemical foods, and grains sprayed with pesticides are the daily fare of beef cattle, and that these toxic residues build up in the bodies of those of us who consume the beef.[23, 24] We note further that among populations where meat consumption is high, mortality rates from a variety of cancers are correspondingly high.[25]

In the U.S., the Seventh Day Adventists, a religious group whose members do not eat meat, offer living proof of the health benefits of vegetarianism. Studies in this group indicate their general health is far superior to that of the rest of the U.S. population. This supports the fact that meat protein is not essential.

Experimentally, we find a problem with the typical meat-centered diet because it is heavy—that is, filling—and discourages children and adults from eating more vegetables. It also necessitates the use of large land areas for grazing and growing food for cattle. One-half of the harvested agricultural land in the U.S. is planted with feed crops; 78% of all our grain is fed to animals. Grain fed to cattle is not being fed to people. And the world is starving. Once again it is a question of balance.

It is paradoxical that we, who may be so cautious about taking risks in other aspects of our lives, would be willing to run such high ones when it comes to the foods we eat and feed our children. In teaching and conducting workshops we are continually amazed at how much our students and participants know about what they shouldn't do. What is lacking most of all is the motivation to attack the problem.

Knowing all this, we offer the recommendations of the McGovern committee about dietary goals for Americans, a few important recommendations for pursuing personal nutritional awareness, and some encouragement to help you in your wellness process.

Eating for High Level Wellness

General Recommendations

This book won't prescribe systems everyone can or should follow. This would undermine the concept of self-trust which has been its underlying thesis. However, some consideration of the components of basic nutrition is needed to develop an intelligent, broad-based awareness of the role that food plays in

your well-being. Moreover, in the midst of the confusing data surrounding this subject, some common recommendations continually surface from almost every source consulted. While it would be foolish to latch on to this or any other plan as the final word, we do believe that the guidelines offered by the McGovern Committee on Nutrition and Human Needs represent a balanced approach. They are presented here for your consideration.

U.S. Dietary Goals
1. Increase complex carbohydrate consumption to account for 55% to 60% of the energy (caloric) intake.

2. Reduce overall fat consumption from approximately 40% to 30% of energy intake.

3. Reduce saturated fat consumption to account for about 10% of total energy intake; and balance that with poly-unsaturated and mono-unsaturated fats, which should account for about 10% of energy intake each.

4. Reduce cholesterol consumption to about 300 mg. a day.

5. Reduce sugar consumption by about 40% to account for about 15% of total energy intake.

6. Reduce salt consumption by about 50% to 85% to approximately 3 grams a day.

The Goals Suggest the Following Changes in Food Selection and Preparation
1. Increase consumption of fruits and vegetables and whole grains.

2. Decrease consumption of meat

and increase consumption of poultry and fish.

3. Decrease consumption of foods high in fat and partially substitute polyunsaturated fat for saturated fat.

4. Substitute nonfat milk for homogenized milk.

5. Decrease consumption of butterfat, eggs, and other high cholesterol sources.

6. Decrease consumption of sugar and foods high in sugar content.

7. Decrease consumption of salt and foods high in salt content.

For the full report, *Dietary Goals for the United States*, write: U.S. Government Printing Office, Washington, DC 20402. Price: $.95.

We would add two more recommendations to this list. There is strong evidence that caffeine has addictive properties, and contributes to erratic blood sugar levels. Coffee, black teas, colas, and chocolate, which are all high in caffeine, should therefore be approached with caution.

Many urban water supplies are contaminated with toxic pollutants

• • • • • • •

It is likely that those most influenced by food advertising are low-income and elderly consumers who are least capable of comprehending written guidance on food selection and least able to make comparisons between foods based on the nutrition labeling and price.

—DIETARY GOALS FOR
THE UNITED STATES

• • • • • • •

such as lead, asbestos, and mercury. Because large amounts of water are filtered through our bodies, even small traces of these toxins will accumulate over time. Consider using bottled spring water, or attaching a high-quality filter to your spigot.

Check Those Labels

If you don't already do so, start reading the labels on cans and packages of food products. You may be in for a real shock. Ingredients are listed in order of their amount, that is, the main ingredient is listed first, on down to the smallest. Comparative shopping often reveals that while one product contains sugar and/or strange sounding chemicals, another brand may not. Keep in mind, however, that ingredient labeling has some limitations. There are numerous additives that the F.D.A (Food and Drug Administration) does not require to be listed on labels. Some ingredients must be listed on some products but not on others. Incomplete or inadequate labeling is also evident, e.g., certified food coloring may be listed, but the specific type is not indicated. Ingredient labeling is not required at all on some products. For instance, due to powerful lobbying the dairy industry has been exempted from listing most additives.

Also realize that the processed food industry may use wording in the labels and techniques in their advertising which can cause you to be confused, deceived, and downright pressured. To give you a few examples:

• "Enriched" or "wheat" flour means white flour. White flour

The McGovern committee's report was less than enthusiastically received by the meat producers and dairy industry officials. Just to give you some idea of the response:

Any set of national dietary goals will have far-reaching effects on all segments of society. It is, therefore, essential that the professional community and the food industry at the highest levels be involved in the formulation of these goals. . . . The dietary goals as formulated by the staff of the Select Committee on Nutrition do not now have such support. We, therefore, urge that they be withdrawn.

National Dairy Council

It appears to us that many doctors and nutritionists have been spending too much time and money trying to prove a preconceived notion that diet is the main problem in this country. Meanwhile, the real problem—more likely lifestyle and physical condition as well as heredity—has been mostly ignored.

The situation reminds us of a sheriff back home who couldn't find the real cattle thief, so he browbeat an innocent man almost to the point of making him say he was guilty. In the meantime, the real culprit was free.

We concur with the Senate reorganization plan calling for elimination of this committee and incorporation of its functions into the Agriculture Committee.

American National Cattlemen's
Association and the National Livestock
Feeders Association, March 24, 1977

To summarize the position of the Salt Institute, we feel that there is definitely no need for a dietary goal that calls for the reduction of salt consumption.

Salt Institute, June 24, 1977

. . . .*Exercise*. . . . .

Match the Number of the "Food" to Its Ingredients

1. Fruit Drink Mix

2. Instant Tomato Soup

3. Imitation Maple Syrup

4. Instant Mashed Potatoes

5. Diet Soft Drink

6. Non-dairy Coffee Creamer

7. Canned Dog Food

8. Canned Cake Frosting

A. Corn syrup solids, hydrogenated coconut oil, lactose, sodium caseinate, dipotassium phosphate, mono and diglycerides, sodium silico aluminate, artificial colors, lecithin, artificial flavor.

B. Potato flakes, mono and diglycerides, sodium acid pyrophosphate, sodium sulphites, citric acid, BHA, BHT.

C. Sugar, dried tomato, modified corn starch, salt, hydrogenated cottonseed and soy oils, natural flavors, dried onion, lactose, dried garlic, artificial flavor, sodium caseinate, monosodium glutamate, dipotassium phosphate, soy flour, artificial color, chicken fat, dried chicken meat, thiamine hydrochloride, disodium inosinate and disodium guanylate, turmeric, spices.

D. Citric acid, monocalcium phosphate, artificial flavor, vitamin C, artificial color, BHA.

E. Sugar, hydrogenated vegetable oils, BHA, BHT, water, corn syrup, cocoa processed with alkali, salt, natural and artificial flavors, wheat starch, polysorbate 60, citric acid, potassium sorbate, lecithin, cellulose gum.

F. Carbonated water, caramel color, phosphoric acid, sodium saccharin, sodium citrate, caffeine, natural flavor, citric acid.

G. Meat by-products, chicken parts, poultry by-products, wheat flour, soy flour, whole egg, salt, dried yeast.

ANSWERS: A6; B4; C2; D1; E8; F5; G7

is made from wheat, except that the bran and wheat germ have been removed. The label should read "stoneground" *whole* wheat or rye to be certain you're getting a true whole grain product. "Natural sweetener" usually means sugar (as opposed to artificial sweetener).

- Supposedly knowledgeable professionals or celebrities may be used to recommend a product.

(Perhaps you have seen the television ad showing a nutritionist and then an astronaut extolling the virtues of a powdered, citrus-flavored drink. The major ingredient of that product is sugar.)

- Labels may list the vitamins and minerals with which a product has been enriched. This usually means that a minimal amount of vitamins has been added to a deficient ("junk") food product to make the label look good. The product is often high in sugar, white flour, and/or fat.

Food producers spend about $1.15 billion annually on advertising. This represents 28% of total TV advertising spending. The greater proportion of this money goes for the glorification of non-nutritive beverages, sweets, and other snack foods which are low in nutritional value and high in calories. As products of our environment, most of us are strongly influenced by these ads, and consequently are lacking in both nutrition education and nutritious food.

Explore Your Own Uniqueness

The concept behind nutritional individuality based on biochemical individuality is certainly not new. Everybody knows that people are different. Every age has had its ways of classifying bodies and personalities: the ecto-, endo-, and mesomorphs . . . the phlegmatics and sanguines . . . the type A's and the type B's . . . and now Metabolism type 1—Metabolism type 10 . . .

The realization that differences exist in the ways our bodies metabolize food was offered by Dr. George Watson of the University of Southern California in the 1960s when he observed the different effects that foods had on people's emotions.[26] Around the same time, Dr. Roger J. Williams was developing his theories along the same lines and expressing them in his book, *Biochemical Individuality*.[27]

Williams believes that we all come into life with unique biochemical needs which can be met only with a proper balance of nutrients. Failure to supply these nutrients in the right amounts results in disease. And what is excess for one may be insufficient to another. There is no such thing, according to Williams, as the "average man."

. . . .

If we continue to solve such (nutritional) problems on the basis of the average man, we will be continuously in a muddle, because the concept of "average man" is a muddle. Such a man does not exist.

—ROGER J. WILLIAMS, PH.D.

. . . .

Unfortunately, our education about nutrition is filled with "norms," "minimum daily requirements," "average weights," and "ideal diets," many of which compound our problems and add to the

. . . . *Exercise* . . . .

A Martian View

Observe TV for several hours and attempt to put yourself in the mind-set of an impressionable child, or naive extraterrestrial alien.

What do you learn about how to eat, what to eat, where, why, etc.?

Record Observations Here: (try to put them in the form of generalized statements and enjoy a good laugh as you share these with others)

Example: Good mothers give children cupcakes after school.

. . . .

general confusion about nutrition. The response to this muddle has been the introduction of the personalized health plan, the personally designed diet, the nutritional analysis, the metabolic profile. Far from being satisfied with recommending calorie limits based on sex and weight, many of these methods use in-depth surveys to determine lifestyle factors which affect nutritional needs. Others test pulse rate, saliva, blood, hair, and urine.

While there are definite values in such detailed testing, the appreciation of biochemical individuality demands that we develop awareness and trust of our own bodies above all else. Ultimately, you are the one who is responsible for the health and well-being of your own body—not a chemist, a computer or a physician.

Awareness and Self-Trust

Listening

Nutrition is a subject as highly charged as politics or religion. Each person has a point of view, (which of course is the right one). No wonder there is so much confusion and disagreement in the field. Start to survey a few books on the subject of nutrition and you soon realize how contradictory the "facts" are. For just about any belief substantiated by one group of studies, you will find a comparable number of articles and experts which will refute it.

- Sugar is poison vs. sugar is a quick energy food.

- Meats are the best source of protein vs. meat is harmful.

- Vitamins and mineral supplements are a ripoff vs. commercial croplands are so depleted, supplementing is essential.

- Distilled water is best vs. hard waters are associated with low incidence of heart disease.

Confusing? Well, before you abandon your search, remember that there is one "expert" who does have answers for you—and that authority is you. Learning to "listen" to your own body will help you in piecing together the parts of your own nutritional puzzle.

"To listen" in this context means to be aware, and it requires honesty and thoroughness if it is to be effective. You may crave sweets because they have been your sustenance and reward throughout life. If you listen only to this craving and set about satisfying it in all circumstances, then you will end up in more trouble. A craving may be an indication of metabolic need, or it may be the result of an addiction. There are lots of other signs which must be attended to if you are to practice self-trust correctly. Let's consider some of these.

The condition of your teeth and gums will be strong indicators of just how well you are eating. Frequent cavities and bleeding gums are not normal, and changing your brand of toothpaste will do little to alleviate them.

Look at your tongue. Is it discolored and coated? Do you have a sour taste in your mouth, and consistently bad breath? Your mouth is trying to tell you something.

Despite what the TV advertisements may lead you to believe, a headache is not something to treat with aspirins and dismiss. Headaches are loud and clear messages that something about the organism is amiss. Commonly they are indicative of general stress, but they may also be the accompaniment to a host of dietary imbalances such as hypoglycemia (low blood sugar) and alcohol consumption. In any case, those long-lasting, fast-acting, extra-strength pain relievers can only muffle the warning sounds temporarily.

It doesn't take too much nutritional sophistication to appreciate the connection between overeating, indulging in spicy, rich food, drinking alcohol, and acid indigestion and upset stomach. To listen to your body on "the morning after" can provide you with lots of valuable information about what doesn't work for you. It can also be a great motivator for change.

Physical strength, endurance,

Stamp Out Food Faddism

"Food faddism is indeed a serious problem. But we have to recognize that the guru of food faddism is not Adelle Davis, but Betty Crocker. The true food faddists are not those who eat raw broccoli, wheat germ, and yogurt, but those who start the day on Breakfast Squares, gulp down bottle after bottle of soda pop, and snack on candy.

"Food faddism is promoted from birth. Sugar is a major ingredient in baby food desserts. Then comes the artificially flavored and colored breakfast cereals loaded with sugar, followed by soda pop and hot dogs. Meat marbled with fat and alcoholic beverages dominate the diets of many middle-aged people.

And, of course, white bread is standard fare throughout life.

"This diet—high in fat, sugar, cholesterol, and refined grains—is the prescription for illness; it can contribute to obesity, tooth decay, heart disease, intestinal cancer, and diabetes. And these diseases are, in fact, America's major health problems. So if any diet should be considered faddist, it is the standard one. Our far-out diet—almost 20% refined sugar and 45% fat—is new to human experience and foreign to all other animal life . . .

"It is incredible that people who eat a junk food diet constitute the norm, while individuals whose diets resemble those of our great-grandparents are labeled deviants . . ."

Editorial, *Nutrition Action*

and flexibility are other factors to be considered in developing awareness of the relationship between the food you eat and the foods you need. While it is difficult to quantify the changes that happen in strength level as a result of eating different foods, most people if asked will tell you that some foods make them feel heavy, bloated, bogged down, or sleepy while others induce a feeling of lightness. Eating for lightness is an excellent criterion to use in changing your dietary patterns for the promotion of high-level wellness. Christina sums up her approach to nutrition by saying, "I eat what makes me feel light and what makes me feel strong."

The list of signs and clues goes on and on. They include: condition of the skin, hair, and fingernails; frequency of colds; susceptibility to flu and other contagious diseases; and difficulty in sleeping. By now you are probably getting a clearer picture of what it means to be your own food expert. Sure, go on reading and learning what others have to share, but balance this with quiet reflection in which you courageously face the question: "How do I feel?" In addition you may wish to set up experiments with certain foods or ways of eating. Allow enough time in each experiment to really experience the effects. Add a food or abstain from a food for awhile and keep a nutritional journal, recording each day what you have done and how you feel. Above all, resist the temptation to criticize the diets of other people as your own food-awareness grows. Redirect this energy as loving acceptance of your fellow beings, and offer a hug instead of a lecture.

Slowing Down

If you are intent upon developing a more generalized sensitivity and awareness for a richer and more fulfilling life, there is no better place to start than at your table. The key to awareness about eating is to slow down. To eat fast is to offer a disservice to the cook who prepared the food, your companions at the table, and primarily to your own body. Ask any weight-control expert and you will learn that slowing down your eating speed will cause you to eat less. It makes sense. When you allow time for the food to reach your stomach, and for the digestive juices to begin the breakdown process, hunger sensations will begin to diminish. It will take a smaller amount of food to satisfy you, and that is not only a help in maintaining your ideal weight, but also in sustaining a longer life.

To appreciate food requires the varied use of many senses and organs besides the mouth, tongue, teeth, and taste buds. Many cooks will complain that they have little hunger left after looking at and smelling food for hours in the preparation. While this condition is far from desirable to most of us, it illustrates the important role that sight and smell play in the whole drama. And that is just what eating can become—a drama. Imagine

Challenging the Sacred Cow

Next to meat and refined sugar products, Americans probably eat more dairy products than any other food items. Millions of dollars are spent each year extolling the virtues of milk. It ranks right up there with Mom and apple pie. The fact is, though, that in some instances, milk itself can be harmful, and in others, problems arise from excessive intake or from the way in which it is processed.

For infants, cow's milk is a poor substitute for mother's milk. Many adults, especially those of Asian or African origin, lack the enzyme used to split the lactose present in milk. The result is that milk ferments in the gut rather than being absorbed as a nutrient. The amount of phosphates present in milk is so great that it may prevent the absorption of other minerals, such as magnesium, zinc, and copper. The milk protein, casein, binds up much of the iron in other foods which may be in the digestive tract (milk itself has little iron), causing iron deficiencies to occur.

With these problems inherent in the use of cow's milk, we then can look at what happens when we alter the milk. First, we pasteurize it, destroying vitamins and helpful bacteria in order to enable it to sit longer on the shelf without spoiling, and to ensure no harmful bacteria have infected it. Then, it is usually homogenized, a process whereby the large fat molecules of the cream are smashed up into a smaller size so they will stay in the solution rather than rising to the

your disappointment, even anger, if you had spent ten or fifteen dollars for front and center theatre seats to witness a famous production, only to have the actors and actresses race through their lines, as if they were reciting grocery lists or multiplication tables, on a stage devoid of sets with no complementary lighting. To eat purely out of habit or in a race against the clock, is to participate in a similar travesty.

Food has aroma, and texture, and color, and form, and temperature, and weight both on the plate and in your mouth. How often have you allowed these characteristics to enter your awareness? To do this you simply have to slow down.

In many cultures and religious traditions it is common to offer a prayer before a meal. Whatever your particular spiritual orientation may be, you can undoubtedly appreciate the wisdom of this practice. The body is given a few moments to rest, to orient itself in preparation for the task of eating. The eyes are temporarily closed, shutting out distractions and allowing one to focus awareness on breathing. A few deep breaths will facilitate general relaxation of the entire organism. Reflection may be made about the love and caring which went into the preparation of the meal, the richness of life in general as symbolized in the richness top. This causes biochemical changes in milk which are poorly understood. Also, the fluid is bombarded with ultra-violet radiation, which converts some of the naturally-occurring ergosterol into vitamin D to make up for the vitamin D we don't get from the sun. This source of vitamin D has been a very useful crutch to our indoor society in recent years.

We process much of our milk into cheese, butter, ice cream, or yogurt. In their natural form, yogurts are one of the best dairy products we can eat because the lactose is pre-digested in the yogurt culture. However, what is actually chemically added as it is processed, we can only begin to tell from reading the labels, because the dairy industry has special exemptions from many of the labeling disclosure laws. The yogurt you eat may have so much gelatin, sugar, corn starch, and preservatives in it that they cancel out any of the beneficial effects of the acidophilus culture. Do you know what's in the ice cream besides petrochemicals and air? Certainly little ice and no cream! (I welcome the notable exceptions now available.) Can you imagine what the dairy industry would say if I were to suggest the sacred institution of milk-drinking were a bit over-played? How dare I contradict those wholesome lads and lassies who extol the virtues of this wonder food. Why, that would be downright unAmerican.

—J.W.T.

Fasting

Throughout history people have fasted, either through lean times when food wasn't available, or in connection with religious beliefs. When the constant steady flow of food into the body is interrupted for brief periods (several days to weeks), major shifts in biochemical processes occur. The major benefit of these changes seems to be the release of toxins (preservatives, sprays, etc.) which are stored in the fatty tissues of the body and can be eliminated when these stores are liquidated. An analogy can be made to backwashing a water filter, cleansing it of the impurities it has collected.

With the proper education even thin people can fast for many days without danger to their health. There are two major approaches to fasting—water fasting and juice fasting—and, naturally, the expected controversy over which is better. Before embarking on a fast, be sure to become knowledgeable on how to start and break it. Consult Airola, P. *Are You Confused?* for one approach.

and abundance of the food, and the resolution made to eat with reverence and awareness. Not a bad habit to start, if this is not already a part of your mealtime practice.

The healthiest way to slow down speed-eating is to start chewing—a long forgotten activity in the repertoire of most moderns, adults as well as children. If for no other reason, the prevention of death by choking should serve to motivate us to start masticating. Walt Whitman is quoted as saying, "Drink your solids and chew your liquids." To "drink" your solids is to chew them so well that they pass like liquids down your throat. To "chew" your liquids is to enjoy the sensation of them throughout your mouth. Good advice for the gulpers among us.

Besides the physical effect (the aid to digestion through the breakdown of complex carbohydrates by the saliva in the mouth), the advantages of chewing include a ready outlet for stress, a strengthening of the will, and patience and peace enhanced by conscious eating.

Finally, while there is little evidence to prove claims for foods as aphrodisiacs (substances which increase the sexual urge), it is general knowledge that seduction is more readily accomplished in a quiet candle-lit atmosphere than at the corner taco stand. Few would argue that the sensual pleasures of food can be heightened by the proper setting, the mode of preparation and presentation, and the service. There is more to eating than satisfying hunger pains. Why not slow down and allow yourself a greater share of life's pleasures by appreciating food for its sacramental and multi-sensual qualities.

. . . . *Exercise* . . . .

A Nutrition Journal

A nutrition journal can be used as:

1. your personal record of the ways your body responds to the foods you eat

2. a balance sheet to observe the kinds of raw materials/fuels with which you supply your body

3. a place to keep special recipes

4. a diet notebook for weight gain/loss

5. a record of emotions felt, resolutions, etc.

For example:

SUBJECT UNDER CONSIDERATION: *Breakfast*

Day/Time	Breakfast Foods	Immediate Effects/Later Effects
Monday 3/22 9:00 A.M.	2 eggs, bacon—2 strips, toast—2 pieces, butter and jam coffee—2 cups	Left the table feeling stuffed. Too much food. Generally good day. Not hungry until 3 P.M.

Record here your observations for a one- to two-day period.

DAY/TIME   *FOODS*   *EFFECTS*

REFLECTIONS/RESOLUTIONS

Taking Nutritional Action

Rarely do you encounter a person who is completely happy with the weight and shape of his/her body or general state of health. Even more rarely—the person who is satisfied with the parameters of his or her life! It is interesting to speculate about how these two may be linked.

Working off excess weight and dealing with the symptoms of disease carries a much deeper meaning—a preoccupation with getting rid of what we don't like about ourselves. It is much easier to wage war on fat or germs than it is to confront the unmet needs and issues of our emotional/spiritual lives; to accept that we are not perfect. It is only too common for an individual involved in rigorous dieting, a stop-smoking campaign, or an exercise crusade to approach the ideal weight or health, only to realize that the color of life hasn't changed a great deal; the feelings of inadequacy are still there despite the alteration of the appearance or the alleviation of a physical pain. Regaining the lost weight or falling back into old habits, will once again offer "something to do," a place to lay the blame, something to hold on to.

Maxwell Maltz, a cosmetic surgeon, is the author of the classic book on positive self-programming, *Psychocybernetics*. In it he recounts numerous stories of his patients who underwent dramatic physical alterations only to experience the same "ugly self" looking out from behind a beautiful face.[29]

While it is true that the body image has a powerful effect upon the self-concept, it is insufficient to

Myths About Hunger

The Hunger Project is, to me, one of the most exciting ideas on the planet today (see page 145). I was most influenced when I heard one of its proponents shatter two of the myths about hunger that I had always believed.

Myth 1: There isn't enough food to go around.

Fact: Enough food is grown each year for every person on earth to eat the equivalent of an average American's diet.

Myth 2: If you feed "them," they'll just multiply faster.

Fact: Every country that has solved its hunger problem in the past few decades has simultaneously experienced a major drop in its birth rate.

For more specific information on this subject, see *10 Myths About Hunger* and *Food First*[30] and the Hunger Project's newsletter *A Shift in the Wind*.[31]

—JWT

work on the body alone. The ways in which you *think* about yourself—as a good person deserving love, or a weak person deserving blame—are of primary importance. This subject will be developed more fully in later chapters, but for now, you may want to consider this connection between self-love and effective change in view of the critical awareness that many forms of dieting and "crash" programs in general are ineffective in dealing with whole-person health.

The first prerequisite in the establishment of a balanced plan of nutrition, pleasure, and weight control, is to create a loving support system for yourself. Solicit the aid of your mate, a close friend, or a counselor—someone who will encourage you in your quest, listen to you, and hug you. You want this person for courage and for positive strokes, not necessarily for advice. Secondly, start tuning in to your

own body. Face yourself squarely and honestly; admit what you have always known about your particular needs. What foods make you feel good—both physically and psychologically? What foods or

If decisions and actions well within the capability of nations and people working together were implemented, it would be possible to eliminate the worst aspects of hunger and malnutrition by the year 2000. Such an undertaking would contribute immensely to global peace and security, to the welfare of the human family, and to the national interests of all countries.

—THE PRELIMINARY REPORT OF THE PRESIDENTIAL COMMISSION ON WORLD HUNGER[32]

patterns of eating make you discouraged, unhappy, heavy? Get in touch with the compassionate source of wisdom which lives in your own heartspace; listen to its voice frequently. Ask it for guidance and rely upon it for help.

Finally, take action. Read some of the books referred to here, and consult with trusted others for help in designing your personal approach to eating for wellness. Beware of extremes, be careful of absolutes, and be patient with yourself.

Love and Compassion

The saying goes "There is nothing more obnoxious than a reformed ——." Substitute any appropriate word. While this may be a cruel and unjust generalization, you have probably experienced a case in which it has been true. Take the food faddist for instance: three weeks of eating nothing but nuts and figs, a condescending smile, and an unasked for lecture directed at a companion across the table who has made the sorry mistake of ordering a cup of coffee. (Or even a bowl of yogurt— "mucus-producing, you know.") What good will it do you to put perfect food in your body if you use your knowledge to alienate yourself from the love of others?

While this may be an extreme example, it helps to make some important points on the subject of moderation and balance in the area of foods, diets, and nutrition in general. Here, as in many other areas, the key words are patience and compassion. Making radical changes in a very short period of time will more often set you up for failure and disappointment, and

can also upset your system enough that you temporarily feel worse instead of better. So take slow steps, reward yourself for your satisfying changes, and love yourself for being noncompulsive when you choose to break your regimen.

Realize that because something works for you now, it may not always. Neither is it the remedy for someone else.

Remember that your body has an amazing resiliency, and can tolerate just about any foods or beverages for a limited time, or in small amounts. So try to restrain your tendency to set unrealistic demands on yourself, like "I'll never eat candy again."

Whatever you do, attempt to do it with awareness. As long as you've chosen to eat that apple, or that piece of cake, please enjoy it in the process. The reward for a well-balanced and more conscious lifestyle is the realization of high-level wellness.

Growing Your Own

Growing your own food can be a very pleasurable and satisfying experience. Not only will you have tastier fruits and vegetables, you'll save money and get a little exercise and sunshine at the same time. An

added benefit is that you can eliminate or control the chemicals used —the fertilizers, pesticides, and herbicides.

Even the smallest plot of land can yield a fair crop. You might consider tearing out your lawn and replacing it with a vegetable garden. There is probably enough space devoted to lawns in the U.S. to feed its entire population!

Feeding Our Planet

This year about 10 million of our brothers and sisters throughout the world will die of starvation while we pursue the luxury of deciding between steak or pork chops, health food or junk food, a high-protein or a high-carbohydrate diet.

The reasons given for mass malnutrition range from the simplistic and crass to the frightening and complex:

- it's nature's way of population control

- people are lazy and ignorant

- the rich will demand what they have come to enjoy

- we have upset the ecological balance

- food costs have risen with the

. . . .

The woman in the library,
    drinking pop and smoking a cigarette,
        refuses my offer of a vending-machine
            peanut butter cracker
                because it contains beef-fat
                and she is a vegetarian.

—R.S.R.

. . . .

rising costs of oil

- food corporations control the world.

And the situation continues to worsen.

Any decision for high-level wellness as a way of life must take this reality into account. The choices and demands we make will impact all the people who share our small planet. They affect the conditions of our soil, the prices we will have to pay for food, and its availability to others.

Our responsibility is a heavy one. It means that we:

- become informed

- resist waste and greed

- possibly change our diets and eating habits

- work for equitable distribution of food and rightful control of the land, and

- do everything within our power to end starvation.

Nature's way is the way of balance. High-level wellness for any must mean a balanced diet for all.

Suggested Reading*

Airola, P. *Are You Confused?* Phoenix, AZ: Health Plus Publishers, 1971.

Ballantine, R. *Diet and Nutrition.* Honesdale, PA: Himalayan International Institute, 1978.

Bryan, N. *Thin Is a State of Mind.* Minneapolis, MN: CompCare Publishers, 1980.

*This is only a representative sampling. Many excellent books have been omitted. At the bookstore or library, look over the whole selection and choose according to your judgment.

Burns, M. *Good for Me.* Boston, MA: Little, Brown and Co., 1978.

Consumers Guide, eds. *The Vitamin Book.* New York, NY: Simon and Schuster, Fireside Books, 1979.

Duffy, W. *Sugar Blues.* New York, NY: Warner Books, 1976.

Ewald, E. *Recipes for a Small Planet.* New York, NY: Ballantine Books, 1973.

Jeavons, J. *How to Grow More Vegetables.* Berkeley, CA: Ten Speed Press, 1979.

Katzen, M. *The Moosewood Cookbook.* Berkeley, CA: Ten Speed Press, 1977.

———. *The Enchanted Broccoli Forest.* Berkeley, CA: Ten Speed Press, 1982.

Kloss, J. *Back to Eden.* Santa Barbara, CA: Woodbridge Press Publishing Co., 1975.

Lappe, F. M. *Diet for a Small Planet.* New York, NY: Ballantine Books, 1971.

Natow, A., and Hesling, J. *Nutrition for the Prime of Your Life.* New York, NY: McGraw-Hill Paperbacks, 1983.

Orbach, S. *Fat Is a Feminist Issue.* New York, NY: Berkeley Publishing Co., 1978.

Palivy, J., and Herman, C.P. *Breaking the Diet Habit: The Natural Weight Alternative.* New York, NY: Basic Books, 1983.

Robertson, L.; Flinders, C.; and Godfrey, B. *Laurel's Kitchen:. A Handbook for Vegetarian Cookery and Nutrition.* Berkeley, CA: Ten Speed Press, 1987.

Roth, G. *Feeding the Hungry Heart.* New York, NY: New American Library/Signet Books, 1982.

Saltoon, D. *The Common Book of Consciousness: How to Take Charge of Your Lifestyle through Diet, Exercise and Meditation.* Mill Valley, CA: Robert Briggs Associates, 1979.

Schwartz, B. *Diets Don't Work!* Houston, TX: Breakthru Publishing, 1982.

Urs Koch, M. *Laugh with Health.* New York, NY: Holt, Rinehart and Winston, 1981.

Williams, R. *Biochemical Individuality.* Austin, TX: University of Texas Press, 1969.

———. *Nutrition Against Disease.* New York, NY: Bantam Books, Inc., 1978.

———. *You Are Extraordinary.* New York, NY: Random House, 1967.

Notes

1. *Dietary Goals for the United States.* Select Committee on Nutrition and Human Needs, U.S. Government Printing Office, Washington, DC (February 1977), p. V.

2. Lappé, F. M. *Diet for a Small Planet.* New York, NY: Ballantine Books, 1971, p. 5.

3. Duffy, W. *Sugar Blues.* New York, NY: Warner Books, 1976, pp. 1416, 5–46.

4. *Dietary Goals*, p. 49.

5. Szekely, E. *The Book of Vitamins.* International Biogenic Society, 1978.

6. ———. *The Book of Minerals.* International Biogenic Society, 1978.

7. Urs Koch, M. *Laugh with Health.* New York, NY: Holt, Rinehart and Winston, 1981. This is the best treatment of diet, nutrition, and natural foods, and their relationship to life energy that we have found.

8 Airola, P. *How to Get Well.* Phoenix AZ: Health Plus Publishers, 1976.

9. See:

Fein, G. *Child Development.* Englewood Cliffs, NJ: Prentice-Hall, 1978, pp. 64–97.

Looft, W. *Developmental Psychology: A Book of Readings.* Hinsdale, IL: The Dryden Press, 1972, pp. 148–59.

Lugo and Hershey. *Human Development.* New York, NY: Macmillan Publishing Co., 1974, pp. 215–69.

Stone, L. and Church. *Childhood and Adolescence.* (4th ed.) New York, NY: Random House, 1979, pp. 118–31.

10. Haefer, C., and Hardy, M.C. "Later Development of Breast-Fed and Artificially Fed Infants." *Journal of the A.M.A.*, Vol. 96 (1929), pp. 615–19.

11. Kimball, E.R. "How I Get Mothers to Breastfeed." *Physicians Management*, June 1968.

12. Margules, D. "Beta-Endorphin Is Associated with Overeating in Genetically Obese Mice and Rats." *Science*, Vol. 202 (Dec. 1978), pp. 988–91.

13. *The World Almanac and Book of Facts.* New York, NY: Newspaper Enterprise Association, 1979, pp. 953–55.

14. Williams, R. J. *You Are Extraordinary.* New York, NY: Pyramid Books, 1971, p. 25.

15. *Dietary Goals*, p. 1.

16. *Dietary Goals*, p. 1.

17. Feingold, B. *Why Your Child Is Hyperactive.* New York, NY: Random House, 1974.

18. Stevens, L.J., and Stoner, E. *How to Feed Your Hyperactive Child*, New York, NY: Doubleday, 1977.

19. *Dietary Goals*, p. 55.

20. Rueben, D. *Save Your Life Diet.* New York, NY: Ballantine Books, 1976.

21. *Dietary Goals*, p. 33. Testimony from Dr. Gio Gori, Deputy Director of the National Cancer Institute.

22. *Dietary Goals*, p. 55.

23. Airola, P. *Are You Confused?* Phoenix, AZ: Health Plus Publishers, 1971, p. 31.

24. Lappe, F.M., pp. 19–27.

25. *Dietary Goals*, p. 33.

26. *Journal of he Nutritional Academy*, Vol. II, No. II, (August 1979).

27. Williams, R. J. *Biochemical Individuality.* Austin, TX: University of Texas Press, 1969.

28. *Nutrition Action* (March–April 1975), a monthly publication of the Center for Science in the Public Interest, 1755 S Street, NW, Washington, DC 20009.

29. Maltz, M. *Psychocybernetics.* New York, NY: Simon and Schuster, 1960.

30. See: Lappe, F., and Collins, J. *Food First: Beyond the Myth of Scarcity.* New York, NY: Ballantine Books, 1979.

For more information about work and publications write: The Institute for Food and Development Policy, 2588 Mission St., San Francisco, CA 94110.

31. For more information about the myths of hunger write: The Hunger Project, Box 789, San Francisco, CA 94101. And see Chapter 7, Wellness and Thinking, for more about the Hunger Project.

32. The complete report of the Presidential Commission on World Hunger, *Overcoming World Hunger: The Challenge Ahead*, can be obtained for $6 from: Superintendent of Documents, U.S. Government Printing Office, Washington, DC 20402.

Five

Wellness and Moving

EVERYTHING IN US is moving. Heart pumps, blood flows, lungs expand and contract, eyes roll, eardrums vibrate. To be alive is to be moving. Inhibit the movement and you create illness. Stop it and you are dead. Allow it fully and you realize wellness.

In his wonderful book, *Stalking the Wild Pendulum*, Itzhak Bentov takes us on a journey inside the human body. We find ourselves in a sea of atoms ". . . weaving back and forth like a field of ripe wheat blown by the wind. They move in unison and in beautiful rhythm."[1] Moving inside an atom we discover there also that ". . . everything is in a constant, very rapid, but very orderly motion."[2]

Because of this movement, everything is changing from moment to moment. To block movement therefore is to block change. The unmoving water becomes the stagnant pool. The moving river cleanses itself. The unmoving body becomes a home for infection and

> Movement is a most basic expression of energy output in the Wellness Energy System. Nourished and stimulated with oxygen, sensory data, and food-fuels, the body responds with internal movement; lungs expanding and contracting, heart pumping, etc., and external movement; smiling, walking, etc. The ability to move is the basis for more complex bodily activities such as working and playing, creative expression, communication, and sexual activity.

depression. The moving body freely channels the energy of life.

Think about it. Close your eyes for a moment and create a mental picture of an unhealthy person. Your image may include a colorless and drooping face, an overweight body—possibly seated in a chair, or a tired form sluggishly climbing a flight of stairs, puffing at every step.

Now, imagine the opposite. See a person in the peak of health. Chances are you have pictured a pink-cheeked complexion, and a

trim beautiful body in motion—running, or jumping with arms reaching out, or making love, or dancing. Dancing is a great metaphor for living—for being—in harmony, since the whole universe, the sum total of energy, moves as in a dance. The person dancing is the person at one with the universe. The person dancing is fully alive.

. . . .
. . . the waves are really dancing the measure of a tune.
—HAVELOCK ELLIS
. . . .

Without movement you have no dance, no work, and no play either. It's that elementary. Movement changes both the inner world and the outer world. Moving encourages movement. The more you move, the better you move. Energy creates energy—in a continuous, circling process—in a constant dance.

The need for human activity, since the Industrial Revolution, has changed dramatically. Most of us no longer chop wood and carry water. Our work more likely involves sitting for long hours at a desk, or in an automobile; or standing behind a counter, or at an assembly line. Much of our business, moreover, is tedious and stressful. Even if we enjoy the opportunity of working in the out-of-doors, our range of movement is probably limited. Joyce, for instance, stands on the highway all day changing a sign from "Slow" to "Stop."

With few exceptions (such as farm work, or running from our neighbor's dog), our needs to move with vigor are usually few. Otherwise, our cars, and buses, and trains and planes will do the work for us.

While these conveniences lighten the load, they also discourage us from moving. The words of John F. Kennedy, spoken in the early 1960s, still apply today: ". . . the labor of the human body is rapidly being engineered out of working life."

Up to this point this workbook has been pointing out that simply allowing the body's natural processes will tend to keep it in balance. With respect to moving however, survival maintenance will not be enough. If you want to be well you are going to have to do something more. And that something is exercise!

All excuses for neglecting it, like:

It's no fun.

It's for kids.

I'm too busy.

I'm too tired.

I'm too fat.

I look awful in tennis togs.

I can't afford the equipment.

I don't have anyone to play with.

or

I tried it once and it didn't work. I can't keep up the pace.

I don't know how.

and

I'm afraid!

Who knows what might happen if I did!

and

I'm still afraid . . .

can be looked at with compassion, and can be dealt with. When we realize that these excuses have combined with our poor diet habits and stressful lifestyles, and have resulted in overweight, heart conditions, high blood pressure, and energy-robbed lives, we can decide to join the millions of Americans who have recently chosen to get moving!

Exercise—The New National Craze

In 1970 no one would have believed that by 1980 there would be thriving stores which sold nothing but running shoes and accessories.

According to George Gallup, we are witnessing one of the most dramatic lifestyle changes ever measured in the American public. A 1979 survey found that 59% of the adult U.S. population regularly engages in some form of physical exercise. This more than doubles the figures of 24% reported by Gallup in 1961.[3] A 1984 Gallup poll reports that 30 million Americans are jogging. Physical fitness has reached craze proportions, certainly one of the most encouraging fads which has ever swept the population.

The why behind this dramatic increase can only be guessed at. Fitness expert Jim Hickman suggests that rising health costs and growing disillusionment with medical practice have led Americans to use exercise for health maintenance and disease prevention.[4]

Another reason is that as a nation we are growing in our concern for the appearance of the physical body. Fat is an enemy! The models of success and happiness which the TV presents to us are generally young, energetic, slim, and good-looking. Since we average five hours of TV per day per person in the U.S., these images must have an impact on us. Also, the fact that so many of us are constantly dieting supports this guess. The connection between self-image and physical appearance is very strong.

Whatever the reason, exercise is becoming more and more popular. Exercise salons and spas, running clubs and dance classes are places to meet people, to gain a sense of community, to receive the encouragement and support—the strokes—we all need. Besides, exercise makes us feel good—not just physically, but emotionally and spiritually. But—more about this later. For now, consider that the run on exercise and public recognition that coronary heart disease is the number one cause of death in the U.S. are probably related. When a friend suffers a heart

Exercise

Joining The Dance—An Experience

Introduction: This exercise may surprise you with how easy and joyful movement can be.

Directions: Play a record or tape of a slow, gentle piece of music. Close your eyes and simply listen for a few minutes. Now direct your attention to your right hand. Begin to tap or stretch your fingers in any way that the music suggests. Allow the movement to extend itself, to encompass your wrist as well. Stay with this simple experience for a while.

Now direct attention to the left hand and do the same. Imagine that you are directing an orchestra, or splashing in water, or molding a piece of clay to represent what you are hearing. Play with it. Next engage your right arm, and then your left, allowing yourself to move from shoulders to tips of fingers. How many different ways can you find to bend them, to position them, to move them in unison or in opposition?

Keep your arms and hands going, doing whatever they want to, as you give attention to your head. Let the music direct it. Conduct the symphony with a baton that extends from the center of your forehead, from the crown, from your chin.

Your upper body now wants to get into the act. Concentrate on your middle section. Allow yourself to bend and sway from the waist in any ways that feel good. Pretend that your whole body exists from waist to head—forget the rest. Let the hips and pelvis come along whenever you are ready for them. Careful here—they will want to take over.

Imagine yourself as a tree in the wind. Roots are firm. Only the branches and upper trunk sway. Be a fettered bird, wanting to escape, but restrained by a silver thread. Fantasize that you are a belly dancer, write your name with an imaginary pencil that extends from your left hip. Write "I love myself" with the imaginary pencil on your right hip.

Unlock your knees and allow your legs to move without lifting your feet. Challenge yourself with how many ways you can direct them. Ways that you have never tried before. Pretend that you are scientifically cataloguing all the possible combinations of movement which legs can make. Keep your feet still until you can't stand it a minute longer. Go inside yourself and take note of what your body feels like all over. Imagine your blood cells dancing, oxygen dancing, energy dancing.

Now "let go" completely and allow yourself to move totally—head, arms, belly, pelvis, legs, feet. Surprise!

Want another one? This time simply try a different, perhaps more active, piece of music. Or another? Read this exercise to a friend and surprise them.

attack—it makes you take notice. It's likely that many people have been shocked into jogging or swimming or some other activity as a result.

Heart disease is the subject of much research, and there is no one explanation why some people get it and others don't. (Unless you support the notion that we choose our illnesses!) What is known is that the leading risk factors in heart disease are:

1. high blood fats
2. high blood pressure
3. obesity
4. smoking
5. high blood sugar
6. being male
7. family history
8. diabetes
9. lack of exercise[5]

Kenneth Cooper, M.D., reported in the *Journal of the American Medical Association*[6] his findings that those who practiced endurance fitness (cardiovascular exercise) had a lower risk of heart disease. Other studies, comparing populations engaged in active jobs (mail carriers, longshoremen) with those holding inactive jobs (clerks, bus drivers) found a higher incidence of heart disease among the inactives.[7]

Exercise provides a safety valve for stress, helps in shedding unwanted pounds, and lowers blood sugar. Many smokers also cut down significantly or stop smoking altogether when they start a regular program of exercise.[8]

Add to all this the findings that exercise is beneficial in treating some backache, ulcers, arthritis, insomnia, nervous tension, indigestion, and even asthma and diabetes—and you have a strong case in support of exercise.

It is important to understand that the exercise referred to in relation to heart disease is cardiovascular or "aerobic" exercise. There are also other types.

Types of Exercise

Exercise can be grouped into three major divisions, depending upon the body systems it most influences. The first, as mentioned above, is *cardiovascular exercise* (aerobics), which stimulates heart and lungs and builds endurance. The second is *flexibility exercise*, which lengthens, stretches, and flexes muscles and enhances balance and overall grace. Yoga is a good example of this type. The third is *strength-developing exercise*—such as weight-training. While the three do overlap somewhat it is generally agreed that for basic fitness, the first two (endurance and flexibility exercise) are essential. We will deal with these two now.

What are aerobics?

Aerobics are a group of exercises that increase the heart and breathing rates for a sustained period of time, greatly increasing the flow of oxygen and blood to all parts of the body. To be effective, the exercise must raise the pulse rate to a certain level (see chart, p. 100) and keep it at that level for not less than 10 to 15 minutes. (NOTE: Many people who are not in condition will have to build up slowly to a 10 to 15 minute exercise period.)

Examples of aerobic exercises are bicycling, running/jogging, swimming, jumping rope, vigorous walking, etc. Stop-and-go exercises (like golf, downhill skiing, housework, gardening, etc.) and those of short duration (like sprinting, square dancing, calisthenics, etc.) are not effective in producing the desired level of fitness.[9]

It works like this: just as soon as you start moving, your heart starts working harder, pumping more blood with each beat. The blood then rushes with greater speed and force through the vessels, which stretch in order to allow for this increased volume. The working muscles call out for more oxygen. Deeper breathing is the response. In moving to arms and legs, the blood is diverted from the digestive organs. Blood vessels in the exercising muscles expand tremendously, allowing a greater influx of oxygen. The process returns to its starting point as the blood goes back to the heart, faster, and in greater volume, filling it to capacity and keeping the whole operation working smoothly. Stressing the whole system in this way is necessary to keep it strong and efficient.

Circulation is not the only process affected, either. Aerobic exercising will shift the body's energy source from glucose dependence to one of fat usage. Fat stored in body tissues will be released at the command of the central nervous system. It moves to the liver for breakdown and then out to the needy muscles to fuel them. Hormones and enzymes jump in to keep the system in balance, and the chemistry of the brain itself is altered. Incredible!

What are some of the benefits of aerobic exercise?

- Decrease in intramuscular fat and increase in lean muscle, leading to a firmer, stronger body.

- Improved circulation. A trained heart is a more efficient pump. It doesn't have to work as hard. This lowered heart-beat rate preserves the heart and lessens its chance of fatiguing prematurely.

- Improved absorption/ utilization of food.

- Increased energy and stamina.

- More restful sleep.

- Lessening (if not elimination) of depression, nervous tension.

- Improved appearance; more positive self-image and out-look on life.

- People who exercise regularly consume far fewer drugs, coffee, tea, alcohol, tobacco, sugar and refined carbohydrates than non-exercisers. They find these things to be antagonistic to a healthy life style.

Recommendations and Cautions

Don't be in a hurry! You need time to condition your heart and muscles to the new demands. Ignoring this maxim invites trouble—increase your exercise gradually.

Before starting your program. Get a physical and EKG first—especially if you are over age 40.

How often? Regular exercise is imperative. Three times per week is good for a maintenance program. Four or five times a week is ideal for increasing one's fitness or aerobic capacity. The weekend or only now-and-then exerciser places herself/himself in potential danger because the heart and body are not strengthened sufficiently to withstand a really vigorous workout.

NOTE: While regular exercise is important, you should temporarily suspend it whenever you are ill or excessively fatigued.

Warm-up. Just like a car requires a few minutes to warm up before running efficiently, your body also needs a gradual warm-up before strenuous exercise. About 5 minutes is all that is necessary. Calisthenics (such as sit-ups and push-ups) and stretching exercises are particularly good for warming up. These exercises serve to get blood into muscles so they're not operating cold. They also get the heart going gradually, rather than in one quick burst, which can be potentially dangerous. Warm-ups increase flexibility and aerobic workout. (See the book *Stretching* by B. Anderson listed in the bibliography at the end of this chapter.)

Cooling down. After a period of vigorous exercise cooling down is just as important as warming up. A gradual transition is good for the heart. During exercise such as running or cycling, the blood pools in the large leg muscles. While the activity continues, the muscles are squeezing the blood back to the heart and the rest of the body. When the exercise is stopped suddenly and completely, the blood is still pooled in the legs, but now there is no contraction of the leg muscles to return the blood to the heart and brain. Dizziness, fainting, or even more serious consequences can occur. A gradual (3 to 5 minutes) cool-down eases the transition between vigorous exercise and rest. Walking after running is a good example.

How much is too much?

There are several good ways to determine if you are exercising too hard:

Breath Test. If you can still talk comfortably as you are exercising, you are probably not overexerting yourself. If not, you are training too hard and need to slow down.

If you experience faintness, dizziness, nausea, tightness or pain in the chest, severe shortness of breath, or loss of muscle control—stop exercising immediately.

Heart rate recovery. Count your pulse 5 minutes after exercise. It should have returned to 120 beats per minute or below. If it hasn't, you're pushing yourself too hard. Count your pulse again after 10 minutes—if it isn't back below 100, ease up a little on your exercise program.

Breathing recovery rate. If you still find yourself short of breath 10 minutes after exercising, your exercise is too strenuous.

Fatigue. Ordinarily, exercise should be stimulating and invigorating. If you find yourself worn out and tired all the time, it may be a sign that you are over-doing and should slow down on your exercise program.

How much is enough?

To gain the desired effect, you

. . . . *Exercise*. . . . .

YOGA—The Gentle Way to Exercise

Many of us are reluctant to maintain regular exercise because it requires pain, or strain, or special equipment, or others to work out with, or traveling to get to the field. If this has been the case for you then yoga may be just the practice you have been waiting for. The word "yoga" means union. It is a discipline that seeks to unite the body, mind, and spirit. It is therefore an ideal practice for those in search of high-level wellness.

Hatha yoga consists of a series of physical postures (asanas) and breathing exercises (pranayama) which are easily learned and have dramatic effects. Regular practice increases flexibility, balance, grace, breath control and overall health and integration. The exercises provide special stimulation of the endocrine glands and thus promote a rebalancing of vital energy throughout the body. Many people experience a greater serenity about life in general, improved circulation, a firmer, trimmer figure, and less illness, as a result.

In doing yoga you are advised to move slowly and with concentrated awareness, to avoid strain or pain, and to coordinate your breath with your movements. Yoga requires no special equipment. It can be done almost anywhere. And you can teach it to yourself simply by following a book or set of instructions, although a teacher is quite helpful. You can begin this very minute without leaving your chair. Interested? Try this Lion Pose.

"Inhale deeply; then forcefully exhale through your mouth. While exhaling with mouth wide open and eyes wide and staring, thrust out your tongue and stretch arms down with fingers stiff and spread tautly apart. Hold the breath for a few seconds. Then close your mouth and inhale deeply through the nostrils (expanding the abdomen). Exhale again slowly through your nostrils and relax. Repeat three times."

Congratulations—you have done a yoga posture! How do you feel? Here are a few more you may want to try. Remember—do not strain, move slowly, and follow instructions for breathing.

Abdominal Breathing

The key to diaphragmatic breathing is simple: as you inhale, expand the abdomen as you exhale, contract the abdomen.

A. Lie on your back with legs bent, feet close to buttocks, eyes closed. Inhale, expanding the abdomen while keeping the chest still.

B. Exhale, pulling in the abdomen and drawing it back to the spine.

Repeat five times, following this ratio:
Inhale: 5 seconds (expand abdomen)
Exhale: 10 seconds (contract abdomen)

All yoga instructions from Rachel Carr, *Yoga for All Ages.*

. . . . *Exercise* . . . .

Body Roll

Rolling from side to side is a good way to firm thighs and hips, and to release tension knots in the back and shoulders.

A. Lie on your back; clasp hands around bent knees and press them firmly toward chest. Close your eyes. Inhale deeply, at the same time rolling over to your right.

B. As you drop limply to the floor, exhale completely; release arms and legs. Relax for 5 seconds to feel tension knots dissolving.

C. While on your right side, clasp hands around bent knees. Inhale deeply. With your right elbow push yourself up and over to your left side, exhaling as you drop limply to the floor. Let go again and relax for 5 seconds. Repeat cycle three times, rolling from left to right, then right to left.

Four-way Stretch

To gain maximum benefit from the Four-way stretch, hold each movement for 2 seconds.

First, stand with feet together, hands to the sides. Inhale deeply and raise arms overhead. Interlock fingers, palms up. Hold breath and stretch upward on tiptoe, feeling pull in the spine and undersides of arms. Second, exhale and bend forward, touching the floor if possible, with clasped hands. Bring them close to feet, or as far down as you can. Third, inhale and come up to standing position with arms raised. Hold breath. Bend to the left and to the right without bending elbows. Hold each time to feel pull along the sides, then stretch upward on tiptoe. Lower arms. Exhale and relax. Repeat twice.

······Exercise······

A

The Hare

Simple as this posture may appear, its benefits are many. When the head is lowered to the floor (with chin touching the jugular notch), and the pose held for a few seconds, a fresh supply of blood is sent to the brain. Also, when the body is in this pose, the spine is stretched and limbered. Hands remain grasping the feet throughout the exercise. This is a good exercise for both children and adults.

A. Sit on heels with legs together, spine straight. Hold feet with hands.

B. Inhale and slowly bend forward until head is lowered to the floor near knees. Chin should touch jugular notch, or close to it. Arms are still stretched to grasp the feet. Exhale, breathe freely, and hold the pose a few seconds, then return to the Kneeling Hare position. Repeat three times.

The Stork

This is a simple lesson in balance and concentration.

Stand on right foot with left knee bent so that foot is at knee level from the floor. Bend elbows, with palms touching close to chest (left). Then bring head down to meet palms, symbolizing a sleeping stork (right). Balance for a few seconds, keeping perfectly still. Repeat standing on left foot with right knee bent back. When balance is secure, this posture should be done with eyes closed and balance held for a few seconds.

Exercise

The Cobra

The slow uncoiling movements of the Cobra will develop strong back muscles as spine rolls back, vertebra by vertebra. Adults should do this exercise with elbows bent for additional toning of the spine. Hips rest on the floor.

A. The Sleeping Cobra. Lie face down with forehead touching the floor, arms bent with palms close to chest, legs together.

B. The Striking Cobra. Inhale and slowly raise torso, keeping hips on floor. When arms are almost stretched, arch neck back. Exhale. While breathing freely, hold the pose a few seconds to feel the stretch in the spine. Then slowly lower chest and arms until head touches the floor. Repeat twice.

The Fishhook

Also known as the Triangle Pose, these side stretches will limber the spine and tone arms, legs and waistline.

A. Stand with feet apart and arms outstretched at sides.

B. Inhale; bend body to the left side with left arm holding on to the ankle. Right arm is stretched up in line with the left arm.

C. Exhale; extend right arm straight over head to the left. Breathe freely and hold the pose a few seconds to feel stretch along the underside of arm and waist. Relax, then repeat same movements bending to the right side.

. . . . *Exercise* . . . .

Conclude your yoga exercise, or any exercise for that matter, by doing a total-body-relaxation. Lie flat on your back on the floor, with arms and legs uncrossed. Close your eyes and breathe normally. Starting with your feet, and slowly proceeding up your body, like this:

• Become aware of the space occupied by each body part.
• Attend to how it feels in relation to the ground.
• Mentally tell that part to relax.
• Imagine that tension, pain, and old memories of pain are flowing out and into the floor.
• Surrender your weight totally in every part.
• Talk to yourself in this relaxed state—reaffirming how good and beautiful you are. Congratulate yourself for taking time to exercise.
• Slowly open your eyes, stretch, and get up.
• Proceed on your way.

These yoga postures are only a sampling of hundreds which are used. To learn more about it see the yoga books by Hittleman and Carr cited in the list of suggested readings at the end of this chapter.

should not over-exert yourself, but neither should you go too slowly. The following chart will help guide you in determining that in-between, optimum level. Find your age in the left hand column and follow it across to the second column to determine your recommended training pulse rate. If you have a history of heart disease you should receive clearance from your physician before beginning your exercise program.

but if the dance of the run
isn't fun
then discover another dance
because without fun
the good of the run
is undone
and a suffering runner
always quits
sooner or later.

from *The Zen of Running* by Fred Rohe

HEART RATES: (Based on resting heart rates of 72 for male and 80 for female.)

Age	Recommended Training Rate
20	160
22	158
24	157
25	155
28	154
30	152
32	151
34	150
36	149
38	147
40	146
45	143
50	140
55	137
60	128
65 +	120

If your resting pulse is more than 12 beats per minute slower, determine your recommended training rate from this formula: Your Recommended Rate = .65 x (Recommended Rate in table - Your Resting Rate) + Your Resting Rate. The value you compute from this formula should be somewhat less than the value in the table.

How To Take Your Pulse

With the palm of your hand facing you, locate the place in your wrist where you can feel a good pulse. Place your index and middle fingers side by side in the groove just inside the bone that leads to the base of your thumbs—about 2 inches below the bump at the end of that bone.

Many people (and vampires) prefer to locate the carotid artery pulse in the neck. First locate your Adam's Apple with your index and middle finger. Slide the fingers over to the side of the windpipe and feel deep into the neck for your pulse.

While looking at a clock, begin counting your pulse beginning with the number zero, not one. After 15 seconds, stop, and multiply your results by 4 to get the number of beats per minute. This is your pulse rate.

. . . .*Exercise*. . . . .

A Page From Your Exercise Journal

Exercising is a form of play and we encourage you to use it that way. If you want results of any kind, however, you will need to apply yourself to your practice with some consistency. One way to keep yourself motivated is to use a record or journal to chart your progress. You don't need to do the same type of exercise every day, unless you want to. I vary my morning workouts. I always start with stretching, yet some days I do race-walking, other days I play tennis, and on still others I ride my bike. Here is a sample journal entry:

Date:	*Time:*	*Type of exercise*	*Comments:*
7-25	6:30-7:15	tennis with Jere	clumsy; we laughed
7-27	7:30-8:30	bike ride (5 miles)	magnificent day; good push

Use this page as your journal for one week.   —RSR

Date:	*Time:*	*Type of exercise*	*Comments:*

At the end of the week it is helpful to record overall impressions, insights, accomplishment of goals, and resolutions.
Do that here.

_____
_____
_____
_____

Resolutions:

_____
_____
_____
_____

. . . .

For someone who is terribly out of shape, walking in place may be all that is needed to raise the pulse to the desired level. Another person who is conditioned, may have to run quite hard to reach the same heart rate. Don't try to keep up with someone else—use the table to find your own pace.

The first few times, stop after a minute or two and take your pulse. If it is less than your recommended exercise pulse, you aren't pushing yourself hard enough. If it is too high, ease up a bit.

When to exercise.

The time of day should fit your individual schedule. You may prefer to exercise after work because it is an extremely effective way of revitalizing yourself and eliminating all the day's problems and tensions. It is almost impossible to be "uptight" when you're exercising vigorously. The morning time holds other advantages. In the hot summer months it is a cool time of day. Also, some people find their morning time more disciplined and less likely to vary than their evenings.

You can read more about cardiovascular exercise in Cooper's book, *The Aerobics Program for Total Well-Being.*

One final note on aerobic exercise—IT DOESN'T JUST MEAN JOGGING! And it's a good thing, since many people, ourselves included, have either found jogging boring or too violent for the ankles, feet, and knees. Luckily, we now have a wide range of aerobic exercises from which to choose, including aerobic dancing, "jazzercise," race-walking (which is gaining wide popularity among injured runners), and rebounding on a mini-trampoline. Of course, swimming is a wonderful aerobic exercise, too. Try one, or try them all—until you find a form of aerobic exercise that suits you. Always be gentle, and enjoy yourself.

What Movement Does for the Mind and Emotions

As if the physical advantages of exercise were not enough, its connection to the ways we think and feel about ourselves is remarkable.

Regular exercise can firm muscles, shed pounds, and add a rosy color to your complexion. A body that moves is a body "taking shape." Sometimes, looking in the mirror is enough to invigorate the self-concept. Liking what you see is just one of the rewards. When you think of yourself in more glowing terms, you light up those around you and can approach them with confidence. You are less dependent on other people for approval because *you know yourself,* and *you approve* of what you know.

Keeping to a regular program of exercise is a statement of personal power. It says that you are in control of your own life; that you have endurance, strength, and flexibility. You witness yourself as the chooser, the mover, the changer. *You* are doing it! What you do in your body you can do in your work, your relationships, your dreams, your world at large.

The moving body is the body releasing stress, letting go of pent-up emotions and unblocking channels for energy. In the chapter on breathing we noted that the breath is the life-force. Encouraging fuller breathing through exercise is one of the most dynamic ways of increasing overall vitality.

Time spent in exercising, moreover, is time away from your books, your budgets, and your boss. It is time for your body. Time for a break. As you allow the busy, problem-solving brain a chance to take a back-seat, you give an opportunity for the sensual, creative brain to direct you for a while. Many runners testify to the inspiration that often occurs as they exercise. The change of pace that movement brings can refresh you. Back at work, you are better able to address the challenges of the task at hand.

· · · · · · ·

It is about 7:30 A.M. I have been up since before dawn. I have seen the world at its loveliest moment. I have run more than eight miles, made my body stronger, and enriched my soul. I will shave, have a hot shower that will seem exotic and sensual, eat, and be off to do what all of us do. The difference is—I own the day.

—JOEL HENNING[15]

· · · · · · ·

Pride in the appreciation of a job well done! Happiness at being alive. The chance to release frustrations. Inspiration, clear thinking . . . these are the powers that heal. These are the joys of high-level wellness. What a way to go!

And It's Good for the Soul

At the end of a long, hard push, serious athletes frequently describe moving into an altered state of

. . . . *Exercise* . . . .

Exercising in Water

Here are some simple and enjoyable ways to use swimming pool time effectively for heart-stimulating exercise, as well as for firming and trimming of the body.

1. **Jogging/Cycling:** Keep yourself afloat with arm motions while you tread water using legs to "jog" or to "ride a bicycle." Time yourself. Rest when tired.

2. **Milk Jug Movements:** Secure two empty plastic gallon-size milk jugs, with caps and handles. Put one in each hand. Use them to support you as you kick, do leg lifts, "jog," etc. To exercise arms, play with pushing them under—you'll be amazed at their resistance. Extend arms in front of you in chest-deep water and drag jugs in large circular motions out to your sides and behind you. Have fun being creative with many different movements.

3. **Ballet Practice:** Stand in chest-deep water, holding on to the side of the pool on your right side: Do leg lifts to front, side and back. Bend your knee and bring it up toward your chest. Reverse your position and do exercises with other leg.

4. **Dancing:** Bring along your radio or portable tape player. Play active dancing music. Do water dancing standing up or floating. Choreograph a water ballet. Be creative.

5. **Swim-a-thon:** Challenge yourself to learn how many different ways you can get from one side of the pool to the other without standing up.

. . . .

consciousness—a place in which the rational mind is temporarily quiet, where the sense of separate self is overpowered by the sense of connectedness with everything that exists. It is a feeling, and a deep "knowing" of peace and balance. Similar descriptions are found in religious literature. Many of the techniques used for meditation are present in a good run, or an extended swim, for example. Both exercise and meditation contain a point of focus—a word or chant, the breath . . . or the repetitious act of simply putting one foot, or one arm, in front of the other again and again and again. A rhythm is set. Often the rhythm takes over. The meditator becomes the sound. The runner becomes the movement.

For centuries repetitious movement has been a form of religious ritual in many traditions. The Sacred Dance again! The American Indian, the African tribesman, the Whirling Dervish, the Yogi—all have made use of the moving body in spiritual practice or communal celebration. Shiva, a Hindu god, is often depicted dancing. Taoism, of China, is based upon the flow of the moving universe. The art of Tai Chi which developed from Taoism is a representation, a dance of this flow.

Many who have grown up in Jewish or Christian homes never learned that dance and movement could be a form of worship or prayer. Church was a place for sitting still and listening, or reading.

Singing may have been OK, but moving certainly wasn't. Maybe we heard about Shakers and "Holy Rollers"—more than likely as the subject of jokes. At best we were uninformed about what they did and why.

Perhaps the reason, as Archbishop Phillips puts it, that "Your God Is Too Small"[16] is that you never approached Him/Her with the energy of your whole being. The mind alone will never grasp the fullness of creation. Mind, heart, and body moving in harmony may begin to approximate the totality which is "God."

. . . .*Exercise*. . . . .

Don't Get Out of Bed (before you start moving!)

How you start the day can set the tone for how you live the rest of it. These exercises are designed to get you moving easily, first thing in the morning. Releasing the kinks that you may have built up will energize you and may even make the transition from bed to floor a less traumatic one. Choose among these movements below and develop your own routine.

1. The Rack Stretch—Extend your legs as far as they will go, point your toes, stretch your arms out to either side extending fingers. Hold for a few seconds. Release. Repeat two or three times.

2. Reach for the Ceiling—Lying on your back, reach for the ceiling. Extend and then contract your fingers. Tense, relax, shake your arms.

3. Still on your back, extend right leg over left leg at a 90 degree angle from trunk of body if possible. (Go as far as is comfortable). Repeat several times. Then do the same with the left leg. Rest.

4. Bring your knees up toward your chest. Grasp them with your arms. In this position roll to your left, then back to center, then roll to your right. Repeat as often as is fun. Release knees. Extend legs.

5. To the count of 1-2-3 arch your lower back. Hold.

   Repeat count and lower it to the bed again. Rotate pelvis clockwise three times. Rotate counterclockwise three times.

6. Bend knees placing feet flat on the bed. Raise buttocks off the bed. Hold for count of 1-2-3. Lower buttocks back onto bed. Repeat three or four times.

7. Inhale as you turn your head to the right slowly, lowering your right ear to the bed. Exhale as you return head to center. Repeat turning head to the left. Do this three or four times. Relax.

8. Roll over onto your stomach. Bend knees and bring heels of feet back toward buttocks. Hold. Lower feet to bed again. Repeat twice.

9. Bring knees up under chest, reach back and hold your feet. Tuck head down toward chest. Feel your neck and back stretch with this one.

10. Let go of your feet. Raise head and straighten back, sitting back on your legs and feet. Look in the direction of the sunrise. Smile and greet the day. Get out of bed.

On Behalf of Trust and Compassion . . . or Why Jerry Doesn't Run

With all these good things available to those who exercise, you might be tempted to feel guilty if you haven't yet joined the team. The answers to why we don't move more are as many and varied as the people who ask the question. Take Jerry for example.

He doesn't hate exercise—he just hates boredom. He's often experienced them as one and the same. Left to himself he would rather spend the morning, or his free time listening to music, reading a good book, or doing a crossword puzzle. But his whole world brightens when an energetic friend appears at the door—inviting him to go swim, to play tennis, to take a hike up a nearby mountain.

For Jerry to berate himself for his lack of self-motivation would be a great energy waste. For him to consciously program situations in which he will have others to share with will meet both his needs for emotional stroking as well as his needs for physical exercise.

Roselyn on the other hand is different. She loves to jog alone along the flat country roads near her home. Every morning she does yoga for one hour. Every evening she does Tai Chi, a slow, dancing form of martial art.

For Roselyn to dictate what Jerry needs would be foolish and frustrating. For Jerry to expect Roselyn to react as he does—would be unrealistic. They are unique and extraordinary individuals. Each will be happy only if they trust their own internal messages, and design their environments so that they can lovingly meet their own needs for exercise. The options are almost limitless. Remember that the *one way* to wellness is *your way*. Here are some guidelines to keep in mind as you design your own way.

Eleven Easy Steps

1. *When the Pain Starts, Stop*. Pain is the body's protective feedback system. Use it responsibly to gauge how much to do, how far to go. While it is OK to push our usual limits when we are in excellent condition, beginners should be extremely respectful of the body's warnings.

2. *If It's Not Fun—Avoid It*. Many of us begin exercise programs with vigor, only to drop them just as vigorously. We set ourselves up for failure, and guilt, when we push, demanding that we do something that we do not really enjoy. There are so many different ways to exercise. Be creative in finding one that is both challenging and enjoyable for you.

3. *Whatever You're Doing—Dance It*. Whether you are jogging, or playing handball, all of your movements can be smooth and flowing. From the study of martial arts we learn that movement directed from the *center*—the place of balance below the diaphragm, in the middle of the body—intensifies strength and enhances overall form. Finding this center and moving from it makes everything you do a dance.

4. *Avoid Imitation*. As beginners we have much to learn from the pros. Many of them, however, became great because they tried something different, and it worked well for them. Beware of modeling yourself too closely upon someone else. What works for them may only serve to frustrate you. If it works for you, do it. If it doesn't, find your own way.

5. *Deal Cautiously with Competition*. The challenge of competition can be a great motivation for growth and development in any discipline. It can also be a source of bad feelings and lead to cheating. Become your own competitor. Use opportunities of playing with others as chances to better your last performance. Lose graciously or win graciously, knowing that the only lasting reward will be your sense of accomplishment, your own integrity.

6. *Reward Every Effort*. Realize that it is never too late to begin, and that there are no limits to the number of times for starting over. Congratulate yourself for 2 minutes of exercise done. Avoid being hard on yourself for the 18 minutes not done. Set realistic limits for yourself and promise yourself a treat (a new bathing suit, a night out, an overdue massage) for accomplishing it, or even approximating it. Remember that guilt is an enormous waste of precious energy.

7. *Follow Spontaneous Impulses*. When the urge to move arises, use it! If you feel like dancing—get on your feet. Close your office door and jump rope. Hang up the phone and run around the house.

Turn off the TV set and walk across the room on your hands! These impulses are jewels—don't pass them by.

8. *Use Every Means to Stay Inspired.* Especially in the initial stages of an exercise program, it is easy to forget why you started this in the first place. You need to create inspiration for yourself. Start by scheduling your exercise time as if it were a high priority meeting, which it is. Mark it on your calendar or in your date book. Find a partner or a group to exercise with. You will keep each other inspired. No friend? Invite your dog to be your exercise companion. Set short-term goals for yourself. Short-term means no longer than 2 weeks ahead. If you are walking for 15 minutes a day, 4 days a week, what can you expect of yourself 14 days from now? Be realistic, and challenge yourself, too. Keep a daily log and a weekly summary of what you did and how you felt about yourself. See the exercise: "A Page from Your Exercise Journal" on p. 101.

9. *Respect the Earth You Move On.* If your exercise takes place in the outdoors capitalize on the opportunity to celebrate the sun, the sky, the fresh air. Don't miss the flowers as you run along the path. And leave the environment unharmed in your travels.

10. *Breathe.* As you move and exercise you may notice that you are holding your breath. This is a sure sign of unnecessary straining. Inhale as your movements expand. Exhale as they

Balloon Walk

B ecause there is entirely too much seriousness attached to many forms of exercise, most exercise ceases to be play. The following piece was created by our friend Kenneth Maue and is used here with permission. We offer it to you as a playful reminder, an alternative.

Go on a balloon walk. Start anywhere, with a sturdy balloon and some extras. Blow up the balloon, then release it, letting it scoot wherever it goes. After the balloon lands, walk to that place. Then do the process again—blow up the balloon, release it, walk to where it lands.

You may also add some-thing specific to do at each place the balloon lands, such as touching your toes or jumping into the air.

If you are a musician, you may take your instrument and play for a bit at each spot.

Continue until you are finished, then end.

used with permission[17]

contract or move back to center. Allow the breath to flow naturally.

11. *Love Yourself.* Compose a little song or lyric for yourself and sing or recite it as you exercise. "I am moving with grace and beauty." "I love myself as I grow in strength and agility." "Look at me, I'm beautiful." And believe it because it is true!

Moving on the Planet

If you have ever been caught in a traffic jam on a hot, summer day you know first-hand about the stress and pollution which is created by dependence on the automobile. The situation will only get worse unless we each decide to do something about it. If you start using your body to take you places instead of your car, you are rewarded many times over. Jogging, bicycling, walking, and roller-skating do not pollute the air. They increase your own sense of power and also conserve valuable energy resources.

As responsible citizens of Planet Earth we can do much to encourage ecological and healthful alternatives to gas-guzzling and fume-spewing automobile use. We can support efforts to increase public transportation and car pools, especially in our cities. In many places bicycling paths are being designated for both urban and rural use. As a tax-payer and a voter you can promote these actions. This may entail both higher taxes and life-style changes. But so will letting things progress the way they are going now.

You decide.

Suggesting Reading*

Anderson, B. *Stretching*. Bolinas, CA: Shelter Publications, 1980.

Balaskas, A. *Bodylife*. London: Sidgwick and Jackson, 1977.

Balaskas, A., and Strick, J. *Soft Exercise*. New York, NY: Charles Scribner's Sons, 1983.

Benjamin, B., and Borden, G. *Listen to Your Pain*. New York, NY: Penguin Books, 1984.

Carr, R. *Yoga for All Ages*. New York, NY: Fireside Books, Simon and Schuster, 1972.

Chang, E.C. (translator). *Knocking at the Gate of Life and Other Healing Exercises from China*. Emmaus, PA: Rodale Press, 1985.

Cooper, K. *The Aerobics Program for Total Well-Being*. New York, NY: Bantam Books, 1982.

Dychtwald, K. *Bodymind*. New York, NY: Jove Publications, 1984.

Frankel, L.J., and Richard, B.B. *Be Alive as Long as You Live*. New York, NY: Lippincott and Crowell, 1980. (For older people.)

Gach, M.R., with Marco, C. *Acu-Yoga*. Tokyo: Japan Publishing, 1981.

Gallwey, W.T. *Inner Tennis: Playing the Game*. New York, NY: Random House, 1976.

Henderson, J. *Jog/Run/Race*. Mountain View, CA: World Publications, 1977.

Hittleman, R. *Yoga: 28 Day Exercise Plan*. New York, NY: Workman Publishing Co., 1969.

Huang, A. H. *Embrace Tiger, Return to Mountain*. Moab, UT: Real People Press, 1973.

Johnson, D. *Body*. Boston, MA: Beacon Press, 1983.

Katz, J. *Swimming for Total Fitness*. New York, NY: Dolphin Books, 1981.

Kuntzleman, C. *Maximum Personal Energy*. Emmaus, PA: Rodale Press, 1981.

Leonard, G. *The Ultimate Athlete*. New York, NY: Avon Books, 1977.

Lowen, A., and Lowen, L. *The Way to Vibrant Health: A Manual of Bioenergetic Exercise*. New York, NY: Harper Colophon Books, 1977.

Rohe, F. *The Zen of Running*. Berkeley, CA: Random House/Bookworks, 1974.

Schneider, T. *Everybody's a Winner: A Kid's Guide to New Sports and Fitness*. Boston, MA: Little Brown and Co., 1976.

Sheehan, G. *Running and Being: The Total Experience*. New York, NY: Warner Books, 1978.

Solomon, H. *The Exercise Myth*. New York, NY: Harcourt Brace Jovanovich, 1984.

Stevens, J. *Aikido*. Boston, MA: Shambhala, 1984.

Ullyot, J. *The New Women's Running*. Brattleboro, VT: The Stephen Green Press, 1984.

Cassette tapes to guide you in yoga movement are available from: Kripalu Center for Yoga and Health, Rte. 183, Box 793, Lenox, MA 01240.

*This is only a representative sampling. Many excellent books have been omitted. At the bookstore or library, look over the whole selection and choose according to your judgment.

Notes

1. Bentov, I. *Stalking the Wild Pendulum*. New York, NY: E.P. Dutton, 1977, p. 26.

2. Bentov, p. 25.

3. Reported in: Hickman, J. "Sizing Up Exercise," *New Realities*, Vol. 3, No. 2, (October 1979), p. 46.

4. Hickman, J. "Sizing Up Exercise," pp. 46–53.

5. See: Kannel, W. B. "Habitual Level of Physical Activity and Risk of Coronary Heart Disease. The Framingham Study." *Canadian Medical Association Journal*, Vol. 96 (1967), pp. 811–12.

6. Cooper, K., et al., "Physical Fitness Levels vs. Selected Coronary Risk Factors," *Journal of the American Medical Association*, Vol. 236 (1976), pp. 166–69.

7. For a discussion of the studies comparing active and inactive occupations see:

Fletcher, G.F., and Cantwell, J.D.D. *Exercise and Coronary Heart Disease*. Springfield, IL: Charles C. Thomas, 1974, pp. 22–27, and

Hockey, R., *Physical Fitness*. St. Louis, MO: C.V. Mosby Co., 1977, pp. 44–46.

8. See:

Cooper, K. *The New Aerobics*. New York, NY: Bantam Books, 1970.

Kuntzleman, C. *The Exerciser's Handbook*. New York, NY: David McKay Co., 1978, pp. 47–117.

9. The material on aerobics is by: Susan Stewart, R.N., Calabasas Park Center for Cervical and TMJ/Cranio-mandibular Orthopedics, 4766 Park Granada, Calabasas, CA 91302, with additions and updating by: Richelle Aschenbrener, R.P.T., Denver Institute for Sports Medicine, 7180 Orchard Rd., Englewood, CO 80111.

10. Stewart, S., and Aschenbrener, R.

11. Carr, R. *Yoga for All Ages*. New York, NY: Fireside Books, Simon and Schuster, 1972, p. 106.

12. The directions for the yoga postures used here are found in: Carr, R., pp. 22, 24, 33, 120, 122, 127, 137.

13. Stewart, S.

14. Cooper, K. *The Aerobics Program for Total Well-Being*. New York, NY: Bantam Books, 1982.

15. Henning, J. *Holistic Running: Beyond the Threshold of Fitness*. New York, NY: New American Library/Signet Books, 1978, p. 21.

16. Phillips, J. B. *Your God Is Too Small*. New York, NY: Macmillan Publishing Co., 1961.

17. Maue, K. *Water in the Lake*. New York, NY: Harper and Row, 1979, p. 22.

Wellness and Feeling

> The expression of emotion—fear, sadness, joy, anger—is an important form of human energy output. Feelings are generated from within the limbic system of the brain, and serve to motivate both thought and action.

. . . .

FROM THE MOMENT of birth, with the proverbial slap on the behind that starts us breathing, we experience feelings and emotions. They can be intense, or frightening, or wonderful. They can also be the most misunderstood, and consequently mistreated, gifts we have as human beings. We judge them, repress them, discount them, drug them, worship them, and run from them. Yet, what a bore to be without them! Life fully lived is life filled with feeling! Life fully lived is high-level wellness.

Sensing . . . Feeling . . . Thinking

The first distinction we need to make is that *feelings*, as the word is used in this chapter, means *emotions*. The physical experience of heat or cold or hunger are *sensations*—the subject of a previous chapter.

Secondly, feelings are not the same as thoughts, even though we commonly hear them spoken of that way. Actually, thoughts and feelings are experienced in widely different areas of the brain. The limbic system, deep within the brain, is the source of emotions, while thoughts occur in the neocortex, or grey matter, which is the surface of the brain, and is a rather recent development in the evolution of mammals.

For any given event, we respond with both thoughts and feelings. Yet most of us give priority to our thoughts about a subject and sometimes ignore the feelings. If you ask a person how s/he feels about a controversial political figure, and he responds by saying, "I feel he should be recalled," he is really expressing an opinion (a thought), not a feeling. Recalling is not a feeling. Anger, sadness, fear, and joy are. A more accurate answer, then, might be, "I feel angry with him, afraid of what he might do, and I think he should be recalled."

. . . .

Since feeling is first
who pays any attention to the
syntax of things
will never wholly kiss you.

—e. e. cummings
USED WITH
PERMISSION

. . . .

In most cases we have a feeling instantaneously, even though we may have learned to suppress it. Then, a fraction of a second later, the intellectual processes have time to compute, and we decide what

109

position we will take and what we will do. This movement from feeling to thinking or from feeling to acting is described in many different ways by learning theorists and psychologists. It is a very important transition that needs to be better understood. One system which deals with it in an exciting way is Transactional Analysis (T.A.).[1] It is a clear and practical framework which demonstrates the relationship between feelings and wellness.

Primer of Transactional Analysis

The Three Generations Under One Roof

When you watch yourself or other people in action you frequently discover that human beings can change very quickly. Take this case for example:

Gladys is upset because her three-year-old daughter, Marsha, has spilled some greasy food on the new white sofa. She stands over the child, finger waving in a gesture of "you bad girl," and angrily accuses Marsha of being careless and stupid. Just then the phone rings. It is a business partner needing to talk about an important deal. Listening to her now, quiet and reasonable, Gladys sounds like a different person. She thoughtfully discusses the pros and cons of the venture, offers her opinions logically, and arranges a meeting for the following day. Hanging up the phone, she sees that Marsha is crying. Gladys now feels remorse. Gathering the child into her arms, she is consoling, gentle. She may even start to cry herself, touched as she is by the baby's tears.

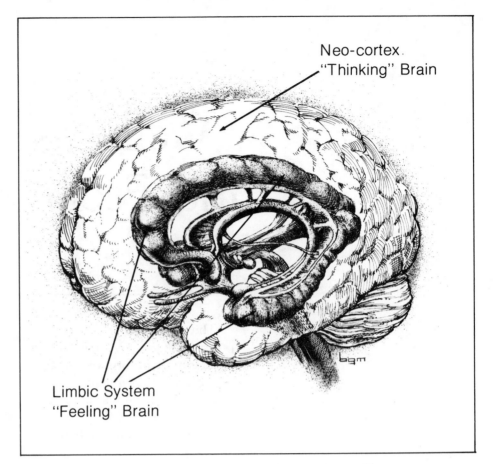

Neo-cortex "Thinking" Brain

Limbic System "Feeling" Brain

Gladys has gone from being angry, to being professional, to being comforting, to being teary—and all within about fifteen minutes' time! The appreciation of these different ways of being and acting form the basis of the theory of Transactional Analysis. The human personality, theoretically, is a composite of three ego states, three separate and distinctive sources of behavior. First, we have an internal Parent—the judging or nurturing part of our personality.[2] When we act as Parents, we are doing and saying things that we heard or saw our parents say or do. We are responding to the way things "ought to be"; we are concerned with the right and the wrong. Then there is the internal Adult. This is the real *thinking* member of the trio. It reasons, weighs the logic of the arguments, makes decisions, and

remains cool, calm, and collected. Last, but certainly not least, there is the internal Child. Here is where the *feelings* happen. The Child is angry, or fearful, or ecstatic, or sorrowful.

This chapter is about feelings—so a good deal of it is about what happens in the internal Child. As we proceed, be aware that feelings start in the Child—but they don't necessarily stay there. We can express them through the Parent, Adult, *or* Child. As a result, we have a good number of options in how we can handle our feelings.

About Strokes

A stroke is any form of stimulation or recognition which arouses feelings. They may appear in bright colored packages as smiles, hugs, and loving words (the positive strokes), or in dingy paper bags as brush-offs, cold stares, and reprimands (the negative strokes). Whenever people acknowledge you in any way—perhaps with applause, maybe with censure—you are moved, touched, so to speak. In T.A. language, these touches are called *strokes*.

To be stroked is to be confirmed in the realization that we exist. And this realization is absolutely essential for survival. If we aren't successful in getting our needs met in life-affirming, positive ways, we seek them out in death-promoting, negative ways, rather than suffer the intolerable condition of being a non-entity. As the saying goes, "Negative strokes are better than no strokes at all."

Let's consider a few examples. Marilyn invests energy in a project to help the poor of the county. She receives the support of her co-workers, the gratitude of her clients, and the powerful self-reward of knowing that she is making some impact on the world. That's stroking! Jeffrey defaces property with graffiti and spray paint. He brags about it and finally gets arrested. In this way he affects his world by frustrating or horrifying others, and receives a short-lived, sensational focus of public attention from his parents, the press, and the police. He too has been stroked. Jeff's alternative—to go through life unnoticed—would be far worse than suffering the consequences of his destructive acts. But he would be the last one to describe it this way.

Matt, at six years of age, starts acting out in school. His work reflects it. He immediately reaps benefits from conferences with the principal and counselor, and lots of attention from his parents. Matt is getting his strokes.

Strokes and Wellness

In Chapter 3 we investigated physical touch as a primary energy input and a necessity for survival. Now as we consider emotional and psychological strokes, the parallels between them become clear. Children and adults need strokes for happiness and health, as much as newborns need physical touch for survival. Eric Berne, the founder of Transactional Analysis, used to say, "If the infant is not stroked, his spinal cord shrivels up."[3] The need for positive strokes, and for learning to cope with negative strokes are each linked with the general state of health.

In his work with cancer patients, Carl Simonton, M.D., of the Simonton Cancer Center in Pacific Palisades, California, finds that it happens all the time. Dr. Simonton states: "The biggest single factor that I can find as a predisposing factor to the actual development of the disease [cancer] is the loss of a serious love object, occurring six to eighteen months prior to the disease."[4] The love object—frequently a child or spouse—is a primary stroke source. When that is lost, it can lead to destructive means of compensation. Nobody wants cancer or other serious disease, but everybody wants strokes!

Sometimes a problem develops because we have collected a deadly supply of negative strokes. We store them up until they eat away at us from within. Hurts, anger, fear, deep sadness—these create an energy which will look for an outlet somewhere in the body if it doesn't get conscious recognition or ex-

pression. Some of those outlets might be:

- a nervous habit such as smoking or overeating
- driving recklessly
- gritting teeth
- "getting" a sore throat or an asthmatic attack, a headache
- an extra rush of adrenalin into the blood stream that makes us feel wired
- a stress-related condition such as constipation, skin disorder, eye fatigue, or ulcer, or
- building defenses, by withdrawal and depression, to keep us from being hurt again.

When we don't understand our real needs or how to fulfill them, we are left with a void which is all too easily filled by illness or dangerous habits. As children, many of us got some of our most nurturing strokes when we were sick. Some of us still use the same tactic as adults. Claudia, at forty-seven, developed cancer, and reported that she never before realized how caring her husband and children could be. Nobody wants cancer or other serious diseases, but stroke-need may be overwhelming. Everybody *must* have strokes!

Are Feelings Good or Bad?

Strokes generate feelings or emotions. From our earliest years we have all received messages that some emotions were "good," others were "bad." It was OK to feel happy. That meant that our needs were being met, and made

. . . . *Exercise* . . . .

GETTING TO KNOW MY CHILD

Here's an exercise that has been invaluable to me. While looking through my baby book I closely examined some of the photos and saw indications of that inner beauty in my child that I didn't know was there. I took some of the pictures out of the book, had them enlarged, and arranged them so I could see those parts of myself, and reincorporate them into my self-image.

Some of them showed me a presence and inner light that I had forgotten.

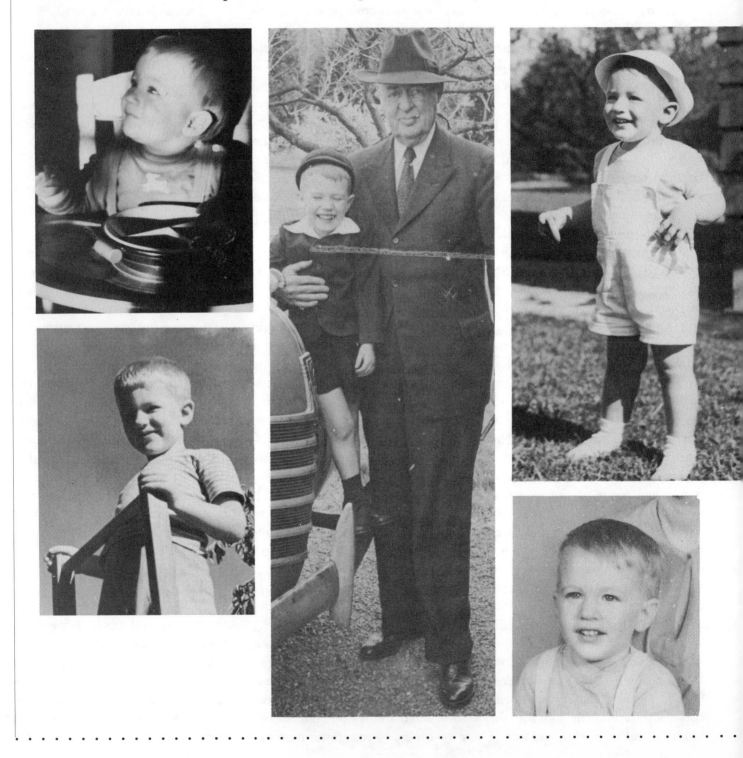

.... .Exercise. ....

In others I saw fear, withdrawal, sadness, pensiveness. Nowhere did I see anger, although I believe that I was really angry when some of them were taken.

In others I found the whimsicalness, silliness and aliveness of my child. I don't easily remember this part of myself. This exercise has helped me to remember.

—J.W.T.

Mommy and Daddy feel good too. But sadness, fear, and anger made people uncomfortable, and so they told us, "It's not nice to be angry," or "Don't be sad," or "It won't hurt; there is no reason to be afraid." At school we often saw smiling, passive behavior being rewarded, and high emotion being punished. It didn't take us long to learn that some feelings were approved of and should be sought after, and others were disapproved of, and should be avoided or denied. The feelings continued, however, and now had fewer and fewer acceptable ways to be expressed.

To help in coping with this confusion, many people have dulled their awareness to emotions in general, accepted the idea that feelings are bad, organized indirect ways of handling them, and lost trust in their own experience. Then they wonder why their lives aren't richer and more satisfying!

The time has come to realize that emotions are not good or bad, they simply are. A loud crash in the middle of the night usually triggers a fear reaction. Watching a tragic movie may result in tears of sadness. The constant interruptions of the telephone in the middle of a project which requires quiet and concentration may arouse anger. How a person chooses to act in the presence of these feelings may be subject to praise or censure, but the important thing to remember is that the emotions themselves are amoral. It is the judgments we learn to connect with feelings—that one is good, that one is bad—which lead to the problem. It is running away from them, or holding them inside which can make us sick.

The Basic Emotions

Children in all cultures evidence four basic emotions. These are anger, grief, joy, and fear, represented here in five-year-old language to make them easy to remember: ·

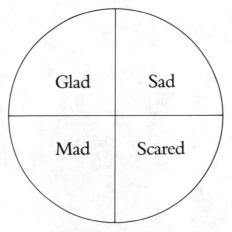

Like primary colors, these basic four blend into the whole spectrum of human feelings. They may be considered separately, but it is important to understand that they are each only part of the whole. The fully alive human being is capable of feeling all the emotions. Increasing our aliveness, our wellness, means becoming aware of our feelings, accepting them as OK, and developing healthy ways of expressing them. Life would be awfully boring without the creative tension of sadness and joy which any moment might hold.

Joy

Let's begin by considering the emotion called *joy*. You experience joy when you realize some gain: anything from finding a dime on the sidewalk, to receiving a compliment, to understanding that "God loves you." It is a state of in-tune-ment, a feeling of expansiveness, a grateful appreciation of the beauty all around. While some see

it as a treasure to be searched for and then carefully guarded, it is actually the natural state of living with your eyes fully open—the gift and grace of being human. If this is true, you may wonder why you don't feel it more often, and that's a very important consideration.

Joy can be easily sabotaged because we often mistrust having too much of a good thing. You have probably observed this scenario happening among young children: laughter and excitement build to a critical level, the energy gets intense, somebody hits or pushes somebody else, and the next thing you know—one of the crowd is crying, or the whole group is fighting. Adults are familiar with this pattern and often caution children: "Calm down now," "Don't get too excited," "Somebody is going to get hurt." And sure enough, it happens!

It is easy to fall into this way of thinking in our adult lives. We often expect the worst, so that we'll never be disappointed. Someplace deep inside, many of us are afraid to open up to joy, because we are afraid of losing it. Sooner or later, we remember, it's got to end. The result of this closing down can be emotional dullness, a grey world, a guarded heart, and a lonely existence even in the midst of abundance.

Much poetry has been written about the joy to be found everywhere—in looking at a flower, breathing sea air, touching a leaf. Yet many of us miss these moments, and the possibility of joy, because we are too busy, too tired, too "intelligent," or too bored. One of the magical benefits of setting our sights on wellness is an opening to this richness—a height-

· *Exercise* ·

Color My World—Glad

Fill the circle with names of people/events which are sources of joy for you.

Joy-Breath Exercise

Color the world with the color that signifies joy for you.

1. Close your eyes and breathe slowly, deeply.

2. Imagine the color of joy filling the room, the air around you.

3. Each time you inhale imagine filling your body with this color.

4. Continue breathing with this color for several minutes.

5. Share with a friend. How do you feel as a result of doing this exercise?

What have your learned about yourself?

ened sense of joy about all aspects of our lives.

It may evolve like this—
awareness of problem
(fatigue, overweight, etc.)

⇩

decision to attack problem

⇩

early morning jogging program

⇩

sense of well-being—sense of joy

Sadness or Grief

The other side of joy is sadness or grief. It is the emotion that arises from a loss, either real or imagined. When someone special, or something important, or some cherished belief is lost, a gap or a hole in your internal reality is felt. This may lead to a variety of physical symptoms from loss of appetite, to tightness in the chest, to insomnia, fatigue, or even hyperactivity. Loss also affects your thinking, and ways of behaving.

In the past few years, new interest has been focused on the psychology of loss, especially the experience of dying, or the grieving for someone who is gone. The work of Elisabeth Kubler-Ross, M.D., in particular, indicates that understanding the stages in the grief process helps us in moving through them.[5] This knowledge can build some sense of security since there is frequently a tendency to fear that you are going crazy, that you are all alone, that no one else ever went through this before, and that there will be no end to it. Realizing that these are very natural responses to loss can provide much

© BRILLIANT ENTERPRISES 1974.   POT-SHOTS NO. 661

YOU CAN ONLY GO HALF-WAY INTO YOUR SADNESS

BEFORE YOU START COMING OUT.

needed encouragement, a tiny ray of sunlight in the midst of so much darkness.

Denial is commonly the first stage in the grief process. You hear yourself, or others saying, "I can't believe it," or "This can't be happening to me." The organism's natural balance is challenged when facing loss or death. Going into shock, withdrawing, becoming numb, or acting feverishly to block out the harsh reality, can provide ways of coping. These are normal reactions in the early stages of grief, since they give the body-mind some necessary distance from trauma. They can offer a chance to awaken more gently to a difficult truth. When the world has been temporarily turned upside down, it naturally takes some time to adjust.

Anger follows denial. People get angry at the employer who fired them, the husband or wife who left them, the God who permitted this tragedy to happen. Since anger may not be an "approved" emotion, it is often swallowed and stored away. This can be

harmful for both physical and psychological health.

After denial and anger, the real grieving takes place. Sadness touches you at the very core of your being and from that place you mourn the loss. The deep sighing or primitive moaning sounds which come with crying are healthy indications that you have confronted the pain right down to its roots. There are two ways of dealing with grief—"hard and fast," or "hard and slow." The healthiest way that you can heal the wound created by your loss is to face it squarely—to cry away the pain you feel. Allowing yourself to curse or scream can loosen the floodgates which hold back tears.

All of these stages lead to the final phase—acceptance. Sadness and grief, like other deep emotions, stir up internal waters which may have grown stagnant, and this can be cause for profound celebration since they call for a reassessment of life values, and raise questions that might otherwise have gone unasked for years.

The Crying Quiz

Questions to spark your emotional memory:
What messages do I remember hearing about crying?

When was the last time I cried?

How do I really feel about crying?

These things make me cry (include songs, movies, events, etc.):

I could cry with these people around:

Because:

I could never cry with these people around:

Because:

What I have learned about me as a result of doing this exercise:

Earn bonus points. Share with someone else!

Anger

Anger is the emotional response to what we see as injustice or frustration. When we think we have been wronged, or that others have been treated unfairly—we get angry. When we are stopped from doing what we want to do, it is normal to strike out at what holds us back.

While society doesn't approve of injustice, it also doesn't approve of anger. As children we heard, "Don't fight," or "It's not ladylike to get angry," or "Hold your temper!" Our parents and teachers probably feared the energy of anger they felt in their own bodies, and so cautioned *us* against it.

Anger-energy is powerful, and ignoring it will not make it go away. Often it will smolder until it bursts into flames, or dam up until it seeps out in ways that encourage illness.

Consider for a moment what you do with your body when you experience anger. Do you tighten your jaw, perhaps grind your teeth? Some people contract their fingers into a fist and at the same time contract the muscles around the stomach and lower abdomen. You have probably noticed a significant change in vocal pitch and intensity in an angry person's voice. These are common physiologic responses which aren't good or bad in themselves. But if being angry is your usual way of dealing with the world, and if repressing it is your habitual response, you are likely to get into trouble. For example, a chronically tense jaw can misalign the bite, induce headaches, destroy teeth, and detract from a person's physical appearance.

Besides the ways it shows up in the body, unexpressed anger can

feed resentment and lead to unpredictable explosions that upset your relationships and your mental balance. Remember this one? You are six years old. You've spilled your milk again. This not unusual childish accident causes a very unusual reaction in Mom or Dad. It is as though a tornado had ripped through the center of your house. You are left with your head spinning, questioning, "Now where

did that come from?" Mom or Dad may have overlooked your annoying behaviors twenty times, but the twenty-first was the last straw. This reaction, while common, is really not helpful for anybody. Kids get confused and hurt. Parents get relief, but often with guilt. Dealing with the little frustrations as they arise is generally much healthier.

Many "nice guys" (and gals)

The Capricorn Incident

It is midnight in April of 1972. Two-month-old Hanne is sleeping in the nursery in the cherry cradle I built for her from plans out of *Ladies Home Journal*. In the next room Sally and I are lying in bed having an "argument." An observer would think it rather a strange argument because Sally is shouting angrily at me and I'm saying nothing, looking very martyred and wondering what the neighbors will think. The subject of her anger is my lack of emotional expression. I feel hurt inside, but am speechless when I try to express any of my feelings. I feel a growing pressure and sense of unreality and suddenly I sit up, yell loudly and ram my head into the plasterboard at the head of the bed (I happen to be a Capricorn—the Goat—but the symbolism eluded me at that point). Stunned, I look at the smashed hole conforming to the size of my head, mentally note that I missed the wooden studs in the wall, or it would have *really* hurt, and collapse sobbing. Sally puts on her overcoat and runs to the next door neighbor, a former campus minister, who returns alone to our apartment. Through my tears I tell him I don't know what's come over me since Hanne's birth. My depressions are getting worse and Sally is spending so much time nurturing Hanne that she hardly has any time for me. David suggests I talk with our mutual friend Ann, who knows several pastoral counselors.

This event marked a major milestone in my personal and professional development as I began one-to-one counseling the next week and started reading *Born to Win*. I discovered a wholly different world of feelings and my own responsibility to deal with them effectively. The implications for my own health and for others were profound, yet nowhere in my previous medical training had I learned to be open to the concept of self-responsibility.

whose behavior in public is exemplary are often hiding intense anger. Instead of sharing openly, they become covertly hostile, smiling as they stab you in the back. Because there are such strong cultural proscriptions against the expression of anger, this passively aggressive activity has become standard operating procedure in many societal institutions. Perhaps this explains, in part, our fascination with violence. Watching the evening news, or a violent movie, we can vicariously experience anger without taking any risks. And risk taking—important risk taking—like speaking your mind caringly rather than provocatively, even in an unsupportive environment, can be exciting and exhilarating. If we were courageous enough to tell the truth about our anger, our world would very likely be a much more honest and peaceful place.

It's OK to feel angry. It's OK to express it. Here are some suggestions for how to use your anger to solve problems, rather than to create new ones.

1. *Decide what you're angry about.* Until you are clear about that, the problem can't be solved. Letting off some steam first may help you to pinpoint the problem. You can beat on your bed with a tennis racket, park your car on a back road and "yell your head off," or have a mock argument with a friend. Discharging some of the energy first clears your head and makes it easier to identify the problem.

2. Once you know what you're angry about, *share your feelings* with the person or persons involved and let them know how

Working With Feelings

Our staff has an agreement that we can call each other day or night and request a negativity session. If the other agrees, the one who has requested it then has full permission to be *totally* negative, without fear of being judged, without worrying. Nothing said in this session is taken "for real." It all goes down the drain with a big flush!

This is the way it works:

One person is a talker (sometimes more like a "ranter") and the other person is a listener. The talker proceeds to lay it *all* out in no uncertain terms—complaints, fears, problems, everything. Genteelness is not the order of the day in a negativity session. It takes some practice to be able to say what you're thinking and feeling without editing, but the more you do it, the clearer you become, and the faster the negativity dissipates.

The listener's job is just to *be there*, without judging or evaluating what is being said. If the listener doesn't hear or understand something, she will let the talker know, but extraneous conversation is discouraged. The talker has the freedom to say anything! And it doesn't even have to make sense! The listener's responses are ones indicating

that the talker has been heard and understood. The only other communications made by the listener other than acknowledgments are things like, "OK, what else?" or if the talker gets into apologizing or rationalizing or philosophizing, the listener can say something like, "Cut the crap and get on with the negativity." The agreement is that positivity is *not allowed* until all the negativity is "dumped." The listener keeps things moving, gently and unobtrusively.

The session concludes when the talker either starts laughing, or says, "Enough!" The listener then says, "Good! Now tell me something beautiful about yourself (or something beautiful that has happened lately)." The session is always ended on a positive note.

The result of using the negativity session for clearing away the unnecessary garbage of our minds has been the establishment of a warmth and a deep trust in our relationships as a staff. The more we can realize that we are all in this together—being human—and the more compassion we cultivate for ourselves and others, the more we can get on with the miracle of living . . . well!

—Barbara McNeill
Wellness Associates

you see the situation. But remember to take the other person's feelings into account. Ask her/him how s/he feels about

it. This is an important step, as it keeps you from assuming that you know how the other person feels and helps to clarify

. . . . *Exercise* . . . .

Angry Answers

Messages I heard about expressing anger:

These things/events/people stimulate anger in me:

The last time I felt anger was:

Is it OK for me to feel angry?

I express it by:

Unhealthy ways I express anger:

Healthy ways I express anger:

What I've learned about myself from these questions:

Share with a friend.

the situation so that you know you're talking about the same thing.

3. After the other person has shared his or her feelings, *decide what you're going to do* so the situation isn't likely to occur again. In this way, you may never have to deal with that problem again. Not all problems or people are easily dealt with. It will help to remember to stay with one issue at a time, to keep your goal in mind and not get sidetracked, and to think of *several* ways of creatively dealing with your problem. You may also choose not to deal directly with the person or situation you're angry about. But to keep yourself in balance, you'll still need to de-energize the feelings in some way. Some people have found a hard game of tennis, or jogging, or talking to a willing listener are helpful ways to deal with anger when it would not be useful to deal with it directly.[6] It's also sometimes useful to just express the emotion, without trying to figure out why you feel it, as long as you do it in a way that doesn't create more problems.

Fear

Fear is the absence of Love.
—FRED MUNN

Fear is a non-specific reaction to a real or imagined threat to our security—physical, intellectual, psychological/emotional, or spiritual. It serves as protection by causing us to retreat and pull back into ourselves so that we may reassess

Fear, Darkness, and Magic

After you understand the "four-feeling view"—glad, sad, mad, and scared—here's an even simpler and more profound one to consider. It is: **there are only two feelings, love and fear.** Actually, only one—love—and the absence of love—fear. My belief is that fear does not exist, but is only an illusion.

Think about a windowless room, with the crack around the door sealed so tightly that no light at all can get in. Now you turn off the light in the room, and darkness fills it. But does it? If darkness is a "thing," and has "come into" the room, you should be able to bring more of it in, and make the room darker. But, hard as you may try, if there is already no light in the room, you can't make more darkness. Magic?

Now suppose you turn on a light so tiny that it emits only one photon—a photon being the smallest possible unit of light. You see it. There is light! Darkness is no longer absolute. "Some of it" has vanished. But, where did it go? Did it fly out the window? No, there is no window. Like magic, everything has changed. Where before there was only darkness, now there is a room with light.

What is darkness? A real "thing," or only a concept, an absence?

I submit that fear is to love as darkness is to light. The quote by Fred Munn, which appears on this page, says it. Fred realized this during a Wellness Associates' seminar several years ago. We were discussing Jampolsky's book, *Love Is Letting Go of Fear*, and reflecting that the title was actually backwards, since you can't let go of something that doesn't exist—like fear. We agreed, however, that you can let go of love, by temporarily forgetting your natural inheritance. In so doing, what you are left with is fear. And fear certainly seems real. (In fact most people would probably bet their lives that it is.) But I say it's only magic. A "magic" we could well do without.

The same reasoning applies in considering other absences like "evil" or the "devil." We give these concepts power over us by making them into "things." Isn't it about time we quit believing in fear, wasting our precious life energy in running from purple-legged, three-headed monsters and other similar fantasies?   —JWT

the situation, and accumulate a needed supply of energy for fighting or running away. For example, in one timeless instant you hear an unfamiliar sound, visualize an attacker, freeze, feel weak in the knees, scan the environment for weapons and exit doors, and turn around with an upraised fist.

Fear happens when we can no longer trust something or someone, or when we anticipate the breakdown of one of our security systems. It can be a physically painful emotion because it involves contraction and constriction of the body. For some (race car drivers, hang glider pilots, etc.) it can be an accompaniment to high exhilaration which can clear and free the emotional channels to allow the flow of life energy. This is one paradox of fear.

People handle their fears in a variety of ways. Sometimes they run from them by transferring out of class in school, or by leaving the cemetery before the casket is actually lowered into the ground. Many children learned to keep quiet about fears because of the angry reactions they got from their parents. "There is no monster under the bed. Now turn off that light and go to sleep!" But the fears remained and sometimes showed up in bed-wetting or sickness, which quickly brought mother to the bedside.

As we matured we engineered strategies for masking our fears. Some people frantically fill their homes with appliances and furniture, their calendars with activities, or their mouths with food when what they are really searching for is a way to deal with fear.

Others withdraw into fantasy or build walls of books and papers to protect themselves from the world of real live people who can hurt them. The paradox is that an immense amount of fear is *created* as we spend our lives trying to escape fear.

Once you are willing to admit to having fears you can begin to "kiss your monsters." Generally you find that the reality is far less scary than the fantasy. One gentle way to begin is by taking a class of some sort that deals with expanding relationships. Assertiveness training is a good one. (See the section on assertiveness in chapter 9.) You can learn to "stretch your comfort zone," meaning take small risks, tiny steps in facing your fears. Every step taken can be reinforced with a little reward. You may start with phoning a business in town to register a minor complaint. Next day you progress to talking with a friend you've had a disagreement with.

It takes courage to confront fears, and that may mean sharing them with others and giving yourself lots of positive reinforcement (strokes, presents, etc.) for each bit of progress realized.

Guilt

Guilt is not one of the primary feelings, but it is so pervasive in the culture that it needs some primary treatment here. We view guilt as a perversion of both fear and anger. Guilt is like an internal smoke screen. It allows us to feel bad about something, but prevents us from seeing alternatives and doing anything effective to change a situation. Regina reports that when she was a regular cigarette smoker she always felt guilty about her habit. She remembers how smokers would often admit to one another—"I hate myself for doing this. I should stop." This little "confession of sins" became almost a ritual which punished and absolved her all in one step. She was then guilt free, until the next nicotine urge struck.

Guilt is rampant among those who are addicted (often since birth) to feeling "not OK" about themselves. It usually covers up anger about all the "shoulds" which have been swallowed that can never be adequately digested; all the demanding and disapproving parental voices, both within and without, which can never be silenced. Those who are preoccupied with guilt miss the opportunity to constructively channel the energy of their rage into actually alleviating or solving the problem. It is much more comfortable to keep one's "familiar misery" and perpetuate the cycle of self-depreciation than it is to risk the unknowns that come along with being effective and powerful.

Learning to say "no" and stand one's ground, rather than over-adapting to others, is a good starting point in breaking an addiction to guilt. The next steps include telling the truth about our anger, admitting our fears, and refusing to encourage negative self-talk which keeps "not-OKness" alive. (See material on internal dialogue in chapter 9.)

Developing Awareness and Support

In order to take the first step in change, you need to be aware that an emotion is present. Learning to be aware, both of what is around us and what is in us, is one of life's great challenges, and results in the ability to freely and responsibly express our emotions. When people are unaware of the feelings they are having, they find it difficult to break old habits. They create unnecessary stress, and consequently illness, by running around in all directions, hitting roadblocks and falling into holes. You can't find something if you don't know what you are looking for. When you

. . . .*Exercise*. . . . .

Stamp Out Oughtism

Used with permission: © 1986 Swami Beyondananda (Steve Bhaerman), 323 E. Williams, Suite 43, Ann Arbor, MI 48104.

Oughtism is a disease of the oughtanomic nervous system where the unfortunate victims oughtomatically do what others tell them they *ought* to do. If left untreated, Oughtism can eventually result in a total loss of the ability to think.

Are *you* Oughtistic?

Take this simple test

YES NO

____ ____ Do you feel obligated to give blood even when you're down to your last pint?

____ ____ Do you put on clean underwear each day just in case you get hit by a car and have to go to the hospital?

____ ____ Are you reading this only because somebody said you ought to?

If you answered "yes" to any of these questions you could be Oughtistic. But don't feel bad. You aren't alone. Forty million Americans suffer from this silent crippler. And most of them don't even *notice*.

• Yes, Oughtism *can* be cured. But first, you must know its warning signals:
• Any involuntary nodding of the head up and down—especially when someone asks for volunteers.
• Sharp pangs of guilt after digesting a single chocolate chip cookie.
• An enlargement of the onus.
• An empty feeling between the ears.
• Constriction of the intestines; that duty-bound feeling.

So join us, won't you? Let's stop this epidemic before we all become oughtamatons.

. . . .

don't know what you are hungry for, you may leave the grocery store overloaded with junk food or empty-handed out of frustration.

You can increase your emotional awareness if you stop and ask yourself "What am I feeling?" frequently in the course of one day. Awareness in general can be enhanced by using any number of creative cues—signs, strings around the finger, colored dots on keys or wristwatch bands—which remind you of the issue that you may be working with at any particular time.

Some people find it helpful to run down a checklist of emotions and determine which one best describes what they are experiencing. The diagram and explanation of the four basic emotions in this chapter may be useful to you. There are a great number of reasonably effective methods for approaching the subject of emotional awareness, and we suggest a few of them among the exercises in this chapter.

You cannot, nor should you seek to avoid painful emotions. What you can do is practice more direct means of expressing them, and establishing a support system to help track them down and deal with them. Do you have at least three close friends with whom you can talk about anything, friends who will support you in being the

. . . . *Exercise* . . . .

Emotional Awareness Trackdown

(Use this several times in the course of a day, or whenever you're feeling unhappy.)

1. What am I feeling?
   Mad/Sad/Scared/
   What is happening in my body?
   How is this feeling affecting my life now?

2. When did this feeling start?
   What was happening at the time/or what occasioned it?

3. What desire/demand did I have which was unmet?
   What expectation was unfulfilled?
   (For example: I expected/demanded that Frank would shower me with compliments for my cooking.)

4. Are you willing to let go of this demand/expectation?
   If YES—go to #5
   If NO—go to #6

5. Congratulations! What are alternative ways of having your needs met, or of releasing these uncomfortable feelings?

6. Congratulations! What do you choose to do about it?

. . . .

best possible person you can be? To create a supportive network may require that you keep extending yourself, meeting new and stimulating people, potential members of your "family." And, it is important to remember that support does not exclude negative feedback, or even criticism from others. It is possible, especially among caring friends, to move beyond the realm of winning and losing, being wrong or being right. It is a mark of greatness to be attuned to the truth, and willing to hear it, no matter how clumsily it is expressed, how painful it may feel.

This is probably the single most important piece of information for you to remember about wellness and feelings. Life is tough anyway. Alone, it is intolerable. Remember, it is absolutely necessary to ask for and be open to help. Just as it is essential to ask for and be open to love.

Love

. . . .

Love is giving someone the space to be who they are and who they are not.

—W. ERHARD

. . . .

What more powerful stroke could there be than to have someone you care about say "I love you"? And

. . . .

Love is a decision to live in a universe which is good, even when there is no proof to validate it.

—BARRY TELLMAN

. . . .

what greater impact could you have on your world than to give your love freely, without reservation, without fear? Unfortunately, few of us dare to open up enough to give or receive love. Typically, we tie up much life-energy in restricting the flow of love because we are afraid—we fear rejection, fear the strong emotions aroused, fear intimacy, vulnerability.

. . . . *Exercise* . . . .

Emotional Awareness "Tune-In"

Ask someone you trust to help you with this exercise.

1. Sit or lie down in a comfortable place.

2. Close your eyes. Breathe slowly and deeply to help yourself relax.

3. Turn all your attention to the physical sensations happening in you as your friend reads aloud the following phrases five times each, slowly. Repeat them silently to yourself.
Phrases to use:
I AM SCARED.
I AM LONELY.
GET OFF MY BACK.
I GIVE UP.
NO/NO/NO!
I WILL.
I'M GREAT.
YES/YES/YES!

4. Share what you have learned as a result of doing this exercise.

. . . .

Like the ground we walk on, love supports us in all we do. Blocking love, whether it be self-love, love for others, love offered, will inexorably have a negative effect on happiness and health. Unfortunately, love is not something you can analyze and define, work at or create. In fact, attempting to do so is likely to keep you from being able to experience it. Suffice it to say that love is letting go—letting go of fears, grievances, judgments. And the secret is simply to allow it to happen.

. . . .

The only thing that is required for healing is lack of fear.

—A COURSE IN
MIRACLES

. . . .

Suggested Reading*

Berne, E. *What Do You Say After You Say Hello?* New York, NY: Bantam Books, 1973.

Bloomfield, H. *How to Survive the Loss of a Love.* New York, NY: Simon and Schuster, 1976.

Buscaglia, L. *Love.* New York, NY: Fawcett Crest, 1972.

———. *Living, Loving and Learning.* Thorofare, NJ: Charles B. Slack, 1982.

———. *Loving Each Other.* Thorofare, NJ: Charles B. Slack, 1984.

Freed, A. *T.A. for Tots.* Sacramento, CA: Jalmar Press, 1973.

*This is only a representative sampling. Many excellent books have been omitted. At the bookstore or library, look over the whole selection and choose according to your judgment.

Gaylin, W. *Feelings.* New York, NY: Ballantine Books, 1979.

———. *The Rage Within: Anger in Modern Life.* New York, NY: Simon and Schuster, 1984.

Harris, T. *I'm O.K.—You're O.K.* New York, NY: Avon Books, 1973.

James, M., and Jongeward, D. *Born to Win.* New York, NY: New American Library/Signet Books, 1978.

Jampolsky, G. *Love Is Letting Go of Fear.* Berkeley, CA: Celestial Arts Press, 1979.

Keyes, K. *How to Make Your Life Work [Or] Why Aren't You Happy?* Coos Bay, OR: Living Love Publications, 1977.

———. *The Handbook to Higher Consciousness.* Coos Bay, OR: Living Love Publications, 1975.

. . . .*Exercise*. . . . .

Variations on a Theme—Clues and Games

Here is a list of feeling states that people often have but fail to identify. It can be used/played with in a number of ways:

• Use it when you're not sure if you're feeling anything, or if you have so many feelings that you are confused and frustrated. Read over the list quickly and check any words that come close to identifying your present state. After you have noted them, ask yourself why you have them, or what has triggered them. For instance, if you identify with "stupefied," record for yourself: "I feel stupefied when all my plans fall apart; and I feel stupefied by my inability to make a decision; and I feel stupefied. . . ." Challenge yourself to come up with as many as possible explanations as you can.

• Use the list with a friend. Ask one another: "Tell me about a time when you felt 'melancholy.'"

• Use it to inspire journal writing. Take one feeling, write it in the middle of a blank page, circle it, and then record all your associations with it. After you've done this for 10 minutes or less, write a little story, or poem, or letter for yourself about this experience. The main thing is to have fun.

The List:	angry	bitter	charmed	conspicuous	desirous
I feel . . .	annoyed	blissful	cheated	contented	despair
I am . . .	anxious	bold	cheerful	contrite	destructive
Abandoned	apathetic	bored	childish	crazy	determined
adequate	astounded	burdened	child-like	cruel	different
adamant	awed	bothered	clever	crushed	diffident
affectionate	awkward	Calm	combative	culpable	diminished
agony	Bad	capable	competitive	Deceitful	discontented
almighty	beautiful	captivated	condemned	defeated	distracted
ambivalent	betrayed	challenged	confused	delighted	distraught

Kubler-Ross, E. *On Death and Dying.* New York: NY: Macmillan Publishing Co., 1969.

LeShan, E. *Learning to Say Good-Bye.* New York, NY: Avon Books, 1978.

Lowen, A. *Bioenergetics.* New York, NY: Penguin, 1976.

Rogers, C. *On Becoming a Person.* New York, NY: Houghton-Mifflin Co., 1970.

Rubin, T. *The Angry Book.* New York, NY: Collier Books/Macmillan Publishing Co., 1969.

Tavris, C. *Anger: The Misunderstood Emotion.* New York, NY: Simon and Schuster, A Touchstone Book, 1982.

Viscott, D. *The Language of Feelings.* New York, NY: Pocket Books, 1976.

Notes

1. See: Berne, E. *Transactional Analysis in Psychotherapy.* New York, NY: Grove Press, 1961.

2. See: James, M., and Jongeward, D. *Born to Win: Transactional Analysis with Gestalt Experiments.* Reading, MA: Addison-Wesley, 1971. (T.A. book we most recommend.)

3. Berne, E. *The Structure and Dynamics of Organizations and Groups.* Philadelphia, PA: J. B. Lippincott, 1963, p. 157.

disturbed	Gay	intimidated	obsessed	remorse	sympathetic
dominated	glad	isolated	odd	restless	Talkative
divided	good	Jealous	opposed	reverent	tempted
dubious	grateful	joyous	outraged	rewarded	tenacious
Eager	gratified	jumpy	overwhelmed	righteous	tenuous
ecstatic	greedy	Kind	Pain	Sad	tense
electrified	grief	Laconic	panicked	satisfied	tentative
empty	guilty	lazy	parsimonious	scared	terrible
enchanted	gullible	lecherous	peaceful	screwed up	terrified
energetic	generous	left out	persecuted	servile	threatened
enervated	Happy	licentious	petrified	settled	tired
enjoyment	hate	lonely	pity	sexy	thwarted
envious	heavenly	longing	pleasant	shocked	trapped
excited	helpful	loving	pleased	silly	troubled
evil	helpless	low	precarious	skeptical	Ugly
exasperated	high	lustful	pressured	sneaky	uneasy
exhausted	homesick	Mad	pretty	soft	unsettled
Fascinated	honored	maudlin	prim	solemn	Violent
fawning	horrible	mean	prissy	sorrowful	vehement
fearful	hurt	melancholy	proud	spiteful	vital
flustered	hysterical	miserable	Quarrelsome	startled	vulnerable
foolish	Ignored	mystical	queer	stingy	vivacious
frantic	immoral	Naughty	Rage	stuffed	Wicked
frustrated	imposed upon	nervous	raptured	stupid	wonderful
frightened	impressed	nice	refreshed	stunned	weepy
free	infatuated	niggardly	rejected	stupefied	worried
full	infuriated	nutty	relaxed	suffering	Zany
fury	inspired	Obnoxious	relieved	sure	zestful

4. Simonton, O.C., and Matthews, S. "Management of the Emotional Aspects of Malignancy," *Cold Mountain Journal*, Spring 1977 Calendar, Cold Mountain Institute, Granville Island, Vancouver, B.C., Canada V6H3M5, p. 6.

For a full treatment of Simonton's work see:

Simonton, O.C.; Matthews-Simonton, S.; and Creighton, J. *Getting Well Again*. Los Angeles, CA: J.P. Tarcher Inc., 1978.

5. Kubler-Ross, E. *On Death and Dying*. New York, NY: Macmillan Publishing Co., 1969.

For practical suggestions for dealing with grief see:

Bloomfield, H., et al. *How to Survive the Loss of a Love*. New York, NY: Simon and Schuster, 1976.

Bozarth-Campbell, A. *Life Is Goodbye, Life Is Hello*. Minneapolis, MN: Compcare Publications, 1982.

Stearns, A.K. *Living Through Personal Crisis*. New York, NY: Ballantine Books, 1984.

6. This material about dealing with anger is from an article by Sara Travis, Mill Valley, CA.

Seven

Wellness and Thinking

THINKING IS THE art and the craft of the human brain. Like the lungs, heart, and stomach, the brain's work is one of transforming energy. We feed the brain with the nutrients carried by the blood, as well as by the energy of great ideas—what we read in books, watch on television, learn from other people, and experience in sights, sounds, and movement. Some of this energy is filed away as data for later use. The rest is available for signaling the body, for creating dreams, and for making connections—for thinking.

Scientific research demonstrates the energy-play of the thinking brain. Hooked up to an EEG (a machine that measures brain activity), the various patterns of thinking or non-thinking are found to produce electrical impulses. Think "hard"—and note an increase in the frequency of energy. Think "soft"—and see that the brain waves slow down. After a day of head work you will feel

> Thinking is a form of electrochemical energy generated in the brain. Thinking is an energy output form. While it requires all the energy input sources, thinking is particularly dependent upon sensory data, and relies heavily on the energy of emotions in creating its internal maps of external reality.

physically tired, because thinking takes energy!

Few would argue that what goes into the mouth will affect the overall health and well-being. Fewer seem convinced that what goes into and comes out of the mind is every bit as important. We are repulsed by rotten and moldy food, by stagnant air, by polluted water, but we tolerate a good deal of rotten, stagnant, and polluted thinking. The images, the energies, which fill our minds will change the body physically, influence the people around us, and move the world at large. Wellness means attuning ourselves to the life-giving or death-dealing energy of our thoughts.

This chapter will focus on the power of your thinking. It will relate thinking to physical and mental health, and offer some creative options for using it to the benefit of your whole system.

Thinking Molds Reality

We see the world through glasses colored by our assumptions of the way things are. When we look at the world through glasses of love and trust, that is what we see. When we look through lenses tinted with suspicion and fear we find the same reflected back to us. "What you see is what you get" is more than an advertising slogan or comedy routine. It is a reality that can be demonstrated in controlled studies as well as in supermarkets.

Again and again scientists find that they prove what they expect to prove, often overlooking the most obvious contradictions. You will hear what you want to hear. You will see what you expect and need to see. When you are hungry or on a diet you see the suggestions of food everywhere. Having finished a satisfying meal, the same magazine you browsed through before dinner will hold a totally different fascination. Before eating, it was the food that jumped out at you from every page. After your meal, you find that it contains many other ideas between its covers.

Man is troubled not by events themselves but by the views he takes of them.

—EPICTETUS,
CIRCA 100 A.D.

Thinking will also color your relationships. Many of us have been involved in one that has begun to deteriorate in some way: the parent losing faith in the child; the wife suspecting the husband of "playing around"; the friend jealous of another friend. The injured party can find scores of "clues" to reinforce the belief that s/he is being wronged.

When we approach the world with suspicions, we find confirmation of those suspicions at every turn. When we approach the world with trust we are rewarded with the same. Rochelle's story makes a case in point here.

Rochelle wanted to buy a Christmas tree and had only ten dollars to spend. Her friends laughed at the prospect, knowing that the price of nice-looking trees had sky-rocketed in the last few years. But she was determined to find one—a beautiful one—for just this amount. She traveled from lot to lot one cold afternoon in Boulder, Colorado, becoming more and

Thinking and Ego Development

After we are born, we continue to be dependent upon Mother, even though the umbilical cord is severed and we must breathe and eat independently. Psychologically we are still connected. Sometime after age one, peaking around age two, we begin the process of separating, and learn to think for ourselves. We set up situations of opposition with our parents (and anyone else around). "NO" becomes the favorite word of the "terrible two-year-old." "Do you want a cookie?" Our automatic response may be "NO." We then notice that we don't get the cookie, and begin to compute the cause-effect relationship. Noticing the consequences of our actions, and deciding when to exert the newfound will, sets the logical thinking process in motion. If this didn't happen we would continue to flow along with whatever Mother or anyone else wished, and would not develop a separate sense of identity, or mind of our own. This stage can be very trying on parents because they must constantly deal with the constant negatives the child must express in formulating his/her independent will. (I want what I want when I want it!) Successful resolution of this stage establishes the Adult Ego State, as described by Transactional Analysis.[1] An understanding of the importance of this stage made interactions with my daughter, when she was two, much easier for both of us.

—J.W.T.

more frustrated when she learned that every tree she liked cost at least twice her limit. Trusting in the power of redirected energy and changed thinking, she pulled over to the side of the road and spent the next few minutes in a concentrated meditation, reaffirming her belief, her trust, her knowledge, of the rightness of things. Resuming her travels she noticed a small hand-drawn sign in front of a trailer, and a few lovely trees leaning against the nearby fence. "This is it," she thought. Finding the tree of her liking she inquired the price. "That one goes for fourteen dollars," the owner remarked. She drew in her breath. "But wait a minute. It seems to have a few stunted

branches here. How about ten?" he smiled. "I'll take it," she sighed. Once again the miracle of grace surrounded her.

We all know people who seem to be similarly graced as a way of life. What is their secret? Can we all have a part in it? Rochelle would say "yes." The world, she attests, is built by our thoughts; and she is not alone in this belief. We mold reality by the energy of our minds.[2]

Thinking Changes the Body

A significant part of "reality" is what goes on inside the body. Thinking changes the body for better or for worse. For example, have you ever gone to bed late one night during the work week, looked at the clock, calculated the hours until you had to get up, and thought to yourself, "I'm going to be exhausted tomorrow. Don't know how I'm going to get through the day"? Upon arising you feel miserable and have to drag yourself to work. All day long you reinforce the situation by repeating: "Am I tired!" Sound familiar?

. . . .

The world is such-and-such or so-and-so only because we tell ourselves that that is the way it is.

—CARLOS CASTANEDA

. . . .

Now replay the same scene, but this time it happens when you are on vacation. You stay out late into the night, dancing, partying. Going to bed you anticipate the exciting prospects of the next day—new adventures, new sights, new people. You remember that some people thrive on only a few hours of sleep a night, and armed with this thought you retire happily. The next day you leap out of bed ready for the magic, barely giving a moment's reflection to the amount of sleep you've had. Your happy thoughts have energized your body.

There are other examples. One night, when we were sharing dinner at John's house in Mill Valley, California, we heard a rumbling noise. John, who had been through three earthquakes in eleven months, immediately labeled the rumbling *earthquake*. The thought of an earthquake was enough to get our hearts beating faster, blood flowing with greater intensity, hormones activated, stomachs and bowels in an uproar. There was no earthquake, but it took a lot longer to convince our hands and stomachs than to reassure our minds. Our bodies responded as actively to the imagined danger as they would have to a real one.

Biofeedback research affirms that we can slow or quicken heartbeat and affect other physiological functions by merely thinking about stressful or relaxing conditions.[3] Early in the century, a Russian, A. R. Luria, demonstrated that imagining running uphill actually increased his subject's pulse.[4] Under hypnosis individuals can create blistered skin when given a suggestion that they have been burned. Simply believing you are in danger, or may be harboring a deadly tumor or virus, will create extreme changes in your body. Bob, who was a medic during the Korean War, tells the story of a young soldier who had a badly lacerated leg. His vital signs were excellent as the corpsmen worked on him. When the doctor arrived on the scene, he took one look at the leg and exclaimed, "Oh my God, this is bad." The young patient immediately died.

Accounts of this nature are common. Doctors and nurses are continually confronted with the reality of the will to live or the wish to die in seriously ill people. Two individuals with the same symptoms. Prognosis for both is the same. One lives. One dies. Why? The Greek philosopher Socrates answered the question in 500 B.C.: "There is no illness of the body apart from the mind." In modern times, Arnold Hutschnecker, M.D., in his book *The Will to Live,* reinforces this: "Anxiety is a whisper of danger from the unconscious; whether the danger is real or imagined, the threat to health is real . . ."[5]

. . . .

Illness
I am ill because my mind is in a rut and refuses to leave.

—KAREN GIARDINO

. . . .

If you can relate to these examples, then you have a good appreciation for the vital connection

. . . .

Mosquitoes

I used to be prime bait for mosquitoes. They had a personal vengeance toward me. One day in 1970, the year of the beginning of my awakening, I was telling this to my colleague, Marc Sanders. He said that they used to eat him up too, but then he began practicing loving them and they seemed to respond by not biting him. From then on, I practiced loving them too, instead of concentrating all my attack thoughts toward killing the maximum number possible. I still get an occasional mosquito bite, but it's no longer a problem for me. —J.W.T.

. . . .

A Loving person lives in a Loving world.

A Hostile person lives in a Hostile world.

Everyone you meet is your mirror.

Reprinted from *Handbook to Higher Consciousness,* by Ken Keyes, Jr. Fifth Edition, ©1975 Living Love Publications, St. Mary, Kentucky, 40063.

between thinking and wellness. Let's explore this mind-body connection further now, and address our attention to these four basic assumptions:

- Your thinking is influenced by many factors in the environment and this influence is often a form of hypnotism.

- You have a part in choosing which factors will influence you.

- You encourage illness or wellness by reinforcing the messages learned under these influences.

- You can use positive strategies to become aware of, and to turn around your illness supporting messages.

Beware of Your Hypnotists

Loosely applied, everything hypnotizes, since you are influenced in some way by all the events in life's path—by every word, book, movie, TV show. Your brain operates like a highly sophisticated computer, your memory-banks storing each experience you have ever had. Wilder Penfield, M.D., found that when a certain portion of a subject's brain was electrically stimulated, the subject could describe minute details of an event that had happened when he was four years old. Not only did the subject recall cognitive data, but the emotional responses to the scene were also recalled.[6] Under clinical hypnosis you could probably remember an event that your conscious mind had seemingly forgotten. Aldous Huxley was able to induce a trance-like state in himself, and then recite verbatim the contents of a page in a book he had not read in twenty years.[7]

When you realize how much you are exposed to, and how influential these elements can be, you might be terrified. On the other hand you might also let go of the need to figure out reasons for all your problems. Simply accepting your wonderful complexity may lead to well-being a good deal faster and more efficiently than any scrutinizing, logical analysis. There will always remain much about you that is simply not logical. (But, more about that later.) Let's go on to consider the second assumption, which is the responsibility we hold in choosing our input sources.

GIGO

It's computer-talk, and it stands for Garbage In—Garbage Out. The fact is that the solutions which computers print out are only as relevant and correct as is the data with which they are programmed. Now you are not a computer (despite what the behaviorists try to tell you). Nevertheless, the analogy is a good one, so let's follow through with it.

You have within you an amazing computer and at the same time you are your own programmer. Looking around at all the possible input sources in the environment, you decide which ones to attend to, which ones to ignore. Say you decide to watch television. Turn it on. Ah, your favorite soap opera! The scene is a hospital waiting room. The distraught woman standing

beside the window is being informed by the doctor that her husband has cancer. Symbolically, the woman reaches for the cord of the venetian blinds, closing them. Fade to black. Commercial. Once again you get a message loud and clear ... "Cancer equals death"— the closing of the light. Now if this happened rarely, you wouldn't need to be concerned. But because similar depictions are made constantly, you can easily begin to believe them. The fear of cancer has become a national epidemic.

. . . .

American cancerophobia ... is a disease as serious to society as cancer is to the individual—and morally more devastating. For this state of affairs, many are to blame ... Among the guilty are the media. Because of our society's disease, any news about cancer, no matter how trivial, is ipso facto sensational ... the minor laboratory discovery is heralded as another "breakthrough" in our "war" against cancer. So the vicious circle spirals upward: cancerophobia elicits sensationalist reporting, which in turn fosters the demonology of cancer.

F.J. Ingelfinger, M.D.

Reprinted by permission from the *New England Journal of Medicine*, Vol. 293, (Dec. 18, 1975), p. 1320.

. . . .

Television has become a powerful force in programming thinking. From it we learn that headaches look and feel like hammers pounding on anvils, that acid indigestion eats away at the stomach lining, that when we take some drug the world will look rosy again. In the highly susceptible state, a near hypnotic trance, that TV creates, we can be easily persuaded that we need the remedies offered for our ills. When we enter a supermarket, a similar trance-like state is produced by the repetitious

lines of color and shapes. One study indicated that grocery shoppers exhibited only six or eight eye blinks per minute, when in an alert state they perform this same function about twenty times a minute. So, when you find yourself reaching for the product that you saw advertised, you are possibly carrying out a hypnotic suggestion.

Similar hypnotic suggestions are experienced all the time from the other people with whom we associate. Parents often "program" their children for illness or accident by constantly telling them: "Don't do that—you'll fall, you'll cut yourself, you'll get sick, you'll get hurt ..."

Surrounding ourselves with a negative climate of constant complaints and continual expectations of the worst drains us of energy and fills our biocomputer/brain with "garbage" which will come out in some way—as illness, accident, depression, whatever. Ben, at seventy-five, is confined to his home because of weak legs. He spends hours each day reading newspapers and talking about how bad the world is with anyone who will listen. The lower his spirits get, the weaker his legs become.

What is called for is *conscious selectivity* in choosing the data which we will feed into the computer. If we feed it encouragement, beautiful images, positive input—we will be gifted with positive output—a program for high-level wellness.

Programming Illness— Programming Wellness

Creating negative mental pictures or repeating messages to yourself about illness, or accident, or weak-

. . . .*Exercise*. . . . .

Imaging Flip—For Self-Healing

Your negative thoughts help to keep you stuck in pain, in tension, in depression, but they can be flipped over and used to alleviate the very same conditions.

Focus in on one problem area to which you devote energy. Perhaps it is the chronic tension in your right shoulder, or the nausea you experience riding in a car or plane. Note as many aspects of it as you can:

• Is there a picture associated with the problem or pain? (For instance, tight, knotted nautical ropes, or a murky, stagnant pool.)

• Is there a sound connected with the problem or pain? (For instance, a grinding or gurgling sound.)

• Is there a texture associated with it? (A sore throat, for instance, might feel like rough sandpaper; an upset stomach might feel slimy.)

• Is there a temperature associated with it? (A headache might feel hot; a broken arm might feel cold.)

• Is there a smell or taste associated with it?

• Is there a movement associated with it? (Churning, pounding, stabbing?)

Now comes the "flipping" part. The essential question here is what will the problem or pain look, feel, smell, sound, taste like *when it is alleviated or cured.* For the image, substitute its opposite.

• Knotted ropes are slowly untied and loosely laid out on the deck.

• A stagnant pool is drained and filled with clear, sweet water.

• A dark cloud of pain in the head is penetrated with sunlight.

• A pounding sound is replaced by the sound of a waterfall.

As you relax, substitute a positive, healing image for each negative, painful one. Use words if necessary to reinforce the stimulus. Like: "My head is filled with billowy, white clouds."

Put up reminders for yourself around the house, in the car, at your place of work. Whenever you see them, flip into your new set of images.

Don't be discouraged if you can't conjure up all the images we have suggested. Use the ones that are strongest for you. Be patient with yourself in anticipating results, but know that other people have used this exercise to great advantage. Give it a try.

ness of any kind, will have an effect upon your body and influence the reality you create.

Worrying about illness wears down the body's natural defense mechanism because of the connection between mind and body. Remember the experience of a severe headache? Say, for instance, you wake up with it. "Damn, headache!" Repeat over and over "I've got a headache!" and you'll have it all day. We've all done this. These messages from the conscious mind create a whole range of responses which become established in the body. The job interview presents another clear example. You know that on next Tuesday you will be meeting a prospective employer. You immediately create a mental picture of him or her, design the office in your mind, visualize yourself seated opposite your inquisitor. If your self-concept has suffered some harsh blows lately, you probably start worrying about your inability to answer the questions asked. You actually hear yourself stumbling over words, moving your hands nervously, drawing a blank. The face that looks across the desk from you is frowning, or aggressive, or smiling condescendingly. The whole experience is one of anxiety, and you will have four days in which to anticipate making a total fool of yourself. If this continues, that is precisely what will happen. There is no magic involved. The power of your negative thinking has produced its intended results. Your whole presence will communicate the invisible message on your T-shirt—"I'm not OK."

Positive worry is our phrase for "the power of positive thinking" and a score of similar techniques. It is a technique for replacing negative thinking with "well-thinking" about a problem or a condition in your body. Here's how it works:

- First of all, focus in on the negative pictures you have been making.

- Then create pictures of wholeness, and healing, to replace them.

- Each time you realize that you are thinking about the problem, or making a negative picture, use this as a cue to substitute the positive image as you take a deep breath.

- Write out or draw the positive picture. Make several copies and place them around where you will see them often.

- Spend several short relaxation periods each day recreating the positive healing image.

- Put other cues in your environment to remind you to plug in the positive. (Colored stickers or dots are good for this.)

- Instead of becoming preoccupied with the future or worrying about the past, tune in to the present moment in all its richness. Attend to the gifts and graces around yourself all the time.

- Finally, forgive yourself for any failures, difficulties, compulsions attached with trying to change. In short—love yourself unconditionally.

Kay's story testifies to the value of this approach. Kay had a lump in her breast which would have to be removed by surgery. She reported that the picture in her mind was of a black mass with tentacle-like arms. She thought of it as cold and hard and evil. She played that picture over and over, day in and day out, becoming more and more fearful as she actually imagined the lump growing in size, eating up everything in its path. When instructed in the process of "positive worry," she drew a picture of what a healthy, clear breast would look like. She used yellows and golds and wide, free, circular, spiraling movements. She placed copies of the picture everywhere. This was the picture she used in breaking her negative programming. Each time she noticed it, she paused momentarily and allowed it to sink into her. She did this for two weeks. When she next saw her doctor, he examined the lump and, in amazement, reported that it simply seemed to dissolve under his fingertips. He had no rational explanation for it. But Kay knew why.

Right Brain—Left Brain

Some of the most exciting research findings of late deal with the diverse functions of our two brain hemispheres. In the 1960s, at the California Institute of Technology, and at the California College of Medicine, a group of severe epileptic patients underwent operations in which their brain hemispheres were surgically separated. The nerve fibers, known as the corpus callosum, which join the two halves of the brain, were cut in an attempt to keep seizures isolated to one hemisphere. As a surgical and

························ *Exercise* ·················

A Private Place—An Exercise in Creative Imagination

This exercise serves a number of useful purposes. Doing it will take you into a state of relaxation. The images you form will stay with you for a long time, and provide you with an imaginary place to retreat to for refreshment and healing. Then too, it will exercise your imagination, and excite you as you realize how resourceful you can be. Finally, it may suggest some possibilities for changing your real environment.

Find a quiet, relaxing place, and give yourself thirty uninterrupted minutes to do this exercise. It is helpful to have a friend read it to you so you can close your eyes and give your imagination free rein. You could also tape-record it and play it back to yourself. Now, in your mind, journey to your bedroom. See it as vividly as possible. Look it over, wall by wall, remembering what is there. Notice that a new door has appeared on one wall. The door has a door knob. Approach it and put your hand on the knob, notice its texture and temperature. When you open the door, you are going to find yourself in a new room, an addition to your house, a room that you have never seen before. The room will be empty, except that it will have several windows. Go inside now and survey your space.

First, decide upon the light in the room. Where are windows placed? Determine what views you would like to have out of each. (One woman looked out upon the ocean from one, a redwood forest from another, and a snow-covered mountain from a third.)

Now cover the floors if you wish. Next attend to the walls—color, paintings, murals, shelves? Now furnish it for yourself—include a special chair or pillow or couch on which you can rest and dream. Want a work space? an art studio, a dance floor, a writing desk? Make it happen immediately. If you like music, listen for it. Or add a piano, organ, flute, and music stand. Many people who have done this report that they added elements of the outdoors into their environments—an indoor waterfall, a floor-to-ceiling bird cage, a tree in the middle of the room.

Be as courageous and as outrageous as you can be. Remember there are no limits. Now sit back and enjoy your place. Tell yourself that you can go to it to solve your problems, to relax in the midst of a hassled day, to prepare yourself for sleep. The uses are as many and as varied as your needs. Have fun with it.

Now you may wish to draw or paint what you have created in your mind. Share it with a friend. Build an addition. It's up to you.

P.S. (from Regina)

I first created my private place in 1977. It is as vivid to me today as it was on the day I constructed it. Reviewing it recently I received the motivation to remodel and redecorate the office in which I am now working. In reality I have designed a nurturing space for myself, one which reflects me— my music, my pictures, my tea service, my live plants, my light and color.

therapeutic technique it was effective. What was learned as a result continues to have a profound impact on our knowledge of the human brain and is gaining wide application in the treatment of psychological, educational, and physical problems as well.

The "split-brain people," as they came to be known, acted quite normally, but exhibited some curious behaviors when subjected to one series of tests. Seated behind a screen which blocked their view of the objects on the table in front of them, they were asked to identify an item placed in one hand. If a comb, for instance, was put into the right hand, it was recognized as such and verbally labeled. If, however, the comb was first placed in the left hand, the subject could indicate how it might be used, and recognize it from among other items, but drew a blank when asked to name what it was.

We know that the right hemisphere of the brain controls the left side of the body, and the left hemisphere controls the right side of the body. What was happening in the experiment with the "split-brains" was that the left hand was sending information to the right hemisphere, but the right hemisphere didn't have a word for it. With the object in the right hand, however, the left brain recognized it as "comb" and named it as such.

The left hemisphere of the brain seems to be the verbal genius, the logician, the researcher, the mathematician, the scientist who looks to cause and effect. The right brain gets the credit for the opposite traits. Not irrational or illogical, mind you, but non-rational or non-logical—*intuitive*. This is the side of the brain in which the artis-

tic, the creative element, dwells. This is where "I don't know why I thought of putting those two things together, but isn't it wonderful that I did?" comes from. Or "Don't know how I knew it, just had this weird feeling in my gut!" Music, art, dance, psychic impressions, seeing the whole picture in an instant, the symbols, the metaphors, the grasping of the fullness of the present moment, experiencing the sunset without the need to analyze its component colors or talk about it—this is the stuff of the right brain.[8]

Split-brain research indicates that we may have been correct in thinking of different sides of our bodies as being distinct in some ways. The right side of the body, controlled by the left hemisphere, dominant in most of us, is generally stronger. In French it is *droit* from which we get "adroit," meaning "skillful." In Latin it is *dexter*—"dexterity," "dexterous" in English. The left side of the body, ruled by the right hemisphere, has perennially been associated with the darker, more mysterious, aspects of the personality. The French word for "left" is *gauche*. In Latin it is *sinister*.

Research in this field is really only beginning, and much of it is seriously questioned. Nevertheless, regardless of the ultimate verdict on the subject, few would deny that most of our education was sorely lacking in "right brain" training. Some of us were lucky to get art class on Friday afternoons after the really important work of reading, writing, and arithmetic was exhausted. Those of us who did get art lessons were often asked to color between the lines, cut out the picture and paste it neatly into

our notebook—the logical, imitative approach once again.

Since wellness means an integration, we will need to start paying more attention to the right brain. Tapping the latent powers of the neglected half of ourselves will provide us with exciting new approaches to education, to creativity, and even to self healing.

Whole Brain Wellness

Over and over you hear it stated that we use only about one-tenth of the brain. If this is true, then the fraction that we do use is largely taken up with the verbal and rational business of living. Reflect upon what you have been doing in the course of this day. Chances are that most of your activities have focused around planning. communicating verbally, following directions, staying on the proper side of the road. Our educational institutions have done a reasonably good job in training us in these skills. But the question is: "At what expense?" In the feeding of the mind we have often neglected the body. In nourishing logical reasoning we have often starved our intuitive and creative faculties. We are only half alive as a result.

Attention to the neglected half means greater wellness for the whole. Encouraging signs are appearing everywhere that this knowledge is having a wide impact because it is producing results. When American business realized that worker productivity could be increased through stress-management techniques, programs to teach it began to spring up. Some of these methods require people to do very non-rational things, such as repeating a meaningless sound.

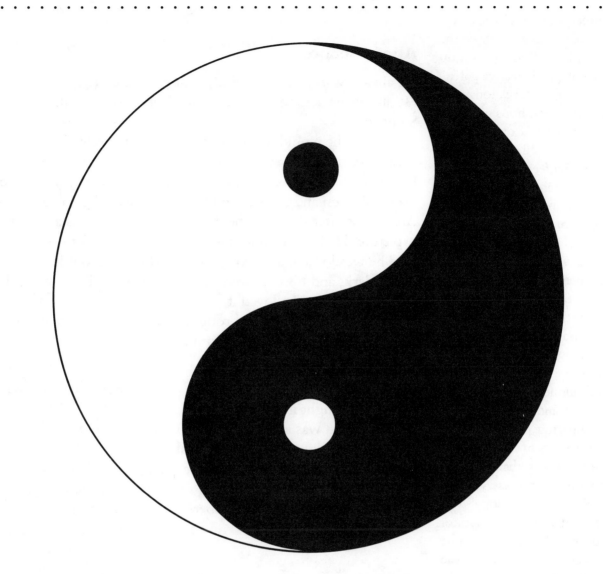

This is an ancient Chinese symbol called the T'ai-chi T'u, which means the "Diagram of the Supreme Ultimate." It is often simply called the "Yin-Yang." It is a representation of the way the world works, from an Oriental point of view. Notice first of all that it is a circle. There is no point at which it starts, no point at which it stops. Half of it is black or darkened; the other half is white or light. These areas represent the opposites—night and day; darkness and light; wet and dry; male and female; attraction and repulsion; expansion and contraction; right and left; sun and moon; heaven and earth . . . the list goes on and on. The dichotomies are separated from each other, but at the same time blend together, one flowing into the other. What it says is that the whole is made up of the opposites. The force of life, of creation, is one of dynamic tension created by the union. It is in the coming together of the male and the female that new life is created. The mysterious play between sound and silence creates the rhythm that we recognize as music, as intelligible speech. One side represents all that is scientific—the logical, rational, mathematical, the verbal. The other is the artistic—musical, intuitive, sensual, non-verbal. Put the two together in one person and you create a genius—the "erotic scientist"—the Einstein who was both physicist and poet; or more commonly, the balanced, integrated female who is both strong and gentle; the male who is both nurturing and powerful.

Quieting the "thinking" brain was found to have relaxing effects on the whole body, as well as to open up previously untapped creative potential.[9] Top-level executives today are signing up for workshops in which they meditate and exercise their way to new and livelier ideas.

Through biofeedback training, people are learning that lowering blood pressure may be as simple as imagining vapors rising from a sun-warmed lake. Migraine headaches are often relieved when the subject creates a mental picture of heat flowing into finger-tips. The practice of eurythmy, as taught in Waldorf education, involves children in learning to read by moving their bodies in a dance that corresponds with phonetic sounds. In *Superlearning*, Ostrander and Shroeder report the amazing possibilities for gaining proficiency in a foreign language, often in less than half the time previously necessary. The method called "Suggestology" was developed by a Bulgarian educator named Lozanov. Subjects, reclining in chairs, listen to vocabulary read to classical music in a unique rhythmical cadence.[10] Artistic development explodes when students are taught to draw and paint from the right side of the brain. This work is discussed and illustrated by Betty Edwards in her remarkable book *Drawing on the Right Side of the Brain*.[11] The book by Tony Buzan, *Use Your Perfect Memory*, suggests similar possibilities in other areas.[12] So what about the field of health?

Previous discussions have singled out stress as the great killer, the imbalancing condition which makes us ripe for disease and accident. Learning to calm tensions creates a state of mind which is re-

About School

He always wanted to say things. But no one understood.
He always wanted to explain things. But no one cared.
So he drew.
Sometimes he would just draw and it wasn't anything. He wanted to
　carve it in stone or write it in the sky.
He would lie out on the grass and look up in the sky and it would
　be only him and the sky and the things inside that needed saying.
And it was after that, that he drew the picture. It was a beautiful
　picture. He kept it under the pillow and would let no one see it.
And he would look at it every night and think about it. And when it
　was dark, and his eyes were closed, he could still see it. And it was
　all of him. And he loved it.
When he started school he brought it with him. Not to show any-
　one, but just to have with him like a friend.

It was funny about school.
He sat in a square, brown desk like all the other square, brown desks
　and he thought it should be red.
And his room was a square, brown room. Like all the other rooms.
　And it was tight and close. And stiff.
He hated to hold the pencil and the chalk, with his arm stiff and his
　feet flat on the floor, stiff, with the teacher watching and watching.
And then he had to write numbers. And they weren't anything. They

ceptive to healing visualizations and suggestible to new and more positive mental programs. Let's note some examples here. The Simonton approach makes use of periodic relaxation coupled with visualizations of healthy, energetic cells fighting and destroying the weaker and disorganized cancer cells.[13] In his work with children with learning disabilities, Dr. Gerald Jampolsky asks them to relax deeply, and then to "wash out" the failure pictures in their minds. The void created is filled with "success pictures," inhaled into every cell of the body. The results are dramatic. These children increased their reading ability by several grade levels in the course of a few months of such therapy.[14] Silva Mind Control, the "Power of Positive Thinking" methods, and devotional prayer, to name only a few, make use of positive-thought programs, repeated over and over while in a relaxed state. Emile Coué, a French physician in the early 1900s, the developer of auto-suggestion, recommended the phrase "Every day, in every way, I'm getting better and better!"[15] Now you may dismiss all this as being hokey, but you'd be foolish were worse than the letters that could be something if you put them together.

And the numbers were tight and square and belated the whole thing.

The teacher came and spoke to him. She told him to wear a tie like all the other boys. He said he didn't like them and she said it didn't matter.

After that they drew. And he drew all yellow and it was the way he felt about morning. And it was beautiful.

The teacher came and smiled at him. "What's this?" she said. "Why don't you draw something like Ken's drawing?

Isn't that beautiful?"

It was all questions.

After that his mother bought him a tie and he always drew airplanes and rocket ships like everyone else.

And he threw the old picture away.

And when he lay out alone looking at the sky, it was big and blue and all of everything, and he wasn't anymore.

He was square inside and brown, and his hands were stiff, and he was like anyone else. And the thing inside him that needed saying didn't need saying anymore.

It had stopped pushing. It was crushed. Stiff.

Like everything else.

—Anonymous

not to try it first. Close your eyes for a moment and slowly repeat to yourself—"Ease and peace, ease and peace, ease and peace." Try doing it for a few minutes and see if it doesn't relax you.

A humorous and appropriate variation of a childhood limerick goes: "Sticks and stones can break your bones, but words can kill you!" The *word* is not the *thing* but people behave as if they are one and the same. Labeling a child "dumb" will change his/her world dramatically. Reinforcing the "cancer is terminal" connection has speeded up the end for many.

Creative Thinking and Wellness

So many of the challenges of life are involved in getting unstuck. You may find yourself stuck in a job that is unstimulating, in a relationship which has ceased to nourish you, on a vacation which promised excitement and developed into boredom, with a headache which no longer responds to two aspirins. "Stuck" is the state of finding a brick wall in the maze, and then retracing your steps only to take the same path again. It happens because you believe your op-

tions are limited to what has worked in the past, or because you feel that you have no other alternatives. You may choose to stay there because it is safer. It is the known, the home court, the back yard. Afraid of uncertainty, ambiguity, dynamic tension, you try again and again to apply the old solutions to the new problems, and end up frustrated, or at least dissatisfied with the results. William James defines genius, or creativity, as "the faculty of perceiving in an unhabitual way." Habits can keep us stuck. Breaking habitual ways of thinking gets us unstuck. The process is essentially one of making new connections. Two previously related elements are brought together in an uncharacteristic way, and a new form emerges. Or, we open our eyes for the first time and really see something else, and we're off and running on a new track. Sandburg feels the fog and watches a cat move and writes a poem that connects the two. Picasso likes blonde women and baskets of fruit and so paints the two together. Newton gets hit on the head with an apple. You eat raspberry and tangerine ice cream and go home to repaint your bedroom in pink and orange. It happens everywhere.

When we examine some of the characteristics of the creative process we find some very strong similarities to those of the wellness process. The creative process is often ambiguous and almost always incomplete. The artist and writer and choreographer are sure that they could always do more to the work, that it could always be improved, but at some point they must declare, "enough, already" and determine to "put it on the mat," as our friend George Leonard, the author and Aikido instructor, loves to say. It is moreover a sensuous process, one that incorporates mind and body and spirit. Yeats has stated: "Art bids us touch and taste and hear and see the world, and shrinks from . . . all that is not a fountain jetting from the entire hopes, memories and sensations of the body."[16] Wonder, awe, and curiosity—those traditionally childlike qualities of mind—these are the characteristics of creative thinking. It is playful and energetic and passionate. The exact opposite of the closed, indifferent approach to life—creativity means openness and receptivity. The great achievements in both science and art have often been serendipitous. This wonderful word means the "chance" mistake which revealed a new door which wasn't seen before. For example: the laboratory is scrubbed, the technicians follow the assigned procedure, the computer is precisely programmed, the experiment is run again. Nothing! Then one day, somebody goofs, something unplanned enters the scene—mislabeled chemical, mistyped instruction, a temperature inversion in the weather outside— Surprise! "Now why didn't we think of it before?" "But of course!"

Finally, the creative process is courageous. The ability to be creative is an ability to be analytical and critical of yourself in the most positive sense of the terms. It takes knowledge of the self, an ego-strength, to be able to reveal your dreams and visions and thoughts to the world at large, to stand by them in the face of opposition. And it requires persistence to stick to

something for long periods of time, to pursue a goal without the guarantee of results.

We all possess the potential to be creative, but some of us have simply never been asked to use it, or have never tried. Learning skills of creative thinking is learning to improve ourselves and our world as well. You are invited to accept this challenge.

A New Way of Thinking—Beyond War

> The unleashed power of the atom
> has changed everything
> save our modes of thinking
> and we thus drift
> toward unparalleled catastrophe.
>
> —Albert Einstein, 1945

Our precious lives, and the fate of our planet, are at stake in every moment. The ongoing development, stockpiling, and threatened use of nuclear weapons has involved us all in a deadly game in which there can be no winners. Even if we eliminated all the weapons tomorrow, we would only have bought ourselves some time. We will always know how to build nuclear weapons. We will always be able to discover new weapons if we want them. The only permanent solution is to change our thinking to see that war of any kind is no longer an acceptable method for resolving conflict.

The Beyond War movement began in 1982 as a grassroots response to the need for a change of heart, and a change of thinking. The commitment to building a world beyond war involves a hard look at the war-making we still carry on in our individual lives, where we are creating "enemies," and the core issue of our oneness—our connection—with all life. We are one planet, one energy, and we share one future.

One individual will make the difference. You are that individual.

For information about Beyond War, and to find out about Beyond War activities in your area, contact: Beyond War, 222 High St., Palo Alto, CA 94301, (415) 328-7756.

Brainstorming

Brainstorming is a thinking process which helps in unsticking. It allows you to tap into your own internal resources, to recall previous experiences, to remember past successes, to fantasize new connections, in short, to play with possibilities without judgment. You can always discard the impractical and unworkable, but without more data you will easily fall back into old patterns, hoping that maybe *this* time they might work out. Here's how it works.

First: formulate a question, or state your problem as simply as possible. "What can I do on my summer vacation this year?" or "How can I cut down on my smoking?" or "I hate my job." *Second*: let go of the need to come up with the "right answer" or the logical, least expensive, or easiest alternative. *Third*: use any effective method for getting yourself relaxed—some deep breathing exercises, a walk in the woods, the visualization of a crystal clear lake, some vigorous exercise. *Fourth*: tape record or write down every suggestion or answer that comes into your head. Doing this with a friend will allow you to speak freely, while the other simply lists what you say. DO NOT JUDGE any suggestion. Do not reject any idea for being dead wrong, silly, impractical, too expensive . . . whatever. *Fifth*: continue throwing out ideas as fast as you can for a limited period of time—say five minutes. This will force you to think fast, and will help to eliminate evaluation. *Sixth*: put the material away. Let it rest, simmer, gestate for a while. *Finally*: go back and review your data with new eyes and an open mind. What surprises you? What delights you? What hits you hard? What elements can be combined? Which ones are possible, and easy? Which ones generate new ones? Which ones are worth a try?

Here are some of the responses generated around the question,

Regina's Wart Removal System

A number of years ago I was bothered by three or four unsightly warts which had developed on my knee. During a routine physical exam, my doctor had written me a prescription for a chemical wart remover. I never used it. I was convinced that I could use the power of creative visualization to get rid of them, and I did within three weeks of time. Here's how.

Twice a day, once in the morning and once at my evening meditation, I formed a mental picture of the wart, and then imagined taking a large pencil with a soft, pink eraser and gently erasing the warts—a layer of skin at a time. After doing this for about a minute, I would stroke my other knee to remember how the skin should feel. Then I would picture the "wounded knee" in a state of perfection—the warts gone, the skin soft and smooth. Finally, I repeated to myself several times: "My warts are melting away, layer by layer. Every day they are becoming smaller."

It worked.

I have also used visualization most effectively in dealing with an occasional bout of stomach flu, and to alleviate the nausea that I frequently get on airplanes. I "see" my stomach as it feels—green-brown slime dripping from its walls. Then I create a bucket of clear peppermint liquid (like the white creme de menthe that I love). I take a wide, imaginary paintbrush and proceed to paint the stomach lining. I do this slowly, remembering what it is like to paint a fence. As I do it, I keep one hand on my stomach to keep myself focused here. I breathe slowly and fully at the same time. This technique has "saved my life" on very many occasions. I recommend it highly.

P.S. Just before this book went to press, Vicki, one of my students, reported that it worked for her. She had warts all over her fingers and they did not respond to any traditional treatment. Using this visualization method for three months she eliminated them.

"How can I make more time for myself?"

get up earlier	turn back the clocks
go to bed later	buy a dishwasher
unplug the phone	hire a maid
hire a babysitter	shop by phone
quit my job	go on strike
eliminate one meal a day	overlook the mess
break the television	organize the house better

Affirmations

An affirmation is a verbal description of a desired condition. You state your desire for the future in terms of the present, as if the result had already been achieved. You say, "My skin is clear and healthy," not "My rash is getting better" or "My face is going to clear up." Then you use the affirmation to create reality.

Clearly state the full outcome you want, paying no attention to how it will come about. The good which is yours will come to you in perfect timing, in perfect, and often totally unexpected, ways. It is as if you were planting a seed. The seed will germinate and sprout when it is ready to, and it will be what it was meant to be. So do not restrain yourself when making affirmations. Abundance is the natural state of the universe; you are free to change your attitudes from a scarcity consciousness to a state of abundant, positive expectation. Prosperity in money, friendship, health, and opportunities for creative expression comes to those who are willing to have it.

It's important to be very specific in the making of your affirmations—otherwise you may get something very different from what you expected, e.g., "I am prompt" may result in your arriving on time but skipping breakfast or getting a speeding ticket. "I am easily on time" would better state your desired result. Someone who was affirming he had a Rolls Royce in his life, got it by having it crash through his living room window. You might conclude your affirmation with the phrase "I now create this or something better."

How To Do It
1. Write, print or type affirmations on a piece of paper, and read them each evening before you go to bed, and the next morning when you get up.

Brainstorming is a good way of unmasking the hidden needs that are manifesting themselves as health problems. As we have asserted in previous chapters, it is not enough to treat the symptoms. You need to find out *why* you have the problem in the first place, too; you need to interpret the body's messages.

Start by asking yourself, "Why . . . ?" "Why do I have a cold now?" "Why did I sprain my ankle?" "Why does my back ache?"

And proceed from there. Answers may generate new questions—answer them. Questions can be repeated until that lead is exhausted.

Q. Why am I so fat?

A. I eat too much.

Q. Why do I eat so much?

A. Food tastes good . . .
I'm hungry . . . I like being served . . . I like the company . . .

Once you've brainstormed and set the answer aside for a while, reviewing the material may furnish you with valuable clues to your real needs and wants. Don't neglect to use material from your dreams, too. With a little practice and attention (see chapter 12), these nightly brainstorms are readily available for your conscious use. Brainstorming is a powerful way of practicing self-responsibility and taking charge of your life.

Brainstorming a Big Question

If you can accept that your thinking is creating your reality—can you also accept that it is helping create the planetary reality as well?

Fear can be contagious. As it is

2. Imagine a picture in your head of the desired end result happening right now, with you in the picture enjoying it.

3. Paste the affirmation on your mirror, car dashboard, telephone, billfold, and anywhere that you might see it during the day.

4. Chant or sing your affirmations aloud while working, driving, playing, or meditating.

5. Write your favorite affirmation ten times in the first person: "I, Jackie, am radiantly healthy." Then write it ten times in the second person: "You, Jackie, are radiantly healthy." Then write it ten times in the third person: "Jackie is radiantly healthy."

6. Record you affirmations in your own voice and listen to the recording while doing chores, driving in your car, or while going to sleep. This can be very powerful.

7. Make a magnet map. This is a pictorial representation of the desired change which will serve as a magnet to bring about that reality. Using a piece of poster-board, paste on your map brightly colored pictures from magazines (or draw them) and write one or two affirmations on it. Always include a smiling or "good-mood" picture of yourself and a personal spiritual symbol which may be labeled as "source." The spiritual symbol is a reminder that your desire is in harmony with your higher self, and in harmony with the "greater good," cosmic plan, etc. Place the magnet map where you'll see it every day, and watch for results.

For greater detail and background on this age-old technique, consult *Creative Visualization* by Shakti Gawain in the reading list at the end of this chapter.

---

shared with more and more people, panic can result. Panicked people do various things—like selling all their stocks, or arming themselves, or committing murder—things that can affect increasingly larger circles of other people. A "group mind" about an issue becomes an overwhelmingly powerful force. If folks believe that Communists are everywhere, they will find them everywhere, as happened in the early 1950s in the U.S. If we believe that war is inevitable, poverty is unconquerable, cancer is incurable, we easily lose heart in attempting to do anything about them. We feed our feelings of inadequacy and impotency, in the face of unsolvable problems, conditions over which we think we have no control. Thinking, then, molds the reality we will all experience.

What would happen if tomorrow millions of people across the globe started thinking that hunger could be eliminated? What would education be like if thousands of teachers across the country accepted the unique beauty and innate wisdom of each child? Skeptics among us may scoff at these idealistic dreams, and immediately challenge "How?"—and

The universe begins to look more like a great thought than a machine.

—SIR JAMES JEANS

"how" is a very important question. But it is misplaced when it is asked first. The "hows" flow from our beliefs. A better question is "What—What are my beliefs?"—since *what* you believe will play a primary role in determining your way of being and working in the world.

Lateral Thinking

Edward DeBono, Ph.D., has devoted his life's work to the study of the thinking process. His term "lateral thinking" describes a process that attempts to counteract the limitations and errors of logical thinking, but not to replace it—a way of rearranging available information to form a new and better pattern. Others have called it "creative thinking," or, more recently, "right brain thinking." Here are some examples:

Random Input: DeBono says, "A random input from outside can serve to disrupt the old pattern and allow it to reform in a new way." For instance, you could take your question to a variety store, a circus, or an art museum, or try opening a dictionary, Bible, or book of facts at random . . . and look for connections. Intrigued? Try it.

Quotas: We often limit ourselves by wrongly imagining that there is only "one right answer." To use "quotas" means to challenge yourself to come up with a minimal number of alternatives, giving yourself the pressure of a limited deadline, for example, ten minutes of concentrated time.

Rotation of Attention: The man who tries every new diet fad in his attempt to lose weight is placing all of his attention on the one connection of food and flab! One element will naturally monopolize our energy in any given situation unless we consciously attend to the less dramatic, or subsidiary ones. Make *each factor* in the problem or question the focus of attention and learn as much as you can by examining it as if it were the only one.

Reversals: Sometimes it helps to turn a situation completely upside down in order to see it from a different point of view. Often we are not sure of what we want, but are very clear about what we don't want. ("I don't want to have to do dishes every day." "I don't want the full responsibility for the cars." "I get too tired cooking all the meals," etc.) To answer the question of what we want our social club to be—we might do better by listing the things we don't want it to be. In response to the question of what wellness is, we may learn a lot by asking ourselves what we are sure that it is not.

Cross-fertilization: This step involves getting input from a variety of other sources, books and people. Sometimes it is most helpful to talk to someone who holds the opposite opinion to the one you support. Ideas generate ideas. The more input you have, the more discriminating you can become in your choices.[17]

Suggested Reading*

Brown, B. *Between Health and Illness: New Notions on Stress and the Nature of the Body.* New York, NY: Bantam Books, 1984.

Bry, A., with Bair, M. *Directing the Movies of Your Mind.* New York, NY: Harper and Row, 1978.

Castillo, G. *Left Handed Teaching.* New York, NY: Praeger Publishers, 1974.

DeBono, E. *Lateral Thinking.* New York, NY: Harper and Row, 1973.

Edwards, B. *Drawing on the Right Side of the Brain.* Los Angeles, CA: J.P. Tarcher/St. Martin's Press, 1979.

Gawain, S. *Creative Visualization.* New York, NY: Bantam Books, 1982.

Keyes, K. *The Handbook to Higher Consciousness.* Coos Bay, OR: Living Love Publications, 1975.

Lecron, L. *Self Hypnotism: The Technique and Its Use in Daily Living.* Englewood Cliffs, NJ: Prentice-Hall, 1964.

Maltz, M. *Psycho-Cybernetics.* New York, NY: Simon and Schuster, 1960.

Ornstein, R. *The Psychology of Consciousness.* San Francisco, CA: W.H. Freeman, 1972.

Ostrander, S., and Schroeder, L. *Superlearning.* New York, NY: Delacorte Press/Confucian Press, 1979.

Peale, N. *The Power of Positive Thinking.* New York, NY: Fawcett, 1978.

*This is only a representative sampling. Many excellent books have been omitted. At the bookstore or library, look over the whole selection and choose according to your judgment.

Pelletier, K. *Mind as Healer, Mind as Slayer.* New York, NY: Delta, 1975.

Samples, B. *The Metaphoric Mind.* Reading, MA: Addison-Wesley Publishing Co., 1976.

Samuels, M., and Samuels, N. *Seeing with the Mind's Eye.* New York, NY, and Berkeley, CA: Random House/Bookworks, 1975.

Von Oech, R. *A Whack on the Side of the Head: How to Unlock Your Mind for Innovation.* New York, NY: Warner Books, 1983.

Wonder, J., and Donovan, P. *Whole Brain Thinking.* New York, NY: Ballantine Books, 1984.

· ·

The Hunger Project

In October, 1977, I encountered an unusual and creative use of thought energy. A program called the Hunger Project was being introduced by Werner Erhard to several thousand people in San Francisco. I went because of my concern about world hunger, even though I did not believe the problem had any solution.

The program was long and detailed, but one idea stood out above all—that big changes can be brought about by just a few people. The "idea" of the Hunger Project was that if 100,000 people really believed that hunger could be ended by the close of the century, that "thought-form" would catalyze the necessary technical, political, and economic changes. What was called for first was a change in attitude. We were reminded that the Marshall Plan, which helped reconstruct Europe after World War II, was initiated by about 100 people.

In the years since the project began, millions of persons have enrolled in it. Through its newspaper, *A Shift in the Wind*, it has publicized the Cambodian famine problem and kept members informed of other current developments, all to good effect. Using the theme "There is nothing more powerful than an idea whose time has come," my hunger project (taking personal responsibility for the project is important) is working, and I enjoy sharing it with over 5 million other people.

An information packet on the project is available from the Hunger Project, Box 789, San Francisco, CA 94101. —J.W.T.

· ·

Notes

1. Schiff, J., et al. *Cathexis Reader.* New York, NY: Harper and Row, 1975.

2. Many new books from a variety of disciplines speak to this age-old hypothesis. For further reading:

Jampolsky, G. *Love Is Letting Go of Fear.* Berkeley, CA: Celestial Arts, 1979.

Wolf, F.A. *Taking the Quantum Leap.* New York, NY: Harper and Row, 1981.

Attack and Defense

When we perceive another person as "attacking" us we usually feel defensive, and find a way, directly or indirectly, to "attack" back. Attacking always stems from fear and guilt. No one attacks unless he first feels threatened and believes that through attack he can demonstrate his own strength, at the expense of another's vulnerability. As with all defenses, which are designed to keep guilt and fear from our awareness, attack actually preserves the problem.

Most of us cling to the belief that "attacking" can really get us something we want. We seem to forget that "attacking" and "defending" do not bring us inner peace.

In order to experience peace instead of conflict it is necessary to shift our perception. Instead of seeing others as attacking us, we can see them as fearful. We are always expressing either love or fear. Fear is really a call for help, and therefore a request for love. It is apparent, then, that to experience peace we must recognize that we do not have a choice in determining what we perceive.

Many of our attempts to "correct" others, even when we believe we are offering constructive criticism, are really attempts to attack them by demonstrating their "wrongness" and our "rightness." It may be helpful to examine our motivations. Are we teaching love or are we demonstrating attack?

If others do not change in accordance with our expectations, we are likely to regard them as guilty, and thus reinforce our own belief in guilt. Peace of mind comes from not wanting to change others but by merely accepting them as they are. True acceptance is always without demands and expectations.

From *To Give Is To Receive,*
Mini-Course for Healing Relationships.
Gerald G. Jampolsky, M.D., Tiburon, CA

The Love Project

Another creative and successful use of thought energy was manifested at Brooklyn's Jefferson High School in 1970. After several futile years of teaching at this inner city school, Arleen Lorrance decided to confront the violence and fear of students and teachers around her with love. She and a small group of students developed six principles, shared them with others, and began to practice them. Here is what they proposed:

- Be the change you want to see happen, instead of trying to change everyone else.

- Receive all persons as beautiful exactly where they are.

- Provide people with opportunities to give.

- Perceive problems as opportunities.

- Have no expectations, but rather, abundant expectancy.

- Create your own reality consciously, rather than living as if you had no control over your life.

The result of thinking in these ways, even by a few people, had dramatic effects. It caught on! Much of the hate and fear in the environment faded. People were inspired. Love had triumphed.

For more on the subject write The Love Project, Box 7601, San Diego, CA 92107.

Ferguson, M. *The Aquarian Conspiracy.* Los Angeles, CA: J.P. Tarcher/St. Martin's Press, 1980.

3. For a good introduction to biofeedback research and training see:

Pelletier, K. *Mind as Healer, Mind as Slayer.* New York, NY: Delta, 1975.

Brown, B. *New Mind, New Body.* New York, NY: Harper and Row, 1974.

Green, E., and Green, A. *Beyond Biofeedback.* New York, NY: Delacorte Press 1977.

Peper, E. *Mind/Body Integration.* New York, NY: Random House, 1977.

4. For more about Luria see:

Luria, A. *The Mind of a Mnemonist.* New York, NY: Basic Books, 1968.

5. Hutschnecker, A. *The Will to Live.* New York, NY: Cornerstone Library, rev. ed. 1972, p. 24.

6. See: Ornstein, R. *The Psychology of Consciousness.* 2nd ed. New York, NY: Harcourt Brace Jovanovich, 1977, p.71.

7. See: *Altered States of Consciousness.* Tart, C., ed. Garden City, NY: Anchor Books, Doubleday and Co., 1972. pp. 48–74.

8. A clear introduction to "split-brain" research and its implications is found in:

Ornstein, R. *The Psychology of Consciousness.*

2nd ed. New York, NY: Harcourt Brace Jovanovich, 1977, pp. 16–39.

9. Green, A., Green, E., and Walters, E. "Psychological Training for Creativity." Paper presented at the annual meeting of the American Psychological Association. September 7, 1971. (Menninger Foundation, Topeka, KS.)

Richardson, A. *Mental Imagery.* New York, NY: Springer Publishing Co., 1969.

Kamiya, J. "Conscious Control of Brain Waves." *Psychology Today* 1:57–60, 1968.

Adrain, L. *Creativity in Science: Discussion on Scientific Creativity.* Third World Conference of Psychiatry 1:41–44, 1961.

Holt, R. R. "Imagery: The Return of the Ostracized." *American Psychologist* 19:254–64, 1964.

Green, A.; Green, E.; and Walters, E. *Brain Wave Training, Imagery, Creativity and Integrative Experiences.* NIMH, Grant #20730.

Research Department, Menninger Foundation, Topeka, KS. (Paper presented to Biofeedback Research Society Conference, February 1974, by Alyce Green.

Fadely, J.L. *Understanding the Alpha Child at Home and School.* Springfield, IL: Charles C. Thomas, Publisher, Banner Stone House, 1979.

10. Ostrander, S.; Ostrander, N.; and Shroeder, L. *Superlearning.* New York, NY: Delacorte Press/Confucian Press, Inc., 1979.

11. Edwards, B. *Drawing on the Right Side of the Brain.* Los Angeles, CA: J.P. Tarcher/St. Martin's Press, 1979.

12. Rico, G.L. *Writing the Natural Way.* Los Angeles, CA: J.P. Tarcher, 1983.

Buzan T. *Use Your Perfect Memory: A Complete Program of New Techniques for Remembering.* New York, NY: E.P. Dutton, 1984.

13. Simonton, O.C.; Matthews-Simonton, S.; and Creighton, J. *Getting Well Again.* Los Angeles, CA: J.P. Tarcher, 1978.

14. Jampolsky, G., and Haight, M. "A Special Suggestive and Auto-Suggestive Technique Used in Helping Certain Children with Reading Problems." *Academic Therapy,* San Rafael, CA, Winter 1974.

15. For an explanation of Coué's work read:

LeCron, L. *Self Hypnotism.* Englewood Cliffs, NJ: Prentice-Hall, 1964 pp. 69–71.

16. Yeats, W. B. *Essays and Introductions.* New York, NY: Macmillan Publishing Co., 1961, pp. 292–93.

17. DeBono, E. *The Mechanism of Mind.* Baltimore, MD: Penguin Books, 1969, pp. 243–45.

......Eight......

Wellness and Playing/Working

> Playing and Working are complex combinations of more basic forms of energy. Work is focused energy directed towards a goal. Playing is a similar kind of energy, except that it may have no specific goal. Both involve the energy of thinking, communicating and moving. It is in work and play that human beings most commonly interact with one another and their environment, produce goods and services, and structure their time and thus their lives.

. . . .

WORK AND PLAY are the stuff of our lives. Almost all your waking hours are spent doing one or the other. Because these activities are so dynamically connected with self-concept, a sense of meaning and purpose, and, in some cases, with your very survival, they are strong determinants of wellness. If there are significant, ongoing problems in either work-life or play, your state of health will usually reflect it. The list of stress-related diseases grows daily. And many of us are employed in highly stressful jobs. Moreover, we can hardly be living life to the fullest if we have no energy with which to play, no inclination for simply "fooling around."

As we begin our exploration of playing and working, let us make it clear that the two are not necessarily separate categories of activity. What is play to one may be work to another (compare a sandlot baseball game to a major league game, for instance). Some people don't consider their jobs as work at all, because they enjoy them so much. And others make a chore out of their recreation.

. . . .

Life's door, love's door, God's door—they all open when you are playful. They all become closed when you become serious.
—BHAGWAN SHREE RAJNEESH

. . . .

In any case, rather than changing *what* you do for work or play, it is increased awareness and a change in attitude that is important. You may want to stop long enough to examine the roles working and playing take in your life. If they do not enhance it, you may want to make some changes.

Redefining Play

The dictionary refers to play as recreation. This is a very significant word. Capitalize it, hyphenate it and it becomes *Re-Creation*. This is play in the fullest sense of the term: to make new, to vitalize again, to inspire with life and energy. This is "creativity" at its best. Everything that does this is play.

Playing is a form of self-nourishment. Playing is not something you do. It is rather an *attitude* you create at any time, in any place, which transforms the mundane into the divine, the boring into the joyful, the required into the desired, and the present moment into a sacrament.

Take a moment to identify the words that are associated with play: laughter, frolic, fun, sports, crazy, exciting . . . and lots of other

A Different Approach

We got together on a brilliant, sunny day in early December, to work up our ideas about playing. Books assembled, piles of writing paper, pens in hand. We had invited our friend Ken Maue to share the task with us. Ken is one of the most creative people we know—a master of play. His book *Water in the Lake* is a collection of pieces which individuals or groups can play. He had agreed to compose some for our purposes. Ken walked leisurely up the path to John's house at precisely the appointed time. We were ready! There was only one minor problem—none of us wanted to work. The sun kept distracting us. We wanted to play in it—faces, arms, weary back muscles. Not to mention the fragrance of green things. The earth was coming back to life after dry days of summer and autumn. We wanted to be there when it happened. John left for a short while and then called us out onto the deck. He had constructed a place to play—sleeping mats and pillows arranged to form a cocoon-like space. Removing our shoes and socks and jackets we settled into our private playground. We held hands, eyes closed, minds and hearts open. Words and phrases started emerging. We decided that we would remember them—there was no need to write anything down. We told stories. Shared jokes. Babbled like babies. Massaged feet. Said and did whatever came to mind. It was delightful. Lots of good things happened. We accomplished our tasks. We had a great time. We gave ourselves permission to work this way more often. We attracted others into our nurturing space. Their ideas sparked more in us. What follows in this chapter reflects the process.

similarly active words. But play can also be described as absorbing, fascinating, peaceful, beautiful, flowing, restful. Perhaps one of the reasons we don't play more is that we have defined play inadequately. We have looked around at what the society tells us is "fun" to do, and accepted this as the meaning of play. We have remembered our childhood and have sought out swings and slides to give us pleasure. We have forgotten natural abilities we had for enjoying a rock, an abandoned tire, a cardboard box. We frequently consider play as the opposite of work, thus solidifying the dichotomy between the two. Play is given a back seat to purposeful, "meaningful" activity. It is something to be done after hours, or on week-ends, or with children. And it frequently costs a lot. Mary recently posted a list of goals for the new year on her bathroom mirror. One of them was to save more money so that she could do "fun things." This attitude is far from uncommon. Many people are frustrated during their vacation periods and only too glad to get back home. They have accepted the notions that play is something you do, some place to go, an expensive camper or piece of sporting equipment. When it doesn't prove "fun" for them they feel disappointed and out of sorts. ("What's wrong with me, anyway?")

What has happened to us in our maturation process that makes adult play so different from child's play? Let's reflect upon this for a moment.

Our Children—The Natural and the Adapted

No, we don't mean "adopted"—we mean adapted. Transactional Analysis (T.A.) refers to that emotional, fun-loving, and mischievous part of our personalities as the Child ego state.[1] This Child has two faces, two modes of being. One manifests spontaneity about life. It delights. It screams. It loves. It hates. And it does it all easily. This is the Natural Child. The other is dependent upon parental approval and will do just about anything to secure it. The "parents" may be Dad and Mom, or teachers in school, or friends on the playground, who send messages either directly or indirectly about how they want the little person to behave. To be accepted, the child must and will adapt. This Adapted Child performs. It obeys. It agrees. It works to incorporate the many and often conflicting parental mes-

It takes one a long time to become young.

—PABLO PICASSO

Exercise

The Play Report—What I'm Sure Of . . .

Introduction: Sometimes it is easier to say what you don't want, than it is to know what you do want. This exercise will challenge you to assert what you're sure *is not* fun for you, and hopefully motivate you to realize what *is.*

I AM SURE THAT THESE ARE NOT FUN, PLAYFUL, ENJOYABLE FOR ME: (be sure to include activities that other people do that you do not care to do)

example: parachuting from an airplane
    (Barbara thinks it's great, Regina is terrified
    by the thought.)
stock car racing
going out drinking
going shopping

I AM SURE THAT THESE ARE FUN, PLAYFUL, ENJOYABLE FOR ME:

example: shopping for new clothes
receiving a letter from a friend
going out for breakfast
taking a sauna

---

sages in order that it may be a "good boy" or a "good girl."

The individual matures, but the "children" don't leave home. Each of us can find them at work within ourselves no matter how grown up we may have become. One of the areas in which we can see their influences very strongly is on the playground. So much of adult play, or lack of play, is a manifestation of Adapted Child behavior and messages. When the Adapted Child plays there is often:

- a time schedule

- competition

- organization

- a specific environment (football field, dance floor)

- costumes and equipment (from jogging suits to hang-gliders)

- doing it *right*

- huffing and puffing

- seriousness (since after all we *should* take time to play)

- a reward for working hard.

We will examine two of these common characteristics which can create problems out of play—the emphasis on competition and the attitude of seriousness. Both have strong bearings on wellness.

Competition

If you operate from the philosophy that all of life is a game in which

New games with new rules, more in tune with the times, games in which there are no spectators and no second-string players, games for a whole family and a whole day, games in which aggression fades into laughter—new games.

—GEORGE LEONARD
THE ULTIMATE ATHLETE

some people come out winners, then it follows that some people must come out losers. From our earliest years we are taught the connection between playing and games. Children soon learn that winning means bettering someone

Your Child

One of the most important reasons for being alive is the child within us all. Without the sense of wonder, the excitement, the emotions—happy and sad, angry and afraid—life is hardly worth living.

There is a child within each of us crying out:

"Listen! I am sick and tired of being ignored day after day. You go to work, out with your friends, to sleep, to eat, live your life as if I do not exist. Every once in a while you notice me when you are depressed or home sick in bed. But do you really care about me? Do you really ask what I want?

"Here I am sitting around waiting, forever waiting for you to recognize me. First your parents began ignoring parts of me and gradually you continued where your parents left off.

"Remember me? I am your feelings, your dreams and fantasies. I am the one who used to enjoy going to the park. I am the one who likes pizza, candy, mountains, sunshine, and who wants to play: I am also the one who likes to be held and told he is loved: I am the child within you, *I am you.*

"I don't care if you are an adult now. Why does that mean you have to forget about me? Why can't adults enjoy themselves as children do? Why must being an adult mean that the child in you must try not to exist?

"Believe me, living in your adult world of constant struggle is not easy. How do you think I feel when you stuff me with lots of food during dinner while you talk with your important friends, people you really don't like?

"Where am I supposed to go when I am angry and you don't recognize me? Then you wonder why you have indigestion or weight problems.

"Where do you think your problems come from?

"I know you need your important friends. I know you have to make a living. I know you have to take care of others. But have you ever thought if you really became *my* friend, you wouldn't need some things from others so much?

"Have you ever thought that if you took care of your feelings and appreciated your little desires that you wouldn't need so much income to appease me? Have you ever thought that if you were nicer to *yourself,* taking care of others would not be so much of a burden.

"I know you are trying to get a better position so you will have more time to be with me. I have felt the different therapies you have tried which reintroduce you to parts of me. But I want you to know *all* of me. I am tired of others pushing and shoving, fishing around for me. I want you to know *me.*

"I don't expect you to change overnight. I have been waiting for you to recognize me long enough. To be honest, a part of me will never understand how you can treat me the way you do. Why is it so difficult for you to be as you want?

"If I was literally your child, you would listen to me and care how I am. Well, I am literally *your child,* you have just learned not to see *me.*"

From *The Magical Child Within You*[2]
Used with permission

or something else. And winning is praised, rewarded. Losing means being bettered. And losing is failure, inadequacy, making wrong moves; it is undesirable.

The link between playing and competition is a strong one. Competition means rivalry, challenge, and excitement. But it may also mean cheating, pressure, putting down the opponent, agreeing to the decisions of referees, and the privilege of the skillful few. It is sad to realize that much physical education being taught in schools involves training children to take part in competitive sports. And few will ever engage in these in later life.

New Games means everyone playing their hardest and as well as they can—just for the fun of it . . . New Games means the players can shape the games . . . New Games means we can play together more easily knowing we care about each other's safety . . . When a game is fun for everyone, we all win together.[3]

—NEW GAMES
FOUNDATION

The other side of competition is cooperation. We recognize it as an essential part of the curriculum of our education programs and all of life. We ask our children to work together, and reprimand them when they fail to share their things. It is little wonder that they are often confused. The messages they get are so often contradictory to them. "Win this." "Help others with that." "Win that, but share it with the rest of us when you do." As adults we can appreciate that competition and cooperation need not be antagonistic. Young children don't see it quite so clearly.

Defining play as competition, as so many of us do, is not only limiting, but is actually harmful. The attitude that "if I'm not good enough to make the team, I'm not good enough" pervades our lives—in our business and economic affairs; in our education; in our politics; in our modes of recreation. When we achieve our self-concept by contrast with the skills and abilities of others, by judging ourselves by the rules that society has set up, by comparing ourselves with our parents, brothers, sisters and friends, it is very easy to come up wanting. And most of us do it

all the time. "Be the first, the strongest, the best and the brightest." "Too bad, you didn't make it." "You lose."

The pressures that result from playing in this dog-eat-dog world, the realm of cut-throat competition, encourage a wide range of stress-related ailments and are often climaxed with suicide or heart attack. We need to take a good, hard look at these "old games" if we are to survive and flourish individually as well as collectively. But, at the same time, we must be careful of compounding these "serious" problems by getting more serious. The opposite of play is not work. The opposite of play is excessive seriousness.

Seriousness

The weight of the burden is the seriousness with which we take our separate and individual selves.

—THOMAS MERTON

This job of becoming more healthy and moving towards greater wellness is serious stuff. Or so we have been led to believe. Just take a look at some of the books which deal with the subject. (Not to mention the somber pictures of their authors.) What you frequently find are predictions of dire consequences for failure to follow their methods; horror stories of what certain foods, or lack of vitamins, or traditional techniques can do to you; lists of do's and don'ts and diets; warnings about the cancer-causing qualities of this and that and the other thing. It's enough to make you crazy!

And the subject of health is not the only one to be taken "seriously." The same attitudes and beliefs permeate our approaches to religion, education, family-affairs, politics—our whole approach to life in general. Everybody is giving us the same message—"You've really got to start taking this more seriously!" And we do—and that is probably the main cause of our problems.

Seriousness breeds anxiety and creates the tension which is one of the chief causes of the problems we experience in body, mind, and spirit. Seriousness is the parent of fear, and fear is a deadly child. Seriousness is the generator of judgment. It demands that we assign meaning to mystery, that we leave no question unanswered, that we catalogue, evaluate, and institutionalize every aspect of our lives. Even if we are playing we've got to get serious and play hard, always try to win, and above all—do it right.

Whatever breaks undue seriousness opens us to play and to the revitalization that play brings. Bearing that in mind, you may want to try out some of these strategies for breaking seriousness:

"Give Me A Break!"— Strategies for Breaking Seriousness

1. *"Give me a break!"* Choose a humorous phrase which helps you to lighten up, to keep things in perspective. Use it often. (When Regina was anxiously pursuing her college training as a young nun in the convent, she was deadly serious about her studies. Her novice mistress,

Mother Genevieve, used to remark: "Keep it up Regina. You'll be the smartest nun in the graveyard.")

2. *The President on the Toilet technique:* Our fears and anxieties around other people frequently result because we hold the other in higher esteem than we hold ourselves. Remembering that we are all "just folks" may be as easy as conjuring up a picture of the other performing the most mundane of operations, those which everybody has to do. (Or as Mamie used to say to Dwight:—"Ike, for God's sake, will you take out the garbage!")

3. *Mirror, Mirror:* For some people the simple act of looking in the mirror is enough to break a serious mood. Look at the wrinkles you are forming. Mothers frequently tell children: "Watch out or your face will freeze that way." Now make ridiculous faces at yourself. Just try to keep from smiling!

4. *Monkey Meditation:* There is a marvelous Zen Buddhist technique which suggests that first thing in the morning you jump out of bed and spend ten minutes assuming the most absurd postures you can achieve. This is enhanced by laughing at yourself the whole time. Try it.

5. *Get Off My Back:* This exercise is good for you not only emotionally, but physically as well. Form hands into fists, bring them together at the center of your chest. Raise your elbows, on a line with your fists. Thrust elbows back, expanding your

---

Finding Humor Everywhere: (Because Life Is and People Really Are Funny!)

From: The Police Log of the *Greeley Tribune*, Greeley, Colorado.

2:00 p.m.
Persons reported a dead sheep was lying on the roof of a house; residents of house had bought a sheepskin and were drying it out.

10:41 p.m.
Report of kids writing obscene words on the street; most of the words were misspelled.

2:10 p.m.
Vehicle enroute to junk yard fell apart in street; wrecker called.

11:11 p.m.
Report of a man going door-to-door with a beer can and asking for donations.

3:23 p.m.
Man reported his ex-wife pulled his hair a week ago.

12:27 p.m.
Report of horn honking continuously; officer found man had fallen asleep on his car's horn.

12:01 p.m.
Woman reported she was walking on the sidewalk when a man ran up, grabbed her breast and ran away; the incident occurred two weeks ago.

3:25 p.m.
Report of a man who got mad and is attempting to walk home to Greeley from Cheyenne, Wyoming.

3:36 p.m.
Man reported girls were throwing grapes at his car.

3:54 p.m.
Man reported someone took his dog, but left the collar and $20.00.

12:16 a.m.
Report of three persons wearing only aluminum foil and running in front of cars.

---

chest and drawing shoulder blades together. As you do so briskly for several minutes say to yourself, or scream out loud, "Get off my back!" Imagine that you are releasing all the heavy burdens which have been weighing you down—persons, jobs, fears, etc.

6. *Screaming in the 20 MPH Zone:* Roll up the windows of your car and scream, rant and rave at the top of your lungs. Or take a drive in the country with windows open and scream as loud as you can.

7. *Dance Off:* Put on the wildest music you can find. Dance until you exhaust your seriousness. (Also good for weight control and breathing.)

8. *Poor Pitiful Pearl:* Exaggerate your mood, or your fears, to the point of absurdity. Dress up. Act out the most pitiful, burdened, suffering creature you can become. Give yourself

a name. Ask someone to take your picture. Carry this picture in your wallet at all times!

9. *Red-Flag Technique:* This is a method for talking yourself out of getting more serious when you realize that you are on the way. The dialogue:

Helen: Hey Helen, haven't you been down this road before?

Herself: Yes, many times.

Helen: Then you remember where it leads?

Herself: Only too well.

Helen: You realize what a dead-end it is?

Herself: I sure do!

Helen: Do you really want to take it again, knowing what you know?

Herself: No! Let's go make some cookies (or take a shower, or . . .)

10. *Take off all your clothes:* Look at yourself in a full-length mirror. Now take a shower and wash off your seriousness.

The Natural Child Plays

. . . .

The way to reconnect with our purpose is to do things that seem, at first appearance, to lack purpose . . .

—KENNETH MAUE

. . . .

Learning to play again means getting in touch with your Natural Child. When the Natural Child plays, it plays with everything. Picture it:

- joyful experimentation with life

- fascination with anything in its environment—a bumblebee, a ray of sunlight

- unlimited reign of the imagination

- trying out various behaviors; imitation of others

- "being" everything—an airplane, a famous ballerina,

- learning consequences in a protected, nourishing environment

- freedom to be silly, fantastic, wrong . . .

There is no work in the child's world. All is playing, and playing is learning, and playing and learning are fun.

Self-Nourishment: The Healing Qualities of Play

Almost everybody suffers some guilt for taking time for themselves. We are often embarrassed by our enjoyment of pleasure and need to justify it to ourselves and others. Some place deep inside we harbor old tapes which we persist in playing over and over. They say things like; "You're wasting time!" or "Watch out when things are going well," or "This is selfish," or "You *should* be doing something more productive." They have come to us from our parents, our religious leaders, our work-crazed culture, our school teachers. And they are often hard to turn off.

Well, if the fact remains that you need justification to allow yourself to play then try this one:

Nourishment of yourself is the best preventive medicine currently available!

From all sides we are constantly being challenged: Change! Grow! Move! Volunteer! Contribute! Boycott! Picket! Diet! Exercise! But in order to respond to challenge we must have the energy to follow through. The way to gain this energy is to allow yourself nourishment.

What nourishes you may not nourish me. One person retreats into the quiet and comfort of home; another gets energy from moving out into a crowd. Your needs may vary from day to day. But everybody needs to be good to themselves. Wellness means the balancing of challenge with nurturance. When we are loved, cared for, almost anything is easy. When we are deprived, tired, needy, even the smallest detail becomes a monumental task.

The alternatives, the possibilities, for nourishment are limited only by our old habits, by our fear of trying the untried. Nourishing yourself is well worth the risk involved.

Healing Laughter

It was in 1964 that Norman Cousins, the editor of Saturday Review, checked out of the hospital a few short weeks after having been diagnosed with a very serious illness, a rare condition which affects the body's connective tissues. His chances of recovery, he was told, were one in five hundred. Barely able to move, and in intense pain, Cousins made two very important decisions. One was that the pain medication he was receiving was worsening the condition. The other was that the hospital was a bad place in which to be sick. So he stopped taking the medication, and he checked into a hotel and began a regimen of high doses of Vitamin C and "laughter therapy."

His reading of several classic books on the subject of stress convinced him that disease was fostered by the chemical changes in the body produced by emotions—such as anger and fear. Would an antidote of hope, love, laughter, and will to live do the opposite? He was determined to try it and to be *the one* of the five hundred who successfully recovered.

In a remarkably short time he experienced that short periods of hearty laughter, encouraged by watching Marx Brothers movies and Candid Camera TV sequences, were enough to induce several hours of painless sleep. He read books of humorous stories, jokes, and continued his "laughter therapy." It was working. Slowly but steadily he began to regain control of his body. He could move without excruciating pain. He could turn his head. He could live again!

- - - - - - -

Life is too close for comfort.
—LEE LOZOWICK

- - - - - - -

The whole experience created in him an overwhelming respect for the ability of the body-mind to heal itself, when nourished by the conditions, the environment, which allow it to reestablish its natural balance.[4]

Critics of this "mind over matter" approach credit the placebo effect for its positive outcome. If you believe something strongly enough, they say, you will produce it. Hurray for them! If that is what is working here then we all need to learn the skills for fostering such belief. As we begin to understand

Making the World Smaller with Dots

I spend many hours on airplanes and in airports. I can get lost in such an impersonal world—airplanes look alike inside and airports are remarkably similar also. During 1976, I started placing colored stick-on dots around Mill Valley in subtle places. In 1976 I decided to expand my activities to make the world smaller. I began with the interiors of jets by placing a single dot in some out of the way place. It wasn't long before I would board a jet and find one of my dots still adorning the interior. That meant I had been on that same airplane before! I also began "dotting" airports by placing them on signs which hang from the ceilings of the walkways.

About the only interesting thing to me about the O'Hare Airport in Chicago is finding how many dots have survived the intervening months since my last visit. I always place them where they will not draw too much attention to themselves, as my goal is to keep them out there a long time.

Now that I've come "out of the closet" with this game, I'd like to solicit other players, so that we can make the world still smaller and communicate with each other even though we may never meet. It would be fun to see dots in new places in airplanes and airports. For instance, a dot placed in the upper corner of a restroom mirror would be unobtrusive. Each time one of us sees the communication from a fellow player, we can put one of our dots partly overlapping the one we find. That way, if a lot of us play, we won't cover the entire mirror.

If you pass through Denver's Stapleton Airport, look for the nine-color rainbow of dots near the Traveler's Aide Station on the lower level (near United's baggage claim area). It marks the spot where I first met Regina in 1978.★

For those of you who don't fly, highway signs are possible vehicles. I left a few on road signs at the Brighton intersection of Colorado Route 85, the halfway point between Greeley and Denver, a trip Regina frequently makes. I thought it would provide an interesting addition to her trips.

Dots of Luck

—J.W.T.

★The dots are now gone. Travelers' Aide has moved. Dot's life!

- -

the secrets of the brain we learn that our thoughts do trigger the pituitary gland which directs the rest of the endocrine system. The role that these glands play in establishing the body's equilibrium has been known for centuries. Perhaps now we will gain some insight into how it all happens. In the meantime, let's keep laughing.

The Play Report—A Summary

Introduction: This exercise is designed to help you to build upon what you may have learned from the previous pages.

Ways of "playing," enjoying myself indoors:

Outdoors:

Alone:

With one other person:

With a group of people:

Ways of "playing," enjoying myself that are *free*:

Which cost money to do:

Which require time off:

Which can happen any time:

Defining Work

The first definition Webster offers for the noun "work" includes the words: effort . . . exerted . . . to do . . . purposeful activity . . . labor . . . toil. The next few include: employment . . . business . . . task . . . and duty. It's enough to tire you out simply reading about it! It sounds so very *serious* and *hard*—and that's often the crux of the problem with it.

We use work to give structure to our time and meaning to our lives, to earn our livelihood, to express our talents, our dreams, our creativity, to change ourselves and the world at large. As such it is both necessary and desirable. But when it becomes hard and serious to the point of causing excessive stress, or depression, or a sense of personal frustration or worthlessness, it undermines both our health and our happiness. That's why we will consider work in the context of wellness.

People Really Are Funny

The following quotes from accident reports to insurance companies were published in the *Toronto Sun*, July 26, 1977.

- "A truck backed through my windshield and into my wife's face."

- "The pedestrian had no idea which direction to go, so I ran over him."

- "I had been driving my car for forty years when I fell asleep at the wheel and had an accident."

- "I pulled away from the side of the road, glanced at my mother-in-law and headed over the embankment."

- "I was on my way to the doctor with rear end trouble when my universal joint gave way causing me to have an accident."

- "A pedestrian hit me and went under my car."

- "The guy was all over the road; I had to swerve a number of times before I hit him."

- "An invisible car came out of nowhere, struck my vehicle, and vanished."

- "To avoid hitting the bumper of the car in front, I struck the pedestrian."

- "I saw the slow moving, sad-faced old gentleman as he bounced off the hood of my car."

- "The telephone pole was approaching fast. I was attempting to swerve out of its path, when it struck my front end."

The Problems with Work

If you listen to yourself or other people talk about work you get a sense of what it means for vast segments of the population. People describe work as:

- the rat race

- the grind

- the dog-eat-dog competition

- the sentence—publish or perish

- the tread-mill

- meeting the deadline

- killing themselves to complete a project.

When Barry leaves his home each morning to teach at the local school, he talks of entering the "madhouse." When Tina goes to the office she leaves word that she can be reached in the "dungeon." Kids refer to school as "the prison" — and in fact many of our educational institutions look that way.

When work is this serious and this hard it robs energy from mind, body, and spirit and contributes to the creation of an internal environment in which illness can easily develop. Work creates illness when:

- it becomes so serious that we assume we *can't not do it*. ("If I don't teach these poor kids, who will?")

- we allow it to slowly suffocate us because we think we have no choice, no alternatives. ("If I quit this job what else would I do?")

- it is based on unrealistic expectations and demands that neglect the physical, emotional and spiritual needs of human beings. ("My boss expects me to do the work of three people.")

There are limitless real-life examples which illustrate these attitudes and conditions, and what they lead to. Take Denis for instance. He *says* he wants a meaningful relationship with a woman. He would like to settle down and have a family. But for the past

What Nourishes Me—A Poem to Write

This is my poem. I share it as a way of encouraging you to write your own.

—Regina

When I consider nourishment, nurturing myself I think of:

Silence, the mountains at sunset, my friend Ruth.

A whirlpool bath, a mound of soft pillows, some soft music and hot tea.

A gently rocking boat, a rainy afternoon, a fire in the fireplace, and a new novel.

Taking myself to breakfast, some sweet incense, and an overstuffed chair.

A phone call from Mia, a phone call to Lloyd, and a letter from Lee in the mailbox.

The church at midnight, a bus ride from New York to Stockbridge, a warm sweater and socks, and a picnic with Barbara.

Drinking coffee at Patricia's kitchen table, playing my recorder, seeing Eileen again.

A sunrise, a pecan waffle, a walk along the ocean, and meeting Jere at the airport.

A bright clean bedroom, hugging Alaina, and coming home from shopping with a bagful of goodies all for myself.

Your Poem:

twelve years he simply hasn't had the time or energy to pursue this goal. As a case-worker for a social service department in a large rural community he has allowed his work to eat up his life. Even on his day off he is on the phone checking with his clients. If you ask him if he is really happy in his life and work he will candidly, and sadly, admit that he isn't. He just doesn't know how to break the script.

At the end of one long winter, Tom reported that he had had three colds. One just barely cleared up when the next one happened. When a friend asked him if things were going well at work, he was startled by the question. Was his friend really implying a connection? As they talked, Tom went on to admit that he hated his job as a reading teacher in a large city school. It had become increasingly tedious over the past winter, and he was really looking for any excuse that would allow him to quit without feeling guilty.

Gene was employed by the U.S. Department of Health, Education and Welfare, and his own health and "well-fare" were at stake in the job. He suffered a continual battle with stomach ulcers, had hypertension, and had trouble sleeping. The pressures on him were enormous, and he disliked his work. But he liked his large salary very much! He wanted his second car, he wanted his boat, he wanted his financial security. He would have preferred to be healthier—but assumed that since that wasn't possible in his present job he would suffer the consequences.

Mary described herself as "bored to death." She was a bank teller, but she wanted to fly. She wanted to work in an environment

I n Thornton Wilder's famous play, *Our Town*, Emily speaks from the grave and comments upon how much she took for granted. How grateful she would be for one more opportunity to do any of the simple things she had done so routinely while she lived. If you can imagine looking at the world from a similar perspective you get an idea of what a transformed vision means in this regard. Gratitude for everything. Enjoying the *privilege* of doing what now you believe is *required*. Seeing everything new, fresh—the way a child looks at the world. Fantasize how you might approach your day and its tasks if this was to be your very last day. Try putting these new "glasses" on for just a few minutes and looking round you. What changes? Why not try wearing them for a few hours and noticing what happens. This really is the first day of your life, and your last as well. The only time you can be certain of is right NOW.

in which her abilities would be challenged, in which she would be stimulated to grow, in which she could have a chance to develop more in-depth relationships with other people. Most Monday mornings found her with a headache. But what to do???????

Working Well

The realization of good health, happiness, and satisfaction in work

is possible for Denis, and Tom, and Gene, and Mary. And it's possible for you, too! But first you must refuse to resign yourself to the status quo. Some things are going to have to change—but it needn't be too hard, or too serious.

The principles of wellness applied to working mean that you assume responsibility for yourself, and your choices; and continue to love yourself. Wellness means that there are alternatives. There are other jobs. There are ways of dealing with stress on your present job. There are ways of transforming your work by incorporating the attitudes which enhance play. There are ways to give up being so serious—being the rescuer for the whole world. There are ways of discovering your real needs and fulfilling them; of discovering your real talents and using them; of dis-

5 Ways to Prevent Burn-out

1. Self-care—nutrition, exercise, creating a supportive environment.

2. Regular deep relaxation and frequent mini-relaxations.

3. Awareness of rescuing tendencies and feelings of victimization.

4. Asking directly for what you want; increasing your "stroke economy."

5. Allowing your inner child to be creative.

—Barbara McNeill
Former Staff Director
Wellness Resource Center

covering your many options and trying them out.

Accepting responsibility for your own life and health means realizing that your present work is really your choice, however much you dislike it. And it means realizing that if you chose what you are doing now, you can also choose to change it. The emerging field of life-work planning is devoted to helping people clarify what it is they really want to do, what they do best, and how to design a plan for doing it. In two brilliant books, *What Color Is Your Parachute?* and *The Three Boxes of Life*, Richard Bolles presents practical guidance in how to find out about yourself, in how to assess the job market, and how to put the two together.[5]

Continuing education programs through large universities, community colleges, and technical schools list courses in everything from small business management to shoe-making. Thousands of folks just like you are taking advantage of these low-cost (sometimes even free) opportunities to develop themselves in new ways. Daria, for instance, was a dissatisfied typist who took evening classes for less than one year. She went on to open what is now a thriving shoe store where she specializes in custom-made sandals. She loves it—and is currently studying auto mechanics so she'll be prepared if she again wants a change of pace. She is determined not to be stuck again!

For many who want to keep their present jobs, using stress-reducing procedures has been enough to transform their attitudes toward work, and to enliven their state of health. In the chapters on

---

Creating a Supportive Work Environment

Win-Win Integrity Game

This game is non-competitive and self-scoring. Any time you do something that makes you feel good about yourself, assign yourself between 1–3 points, depending on the intensity of the success. Examples may be: telling the truth when ordinarily you might "fudge" a little; communicating something instead of withholding it; accomplishing something you have been stalling on.

Keep track of your successes and points by writing them down. Find another person or group of people to play with you, and share your wins once a week. Really praise each other—applaud, whoop and holler, make a big deal of it, and just enjoy how you feel about yourself at the end of your sharing session. Notice that something that may not even qualify as a success for one person is a three-pointer for another. It is a very individual matter. It is also possible to go off the scale if it is a big win.

A good way to continually build your self-esteem is to persist at something every day that is a "one-pointer," like going jogging instead of letting your lethargy drag you into an old rut, or using your positive self-affirmations faithfully, or not eating too much, etc.

This game has been a wonderful help to us as a staff. If someone says, "Boy, I'm going to get some points on this!" we all understand immediately that it is a high risk. Because we share our wins and validate each other enthusiastically, we've created a safety that nurtures us and supports us in being all we can be.

—Barbara McNeill
Former Staff Director
Wellness Resource Center

---

moving and breathing, some of these techniques were highlighted. In the chapter on thinking we discussed ways of using "positive worry" and creative brainstorming to relieve stressful problems. In the next chapter you will learn more about asserting yourself, and about breaking typical game-playing patterns in communication. All these approaches can help you cope with stress. The concluding chapter on transcending will present a variety of meditation techniques which can be used to get you in touch with

yourself again, and to aid you in dealing with the pressures of life which confront us all.

The material on play as nourishment which is presented in this chapter may help you to get a new perspective on your job. Creativity in bringing a playful attitude to bear on your work may include things as simple as rearranging your office, giving a flower to each of your co-workers, inviting your boss to play tennis, or changing the music station on the radio. One small company in Colorado found that weekly staff meetings could become brainstorming sessions in how to personalize and relax the working environment. Productivity increased at the same time.

Burn-out is an all too familiar phenomenon in all jobs, at all levels. It happens when people are stuck in jobs they do not like, in jobs that fail to satisfy their needs. In the work John did as director of Wellness Associates, he found burn-out quite common among those in the helping professions. The "helpers" often turn out to be "rescuers" who take on unnecessary and unrealistic burdens and actually undermine their own health. Facilitating this awareness has meant real liberation for many who have participated in the seminars on burn-out given by Wellness Associates. (For more on burn-out and "rescuing" see page 176.)

Loving Yourself

There is little doubt that your self-concept and the work you do are intimately connected. Typically when people meet, the first question they ask each other is, "What do you do?" To which each responds with a job description: "I'm a butcher." "I'm a baker." "I'm a candlestick maker."

The trouble is that when we are temporarily out of work, or when we lose enthusiasm for our work, and even when we are merely on vacation, many of us feel that we've lost our identity as well. While it is true that meaningful work enhances your sense-of-self, it is dangerous to tie up all your self-worth in your work alone. As you are more than your physical body, so you are more than the work you do. Regardless of what you do, you are a complex, unique, powerful and beautiful human being. The more you open to your truest self—the more you accept yourself for who you are, not just for what you do—the more open you become to reading the signs that point you in the direction of meaningful and satisfying work.

The Planet At Play

In discussing competition we saw how it can become a destructive force in our personal lives. As a national policy it can lead to devastation. Where is the satisfaction in winning the "Arms Race" if we must live in constant fear as a result? Where is the joy in having the world's highest standard of living if to do so is at the expense of the poorer countries which we exploit? Does happiness mean becoming an island of plenty in a sea of poverty and misery? These are hard questions. But they are real issues nonetheless. If we need to learn to play and work cooperatively on the corner lot, we need to learn to play and work cooperatively on the planet-field if we are to survive.

In Hindu mythology there is a concept called "lila." It means the play of God or the divine play. Creation as we experience it is the result. God, at play, like a great magician, transforms Himself into the world. All, then, is God. All is One. Our confusion, our inability to see the unity which underlies all forms, generates the eternal human problem, the great dilemma.[6]

The concept is not unique to Eastern thought. In Christian the-

The tickets to the play of a rich and happy life are always there, waiting to be picked up. The readiness is all! Preoccupation with fear, with old, stale thoughts, with silly regrets and self recrimination clouds our vision, and prevents us from seeing them.

—R.S.R.

ology we find it reflected in the doctrine of the Mystical Body of Christ. All of creation forms one body, one being, and that being is the Christ—the manifestation of God. The job of salvation is that of evolving realization of this unity— each cell working harmoniously with every other cell towards the perfection of the whole.[7]

Whether or not these beliefs are in accord with your own, the principle they elaborate is hard to deny from even a purely materialistic viewpoint. Your thoughts affect your body. The ways in which you think and feel will influence your family and friends. Our families' involvements create the atmosphere of our neighborhoods. Our neighborhoods . . . Our nation . . . Our hemisphere . . . Our planet . . . "Global Village" and "Spaceship Earth" are being realized by more of us all the time. We are interdependent. We are one.

Try this. Relax yourself, close your eyes, and reflect for a moment about what you have just read. See yourself in the center of a vast series of concentric circles. Each circle represents an expansion of your personal environment. Imagine yourself at work and fantasize the impact which your job has on the

The Wellness Antidote

In May, 1975, 100 questions (which were later to become the Wellness Index) were tested on 25 staff persons at the Department of Health Services Research, U.S.P.H.S. Hospital in Baltimore. Within 24 hours after distributing the questionnaire, the counter-attack was launched in the form of a spoof by the "guys" in the computer division. One William "Mac" Chapin of Annapolis, Maryland, was the chief perpetrator of the creative endeavor. John subsequently labeled it the Wellness Antidote. Regina developed the scoring scale. It will gauge your ability to break your seriousness about wellness. Scoring is an individual matter. One method for doing it is to rate your responses to each question:

0 points—didn't move a muscle
1 point—partial smile
2 points—wide smile
3 points—chuckle in your throat

4 points—chuckle in your belly
5 points—audible laughter
6 points—uproarious laughter
7 points—uncontrollable response, falling off your chair

I. Productivity, Relaxation, Sleep

_____ 1. I enjoy goofing off.
_____ 2. I seldom go to bed before passing out.
_____ 3. My bed is at least two feet off the floor.
_____ 4. I rarely bite or pick my nose.
_____ 5. My room is bolted down to prevent spinning.
A Bonus Point for Strangers
_____ 6. Although not centered, I usually try to stay within the outer limits.
_____ TOTAL

II. Personal Care and Home Safety

_____ 1. I smoke only during and immediately after sex.
_____ 2. I regularly check my sex.
_____ 3. I keep an up-to-date record of all germs in the house.
_____ 4. I wash my hands in the toilet before handling food.
_____ 5. I avoid nuclear explosion like the plague.
Bonus Point for Women
_____ 6. I keep my pap covered in cold weather.
_____ TOTAL

III. Nutritional Awareness

_____ 1. I drink beer instead of water because it's less polluted.
_____ 2. I salt only spoiled food.
_____ 3. I eat labels on packages rather than the contents.
_____ 4. I know the basic types of alcohol and try to keep an ample stock of each.
_____ 5. I avoid eating large quantities of wood pulp.
_____ TOTAL

IV. Environmental Awareness

_____ 1. I recycle my septic system by using it to wash my windows.
_____ 2. I set my thermostat on the windowsill before going to bed.
_____ 3. My car burns less than 3 gallons of oil per 100 miles.
_____ 4. I throw bums into the dumpster.
_____ 5. I use public showers and eat at the "Y."
_____ TOTAL

V. Physical Activity

_____ 1. I jump off buildings rather than use the stairs.
_____ 2. I kick doors down instead of opening them.
_____ 3. I participate in orgies every week.
_____ 4. I yodel at least 20 minutes 4 times a day.
_____ 5. I jog to the liquor store.
_____ TOTAL

VI. Emotional Maturity and Expression of Feelings

_____ 1. I am frequently sober enough to think.
_____ 2. I am able to punch people out without taking it personally.
_____ 3. I am frequently nice to idiots and don't hesitate to use that word.
_____ 4. I prefer to get money, but still accept compliments.
_____ 5. I would seek help from friends if I had any.
_____ TOTAL

VII. Community Involvement

_____ 1. I vote early and often at each election.
_____ 2. If I saw a broken kid in the street, I would put him out of his misery.
_____ 3. I know who my neighbors are and swear at most of them.
_____ 4. I love my neighbor's wife.
_____ 5. I am a member of one or more subversive organizations.
_____ TOTAL

VIII. Creativity, Self-Expression

_____ 1. I enjoy expressing myself. Period.
_____ 2. I like myself because I'm so irresistible.
_____ 3. I enjoy being touched by my hamster.
_____ 4. I am emotionally close to at least five hamsters.
_____ 5. I enjoy spending time doing just about anything with Farah Fawcett.
_____ TOTAL

IX. Automobile Safety

_____ 1. I know what a car looks like.
_____ 2. I do not mind spending $4.50 a quart for oil.
_____ 3. I drive on the road usually.
_____ 4. I check my dome light frequently.
_____ 5. I carry an emergency fifth at all times.
_____ TOTAL

X. Parenting

_____ 1. I allow my kids to play with the fan belt only while the car is idling.
_____ 2. I use what is left over from washing the windows to prepare baby food—it's really organic.
_____ 3. I frequently beat the little bastards.
_____ 4. I do not store loaded shotguns in the crib.
_____ 5. I do not allow any child over 50 lbs. to eat.
_____ TOTAL
_____ GRAND TOTAL

Range of Scores and Evaluations

above 350 points	you'll probably live forever	50-99- points	you need a vacation
above 300 points	add 10 years to life expectancy	25-49 points	you need a long rest
200-299 points	add 4 years to life expectancy	10-24 points	call the hospital
100-199 points	have another drink	0-9 points	call the morgue

world at large. The whole scene is changed by your presence. The whole scene will be changed when you leave. Somebody else will be touched in some way by your pain. There is no way to rejoice alone. Everything will change as a result of your joy.

Suggested Reading*

Bolles, R. *What Color Is Your Parachute? A Practical Manual for Job-Hunters and Career-Changers.* Berkeley, CA: Ten Speed Press, 1987.

Bolles, R. *The Three Boxes of Life, and How to Get Out of Them.* Berkeley, CA: Ten Speed Press, 1978.

DeKoven, B. *The Well-Played Game: A Player's Philosophy.* New York, NY: Anchor Books, 1978.

Fluegelman, A., ed., *New Games Books.* New York, NY: Doubleday, 1976.

Jongeward, D., and Seyer, P. *Choosing Success: Transactional Analysis on the Job.* New York, NY: John Wiley, 1978.

Lakein, A. *How to Get Control of Your Time and Your Life.* New York, NY: Peter A. Wyden, 1973.

Leonard, G. *The Ultimate Athlete.* New York, NY: Avon Books, 1977.

Matt, M. *Human Anatomy Coloring Book.* New York, NY: Dover Publishing, 1982.

Maue, K. *Water in the Lake: Real Events for the Imagination.* New York, NY: Harper and Row, 1979.

Moody, R. *Laugh After Laugh: The Healing Power of Humor.* Jacksonville, FL: Headwaters Press, 1978.

Pelletier, K. *Healthy People in Unhealthy Places: Stress and Fitness at Work.* New York, NY: Delacorte Press, 1984.

Peter, L.J., and Dana, B. *The Laughter Prescription.* New York, NY: Ballantine Books, 1982.

Pirsig, R. *Zen and the Art of Motorcycle Maintenance: An Inquiry into Values.* New York, NY: William Morrow, 1974.

Schutz, W. *Profound Simplicity.* San Diego, CA: Learning Concepts, 1979.

Simon, S.; Howe, L.; and Kirschenbaum, H. *Values Clarification.* New York, NY: Hart Publishing Co., 1972.

Stellman, J., and Henifin, M. *Office Work Can Be Dangerous to Your Health.* New York, NY: Pantheon Books, 1983.

Terkel, S. *Working.* New York, NY: Pantheon/Random House, 1974.

Verdesca, A. *Live, Work, and Be Healthy.* New York, NY: Van Nostrand, Reinhold Co., 1980.

*This is only a representative sampling. Many excellent books have been omitted. At the bookstore or library, look over the whole section and choose according to your judgment.

Notes

1. James, M. and Jongeward, D. *Born to Win.* Reading, MA: Addison-Wesley, 1971.

2. Davis, B. *The Magical Child Within You.* Berkeley, CA: Celestial Arts, 1977, pp. 7–8.

3. Fluegelman, A. *New Games Book.* New York, NY: Doubleday, 1976.

4. Cousins, N. *Anatomy of an Illness.* New York, NY: W.W. Norton and Co., 1979.

5. See:

Bolles, R. *What Color Is Your Parachute?* Berkeley, CA: Ten Speed Press, 1987.

Bolles, R. *The Three Boxes of Life.* Berkeley, CA: Ten Speed Press, 1979.

6. Capra, F. *The Tao of Physics.* Berkeley, CA: Shambhala Press, 1975. pp. 77–78.

7. See: 1 Corinthians, 12, 23–30. *The New Testament.*

Nine

Wellness and Communicating

H UMAN COMMUNICATION IS simply an exchange of information, verbal or nonverbal, between a sender and a receiver. (A rather cold description for what can be poetry or lovemaking.) However, because we humans are so fantastically complex, it is virtually impossible for us to communicate isolated bits of data, despite what you may have experienced from your high school history teacher. Every time you speak to (or write to, or look at) someone you are revealing yourself. You can't avoid it. Your tone of voice, selection of words, facial expression, even the clothes you wear and the way you comb your hair, all these are messages in themselves, messages about *you*. Furthermore, the person you are addressing interprets what you share in the light of his/her own beliefs and values. Sometimes there are so many variables, so many hidden messages, that the original information is

> Feeling and thinking together lead to communication. Communicating is the organization of feeling and thinking energy and their transmission in the form of a message, verbal or non-verbal. Communicating is an energy output which allows us to share our internal maps of reality with others, and thus forms the foundation of culture.

deeply buried, and a map is required to recover it.

When you are not busy communicating with someone or something else, you are carrying on a running conversation with yourself, even though you may not be aware of it. These internal conversations are as vulnerable to distortions and misrepresentations as any other conversation. Because internal conversations direct the way you view the world and the way you view yourself, they have momentous impact on your health and happiness. If you tell yourself enough times that the world is a vicious rat race, if you tell yourself

enough times that you are weak and susceptible, then very likely the outcome will be just so.

In this chapter we will focus almost exclusively on verbal communication, exploring the dynamics of how people talk to themselves and one another. We will also study the breakdowns that can occur. As you come to understand and appreciate this process, you may simultaneously understand and appreciate yourself. The clearer the channel (you), the better the possibilities for a meaningful encounter—a dynamic energy exchange.

Talking to Yourself— Intrapersonal Communication

You communicate with yourself more than you do with anyone else. Talking to yourself is more formally referred to as intrapersonal communication and is synonymous with the process of self-awareness. It includes your intuition, your dreams and fantasies, your problem-solving strategies, as well as your attunement to bodily messages, emotions, thoughts, needs, and wants. Since personal awareness is one of the primary concerns addressed throughout this book, many of these elements mentioned are covered in other chapters. Our attention in this one will focus upon two areas that require special attention because they are so strongly connected to wellness. The first one involves the ways in which you describe and evaluate the world to yourself. These conversations actually structure your reality. Since they will influence what you find out there, they will have an impact on your health and happiness. So beware what you tell yourself.

The second consideration deals with the way in which talking to yourself builds your self-concept. As the sum total of the messages you give yourself about who you are, and what you are worth, your self-concept designs your internal environment. A strong, positive self-concept will create a strong, positive body-mind, and so your wellness depends upon it.

Here we go.

Beware What You Tell Yourself

As children, the world was described for you and you got your strokes for repeating these descriptions. "Nice doggy!" "Bad cold." "Pretty girl." "Ugly mess!" You soon came to understand that words were symbols for things and that some things were good

· · · · · · · · · · · · *Regina's Journal.* · · · · · · · · · · · ·

The Headache Story.

The headaches started in 1973 as I struggled over producing what had to be the best master's thesis the Communications Department was ever to approve. The tension gathered around my right shoulder blade and slowly worked its way up to my neck, the side of my face, the top of my head, and came to rest over my right eye where it proceeded to stay, day and night, for the next three days.

By now I know the pattern well. What is exciting is that I've finally begun to understand why! You see, it's on my right shoulder that my judgment sits, unrelenting and insidious in its constant whispers:

"You should have done that better."
"Not good enough!"
"What a dumb thing to say!"
"What a stupid thing to do!"

Craning my neck, as I turn my head to respond to the nagging, the criticisms, the demands, creates a lot of tightness in the muscles around this area. A few days of doing so and the pain is upon me, wiping out all other considerations and coloring the world grey. I am well punished for my weaknesses.

Lately, I've been able to avert, on several occasions, what used to be the inevitable! As I recognized the tension growing in the right shoulder (as I write this I realize that the bulk of the word "shoulder" is the word "should"), I took to the quiet of my bedroom where I proceeded to talk to myself in a more beneficial way. Flat on my back, with eyes closed, I repeated over and over:

"I am a good and beautiful person."
"I don't have to 'have it all together.' "
"It's OK to make mistakes."
"I'm a likeable and lovable and creative woman."
"I am OK!"

It is working! I have actually begun to listen, and what's more, I've even started to believe.

· ·

and necessary, other things were bad and should be avoided. As you asked "why" and "what is it?" you received not only a verbal message, but a whole range of more subtle, non-verbal cues about what was approved and what was not. Since you didn't comprehend all the words used in these descriptions, you relied more upon the emotional tone that accompanied them. You were very perceptive in picking

. . . . *Exercise* . . . .

Who Are You Anyway?

To help you find out what internalized messages you have about yourself, it may be helpful to write some of them out. First list all the roles you play, then make a list of adjectives that describe the kind of person you are. The faster and more spontaneously you do this exercise, the better. Don't evaluate or edit as you go along. Give yourself a three-minute time limit and go to it. When you're done, look back over your responses.

John Responds:

Roles
I am:
a pioneer
a healer
a stubborn nut
a loner . . .

Adjectives
I am:
sensitive
proud
self-doubting
critical
warm
generous . . .

Your Responses:

I am:

I am:

. . . .

these up. Your parents and others around you used tone of voice, facial expression, and physical touch (a slap on the hand as you approached the stove) to teach you, to protect you, to control you.

As you developed and learned more language, you moved from a simple awareness of a few things, into the process of talking to yourself about everything. You began to describe your world within the limitations of the words you knew. Any white stuff which fell from the sky became snow. You *understood* snow. Or so you thought. The fact that some of it was heavy and very wet, while some of it was light and powdery may have escaped you. Snow was snow, falling, piling up on the fence or trees, frozen into ice, turning black as it was trampled underfoot. All of its textures, its infinite patterns, its many stages—for which the Eskimo has scores of words—may not have been appreciated. Snow was snow! This is what we mean when we say that the way in which we describe the world limits us. Nevertheless, this is usual in the process, and this is what you probably did.

As you look around your room right now, you are talking to yourself about everything you see. Your language is structuring your reality. Furniture and pictures are not good or bad in and of themselves. They become beautiful or ugly, valuable or tacky, based upon your descriptions of them. The "real" world simply *is*, but *your* world is created by *your* judgments. Let's use a common example to illustrate this concept. Remember a time in your life when you were in love? Perhaps you had just met the person of your dreams, or been newly baptized into the love of God, or held your first child, or grandchild. Do you remember what the world was like for you then? Typically, you found beauty everywhere. The sun was brighter and warmer, or the clouds more dramatic. Colors were deeper. You laughed at situations that formerly annoyed you. People in supermarkets let you ahead of them in line. Others smiled at you as you walked down the street. Without effort you found the perfect greeting card, or the ideal restaurant or the best accommodations. We say that "love is blind" not because it diminishes our sight. On the contrary, it usually intensifies it. The blindness referred to is the inability to see what formerly you called bad, or ugly, or meaningless. Love causes you to change your language. The world becomes beautiful as a result, and what's more, you usually feel better too.

If we all really understood this connection then the focus of our attention on health would switch dramatically. Instead of talking to ourselves about germs and flu and headaches, arthritis and senility, we would talk about enthusiasm and strength and balance, energy and joy! If we appreciated that what we find is really a function of what we look for, our sense of responsibility for our own life and health would increase even more.

The Positive Self-Concept

Your self-concept is the sum total of the messages which you give yourself about who you are and what you are worth. Our second point in this subject of intrapersonal communication is that a positive self-concept creates a healthy body-mind environment. Your own experience probably verifies this.

Sad and depressed people are sick more often. Two teachers work in the same classroom. One is continually negative. Failure is his home territory. The other is generally positive. She is grateful for every little success. The gloomy teacher contracts every illness that hits the class during the course of the year. His sick leave is used up in the first six months. The other teacher seems immune. She doesn't miss a day. The crucial point here is that while both are working together on the same project, one continually reinforces the failings, the other capitalizes on the successes. It's a question of attitude, based on the selectivity of perception. (We observed the same phenomenon at work in discussing the will to live in chapter 7.) It's a question of which messages one chooses to repeat: I'm incompetent, frustrated, and not OK, or I'm likable, energetic, and capable!

. . . .

You think it's a secret, but everybody knows.
—FORTUNE COOKIE
MESSAGE

. . . .

Many people have spent a lifetime turning gold into garbage—using what is called the Midas touch in reverse. Someone says, "I like what you're wearing tonight." Internally the other questions, "So you didn't like what I wore last night? I suppose that means I'm not OK?" A supervisor remarks, "This is good work." The "garbage-collector" remarks to him/herself, "So everything else I've done has been bad? I'm just an incompetent person?"

Continually replaying negative programs ingrains them deeply into the consciousness. The more they accumulate, and the stronger they take root, the more the self-concept is weakened.

These inner conversations are often referred to as the "internal dialogue." This is you talking to yourself all day long. This is your judgment of yourself and others which goes on from morning till night, and even in your dreams.

The Fat Man with the Bald Head

There are probably an infinite number of ways in which to describe the same person, the same event. The one we choose to use betrays much about our attitudes, our appreciation of the person or scene. I describe the man I don't like as the fat man with the bald head. To his friend he is the one in the blue jogging outfit, or the heavy-set one with thin grey hair.

Listen to yourself describe things and people to yourself and others.

If you find negative traits as your focus you might want to plug in a more positive description. And while you're at it, try applying this to descriptions of yourself as well.

—RSR

Collecting Gold

What might happen if you were to devote the next three days to listening and looking for the strokes which are aimed in your direction? What if you were to accept them with nothing more than a simple "thank you"? Here are some of the experiences you might notice:

the thank you's of bus drivers
the admiring looks of your children
the comment of a coworker, a client, a student, a customer
a stray dog following you home
an obliging motorist who stops to let you through the traffic
a wink, a whistle, a second look
an acquaintance remembering your name
a letter from home
a phone call from a friend
a hug and a kiss
a discount, a bargain, a dime in the pay phone
a grateful waiter
your newspaper left in a plastic bag on a rainy day
a luncheon date
a sunset more dramatic than any you can remember
a cool evening; a warm fire; a feeling of well-being . . .

Why not try it and make up your own list. You may even find that you have written a poem.

This is your endless creation of categories, boxes, in which to safely place everyone and everything. This is what tires you out. This is what furnishes the stage on which you will act out your personal drama. Changing the tone of it is a process of heightening your awareness. As you realize how frustrating and exhausting so much of this "talk" is, you motivate yourself to let it go. When you can accept what it is doing to you, you decide to do something about it.

Building a more positive self-concept might well begin with learning to accept compliments. These golden nuggets, or strokes, are being handed to all of us all the time. Even if the people in your immediate environment don't seem to be giving them, nature itself is showering them continually—a fresh breeze, a purple sunset, a spring rain. Simply opening your eyes, and cultivating gratitude as a way of being can show you lots of good things to talk to yourself about. It's sort of like making Thanksgiving Day happen every day of the year. (See the section on affirmations, chapter 7.)

Interpersonal Communication

We move now to a consideration of the information-exchange which happens when you talk to other

. . . .

Communication Theory

I know you believe you understand what you think I said. But I am not sure you realize that what you heard is not what I meant.

. . . .

people—*interpersonal* communication.

People talk to one another because they have needs which must be met. They require direction, or food, or relief from pain, or quiet, or touch, or acknowledgment. Getting needs met helps keep us in control, in the most positive sense

The Communication Formula

Communicating with others is more intimate when you are able to share your true feelings with another, rather than merely talking about the weather or hobbies. Since feelings are not always pleasant subjects and most of us have trouble expressing negative feelings, here is a formula you can use when you are upset with someone and want to solve the problem.

1. **State what *you* are feeling (and what triggered that feeling).**
   Mary: "I'm angry at you for running over my cat and not telling me."

2. **Ask how the *other person* feels about the subject.**
   Mary: "How do you feel about this whole thing?"
   Joe: "I'm very sad, I didn't even know I had done it."

3. **Together work out a solution to help both parties feel better.**
   Mary: "Will you help me bury the cat and buy me a new one?"
   Joe: "Sure." or "How about my paying for only one-half the cost of a new one, since he was in my driveway when it happened."
   Mary: "OK."

When this simple 3-step formula is followed, you may be amazed at how much easier communication becomes. Often when we are upset we send "you-messages" to the person with whom we are upset, rather than state how *we* feel. The other person is likely to become defensive because s/he is being judged but would be more receptive if he knew what you were really feeling behind the judgment.

Example of "you-message" with a judgment:

"I think you are awful for forgetting our anniversary."

Example of "I-message" with an emotion stated:

"I'm sad (or angry) that you forgot our anniversary."

Notice how the first can be construed as an invitation to fight, and the second an invitation to share feelings and solve the problem. These methods are effective with those who are invested in having a healthy relationship with you. Some people will probably want to continue playing games and will not respond favorably to your efforts to improve communication. You may want to reconsider having having such persons in your life and decide to change some of your friends.

of the word. Without shared information, you are alone in the world. You don't know what to expect. Without the ability to communicate, learning becomes an almost impossible task. Without mutual understanding, relationships break down. Lacking the needed energy—life becomes imbalanced. What often results then, is a state of "dis-ease."

Our investigation here will highlight some common causes for breakdowns in communication. These include: conversations which are really monologues—and thus don't share energy; failure to express real feelings—resulting in non-assertiveness; inflexibility which shows up in absolutes and generalizations; game-playing—which is a form of dishonest communication; and the failure to listen. We will look at the connection between breakdowns in communication and the potential for illness, and explore ways of using communication in the service of wellness.

Monologues and Dialogues

When a character in a play delivers a monologue, it generally serves an important purpose. When two people in conversation each carry on a simultaneous monologue, very little happens. I tell my story. Meanwhile, you tell your story. Neither of us really hears the other, so we may each start talking louder. When this has gone on for a short time, and nobody is truly satisfied, we often give up on conversation altogether and turn on the TV, or suggest going out for a drink. Anything to change the energy or the environment. *Simultaneous monologues* sometimes sound like this:

A: "I just heard from Bob."

B: "Oh yeah. Have you seen Fred lately? I hear he is looking really bad."

A: "You don't say. His wife sure is terrific through all of this."

B: "Your wife seems happy since she got her new job."

A: "I don't know. Makes me feel like a real loser—her making more money than I do."

B: "I guess. So what did Bob have to say anyway?"

The image which this conjures up is that of a couple running towards each other with outstretched arms and longing looks, and then tripping as they run right past each other.

Despite all that we have in common, we fail to really meet each other time and time again. We may spend an evening, a bus ride, or our whole lives together, and never achieve common ground. These unsatisfying relationships lack the energy needed for life and health. They create boredom and joylessness. We leave them with our needs for intimacy, for caring, unmet. Some of us even use sickness as a last resort in our attempts to make these relationships work because illness demands a response.

It would be far better to use communication for revitalizing, for wellness. To do this we need to make communication an energy exchange, a dialogue.

Every person alive has a story—his story, her story—one more fascinating than the next. When you are open to hearing my story, and I am open to hearing yours, when we are truly aware of one another and sensitive to what each of us needs, then we are experiencing dialogue.

Dialogue is characterized by true presence, nonjudgmental listening, and honesty.[1]

With *true presence*, you attend as fully as possible to the other. You turn your face, your body, in his/her direction. Your eyes are open to more than the movement of the lips. You become sensitive to what is going on inside the words, between the lines. People are giving much valuable information about the world as they view it through the tone of voice, the fluency, the facial expression, hand gestures, posture, and the distance they put between you when they talk.

With *nonjudgmental listening* you try to understand as fully as possible what is being said. If you spend your time calculating your responses, you will miss the full impact of the message being sent. Oftentimes one word or expression triggers your disapproval or disagreement so strongly that a conversation becomes a subtle debate. You get hooked on it and block out everything that follows. When you become aware that this is happening it takes courage to stop and admit it.

. . . .

I sometimes react to making a mistake as if I have betrayed myself. My fear of making a mistake seems to be based on the hidden assumption that I am potentially perfect and that if I can just be careful I will not fall from heaven. But a "mistake" is a declaration of the way I am, a jolt to the way I intend, a reminder I am not dealing with the facts. When I have listened to my mistakes I have grown.

—HUGH PRATHER

. . . .

Misunderstanding is at the root of most of the problems in relationships—personal as well as professional. Yet most misunderstandings can be prevented by dynamic, nonjudgmental listening.

The third characteristic of dialogue is *honesty*. When communication is carefully guarded, when we "walk the fence," when we say "yes" when we mean "no"—we are being dishonest. The result is that our interactions with other people become dry and tasteless. Cocktail party chatter is not bad, but it is generally not all that nourishing. The dishonesty of repressing real feelings isn't bad in itself. But it robs us of energy. Sharing ourselves honestly with another offers both them and ourselves a real gift—a gift of energy.

By sharing your words with me, you share your thoughts, and that means you share yourself. As we learn about each other we learn more about the world at large, and more about ourselves. The ability to view our exchange in this way allows us to be open, allows us to learn and grow.

Assertiveness

In recent years assertiveness training, particularly for women, has become more and more popular. Assertiveness basically means the ability to express your thoughts and feelings in a way that clearly states your needs, and keeps the lines of communication open with the other.

As you listen to people talk you become aware of how often they hint at holding in their real feelings. Perhaps they say:

"I was furious, but I wouldn't give him the satisfaction of seeing me blow up."

"Just swallow your pride!" (Which usually means your anger.)

"What a strong woman—she never cried, even at the funeral."

"No matter how tough things get—keep smiling!"

You can probably list many more. Society doesn't approve of angry outbursts or "cry-babies." Most of us learned this sorry lesson when we were little children. In the chapter on feelings, this point was discussed in depth. By blocking our real feelings, we create tensions which pool in different parts of our

bodies. Eventually, they surface as illness of some sort.

Giving over responsibility to so-called "experts," in so many areas of our lives, has caused us to discount our own intuitions and put down our own experiences and knowledge. Jere tells the story of getting a flat tire recently and watching the service station mechanic at work on it. Jere immediately found the source of the problem and guessed how best to fix it. Nevertheless he stood by, observing the mechanic's futile attempts. Finally, apologetically, he offered his own advice. The me-

chanic took it, and the damage was soon repaired. Jere's mental program was that "experts know best." His reluctance to speak was an example of non-assertiveness.

It's risky to be assertive. People might not like us. They may reject us by saying:

"NO" or

"What gives you the right . . ." or

"Mind your own business . . ."

We tell ourselves that we really don't want to hurt other people's feelings. Our friend might be in-

---

Assertive Bill of Rights

I HAVE THE RIGHT TO . . .

- be responsible for my own life
- support others being responsible for themselves
- create conscious interdependence in my life (we're all here together)
- accept and respect myself and others
- feel happy, satisfied, and to allow inner peace
- take good care of my whole being: my body, my mind, and my spirit
- be imperfect, and to forgive myself and others for our mistakes
- be aware of and fulfill my own needs (and to support others doing so also
- have dreams, goals, and ideals—and to bring them into reality
- have and express all my emotions, without indulgence
- tell others how I want to be treated
- allow people to help me even if I'm feeling guilty, unworthy, or dependent
- set my own priorities for the use of time, money, space, and energy
- get what I pay for
- get paid what I deserve
- have healthy, life-enhancing relationships
- change, emerge, expand in new directions
- free myself from guilt and worry, and trust the goodness of myself
- work together with others to resolve conflict and build a world beyond war

Ruth Sharon, M.A.
Englewood, Colorado

I think that I am of most service to others when I take the risk to express unconventional views, rather than saying what I think people want to hear. I then find a lot of similarly-minded people. My risking is like breaking the ice. Suddenly, others begin speaking out, too.

. . . .

Cornering Questions or "Isn't It True That . . ."

Y ou've probably all seen a TV show or a movie in which a crafty lawyer skillfully uses questions to "trap" the defendant into an admission of guilt. You may not realize it, but many times your own questions "corner" people, or subtly "trap" them. This can set up barriers in the communication process, and may even bring a conversation to a swift close. Here are some examples of cornering questions:

1. Questions which force a *yes* or *no* answer.
   Isn't this beautiful?
   Wouldn't you like to help me out?

2. Questions which are really statements.
   You really hate me, don't you?
   This is awful, isn't it?

3. Questions that require an *all* or *nothing* response; or that allow for only two alternatives.
   Are you joyful or sad?
   Are you religious or atheistic?

4. Questions that take us off the hook by making the other person responsible.
   What do you want to do?

Follow-up: Determine to listen attentively to your own conversations over the course of the next few days. Focus on your use of questions. This awareness may prove valuable in improving your communication skills.

sulted if we were to admit, "I really don't want to go out tonight." So, instead, we smile and say "Sure," or "I'd love to," while inside we churn with anger or sadness or frustration.

It takes a great deal of effort to continually walk the fence, trying to please all the people, all the time. But that's what we must do to remain "good guys" or "sweethearts." We have to swallow hard and breathe lightly and walk on tiptoes and maybe end up with stomach ulcers, or arthritis or cancer. The body will allow just so much repressed emotion to collect. Then—it will have its way.

The reluctance to be assertive often stems from confusing this type of communication with aggression. But they are simply not the same. If someone is talking near your seat in a movie theater the aggressive response is, "Shut up." The assertive response is, "I can't hear the film. Will you please be quiet." The first one is hostile. The second is firm but respectful— and probably does the job much more effectively. Hostility breeds hostility. Firmness with respect leaves the other intact.

Taking care of your own needs, taking charge for yourself, or letting others take charge, as appropriate, expressing an unpopular opinion, saying "No" when that is

what you mean, are among your rights as a human being. To refrain from doing so is to undermine your peace of mind, your self-esteem, and your body's natural inclinations towards equilibrium.[2]

Absolutes as Roadblocks

It is natural to form judgments about the world. We do it continually, whether or not we are aware of it. It can become a problem if we are unable to change our opinions, or if we make the mistake of assuming that everyone else shares our opinions—or would, if they were intelligent enough or better informed.

This rigidity commonly shows up in conversations as absolute statements, generalizations, and "is" labels—

"All teenagers are bad."

"This coffee is the worst."

"There is nothing we can do about it."

"He'll never change."

"Politicians can't be trusted."

Statements like these are communication barriers, and they detour our energies in a number of ways:

• They limit our world view,

. . . .*Exercise*. . . . .

"Yes-But"—A Game to be Played with Yourself

One of the most common ways we sabotage our own efforts is by playing the game of "Yes-But." No matter how, great a job we are doing, no matter how well things are going, we look for pitfalls, weaknesses, and inadequacies, and capitalize on them. Here are the rules for "Yes-But."

1. Accept the fact that no matter what anybody, including yourself, says or does, the situation simply cannot change.

2. Each time a positive alternative is suggested, discount it as being too expensive, unreasonable, too late, idle dreaming, ridiculous, etc.

3. Put down all attempts at pointing out any good in the situation by saying, "Yes-but it won't do any good now" . . . or . . . "Yes-but that's only a drop in the bucket," . . . or . . . "Yes-but that's easy for you to say," etc.

4. Extend your inability to cope or succeed in this experience to the whole of your life in general.

5. Reinforce your negativity as often as possible by talking about it to everyone who will listen, by bringing it up constantly, by calling friends all over the country.

6. Repeat your fail-sure arguments to yourself at least 12 times daily.

7. Have a T-shirt made that reads "I'm Incapable." Wear it everywhere.

8. Resist distractions, time off, vacations, parties—anything that would take your mind off the problem.

9. Practice a look that says "I'm suffering inside, but trying hard to hide it."

. . . .

and also our alternatives. As alternatives decrease, stress increases.

• They set us up for opposition, debate, and confrontation with those who don't agree. As defensiveness increases, so does stress.

• They distance other people or cause them to decide "no use talking to her . . ." And it's difficult to cultivate intimacy and get the strokes we need when the other moves away.

Try listening to yourself to see if you have fallen into the habit of speaking in absolute terms. As you catch yourself in a roadblock pattern, let that cue you to substitute a more open-minded statement. For instance:

J: How was the movie?

R: It was the greatest movie in the world! [the absolute statement]—I mean, I really enjoyed it.

or

J: Have you been following the campaign?

R: Yes, Joe Evans is an idiot! [the absolute statement] Excuse me—I mean I can't follow his reasoning and don't approve of his policy on energy.

Note how these amended responses actually communicate more data, leave the other free to disagree, and therefore keep the lines of communication open. If you're interested in learning more about the effects of communication patterns like these, there are many resources to be tapped. The whole field of general semantics is concerned with them.[3]

* * * * * * *

The advantage of telling the truth is you don't have to remember what you said.
　　　　　—RITA MAE BROWN

* * * * * * *

Games

Many of our communication exchanges go round in circles, leaving us feeling power-robbed, angry, dissatisfied. In the language of Transactional Analysis, we are playing "games."

People play games because they want strokes and games provide strokes, albeit negative ones. Although they provide a payoff, they are really set-ups in which everybody ultimately loses. They drain our energies, often weaken our relationships, leave us frustrated and feeling clumsy, stupid, inadequate, or just plain *not OK*. When this happens, we are thrown off balance, and thus make ourselves more susceptible to disease. Because games don't meet our needs in a positive way, we may resort to accidents or more serious illness to get the attention, strokes, or revenge that we are really seeking.

Another way to describe games is to call them crooked or manipulative communications. They are crooked because the words used hide the underlying message, a message we may be unaware of. You may ask innocently "Where are you going tonight?" when you really mean "I have plans for us tonight." You may ask, "What can I do about it?" when you are already convinced that there is really no way out.

A game begins when one party offers a bait—a loaded question or a message that masks the true intention. It starts rolling when the

The Drama Triangle

This diagram illustrates the variety of position-switches that can occur in the course of a "game" as defined in Transaction Analysis.

The three positions (Victim, Rescuer, Persecutor) are like roles assumed by characters in a drama. For instance villain (persecutor), hero (rescuer), or damsel in distress (victim).

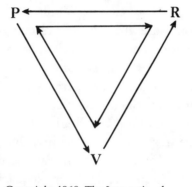

Copyright 1968, The International Transactional Analysis Association, Inc. Reprinted by permission.

other bites the bait. The climax is reached when the initiator switches roles—starting off as the "innocent" and becoming the "belligerent," or starting off demanding, and reprimanding, and ending up whimpering. It concludes with both parties getting a "payoff" of some sort.

Let's use a simple example.

Offering the Bait

Rita: Damn it, Jim, I tripped over your shoes again. You're such a slob. (Rita here is the demanding agent—the Persecutor.)

Biting the Bait

Jim: Well, Rita, you're no queen of neatness yourself. Look at this mess in the kitchen, etc. (Jim has taken the bait and is defending

himself by becoming a Persecutor of Rita.)

Climax Switch

Rita: You know I've got no time to do dishes. I'm working two jobs now, and I have to keep the kids happy. You know how I slave to get your meals on the table. (Starts crying.) (Rita has now switched into an "over-worked housewife" or Victim role.)

Payoff Conclusion

Jim: There, there, I didn't mean it. (Jim becomes Rescuer—his payoff. Rita gets attention—her payoff.)

Sound at all familiar? We all play games at times—when we are afraid to be honest or to reveal true feelings, or when we want intimacy, but fear it. Unfortunately, some people make game-playing a way of life, effectively shutting off any real communication.[4]

If any of these sentences have a familiar ring, you are very likely involved in a game:

My relationship with ———— is going downhill.

Talking about ———— makes me angry, frustrated, uptight.

———— never listens to me.

When I talk to ———— we usually end in an argument.

I'd really like to teach ———— a good lesson once and for all.

Once you are aware that you're playing a game, and aware, too, of just what triggers it, you're in a better position to break the cycle. You can decide not to start the game, or not to take the bait if someone else initiates a game.

Then you can invest the support of your fellow game-player in getting your real needs met. Share your awareness with them. "Mary, every time we talk about visiting my parents we end up deadlocked or in an argument. I think we may be playing or replaying a game here and I'd like you to help me to break it."

If the other agrees, you've got some excellent available alternatives. These may include:

- dropping the subject when it is emotionally overcharged, while agreeing to consider it when you both feel more balanced

- asking a third party to be present, to help you keep the *real issues* on the table

- using "dialogue"—really listening to the other, reflecting back what you think they're saying, until you're both sure that understanding has been achieved

- agreeing that it's OK to disagree

- working together to find out what each person's unspoken *needs* are

- contracting a workable compromise with one another

Throughout the process remember one significant rule: Tell the truth. Honesty is always the antidote to game-playing (and to most of the other "wars" on the planet as well). Our good friend, psychologist Will Shutz, Ph.D., has earned for himself, within the corporate domain, the affectionate title of "Dr. Truth." The secret of business success, he says, lies in simply telling the truth. Sound ad-vice, which we heartily support in every other domain as well. (For more on Will's work see his newest book, *The Truth Option*, cited in the reading list.)

Rescuing

Rescuing is a game strategy, and one of the most energy-draining. A rescuer is a compulsive helper, someone who cannot keep from stepping in to give aid, even when it is not asked for. Whole professions are based on rescuing—doctors, nurses, teachers, social workers, therapists often fall into that category. And parents are notorious for being rescuers.[5]

It might seem illogical to criticize rescuers or rescuing, but a closer look at the dynamics of the interaction reveals the inadequacies in the situation. The rescuer will be left unsatisfied because in attending to others, s/he neglects her/his own needs and becomes stroke-deprived. It is a double blow because the prime reason behind rescuing is to *get* strokes, and more often than not, the rescuer is rejected by the very ones he is trying to help and becomes a victim. (This is one of the chief causes of "burn-out" in the helping professions.) The one being helped is also left dissatisfied because the rescuer's position is "I'm OK, you're not OK—you're so inadequate I have to do it for you." From this vantage point, the victim typically turns on the rescuer with a "leave me alone" or "see what you've done."

This is not to say that you can never help someone. But you need to find out if help is wanted, and you need to find out if what you're doing is beneficial.

If you are a chronic rescuer, you would do well to do some self-examination. You may be projecting your inadequacies or needs onto others, or your primary need may be for strokes, in which case there are more effective ways to communicate your needs and satisfy them.

Here is a comparison of characteristics of both helpers and rescuers:

The Helper:

1. Listens for request.

2. Presents offer.

3. Gives only what is needed.

4. Checks periodically with person.

5. Checks results:
   — functioning better?
   — meeting goals?
   — solving problems independently?
   — using suggestions successfully?

The Rescuer:

1. Gives when not asked.

2. Neglects to find out if offer is welcome.

3. Gives help more and longer than needed.

4. Omits feedback.

5. Doesn't check results and feels good when accepted, bad when turned down.

6. Does the greater share of the talking.

Listening

Since almost half of the time you spend in communication is spent

Rescuer's Checklist

Completing the checklist can help you become aware of ways you may be rescuing people without realizing it. It is taken, with permission, from the *Transactional Checklist*.[6]

Mark each of the statements below as it applies to you according to this code: 0 = seldom or never; 1 = sometimes or occasionally; and 2 = frequently. X = significant others in your life, such as a spouse, boss, parents, friend, or colleague.

_____ **1.** Is it hard for you to take time for yourself and have fun?

_____ **2.** Do you supply words for X when s/he hesitates?

_____ **3.** Do you set limits for yourself that you then exceed?

_____ **4.** Do you believe you are responsible for making (keeping) X happy?

_____ **5.** Do you enjoy lending a shoulder for X to "cry" on?

_____ **6.** Do you believe that X is not sufficiently grateful for your help?

_____ **7.** Do you take care of X more than you take care of yourself?

_____ **8.** Do you find yourself interrupting when X is talking?

_____ **9.** Do you watch for clues for ways to be helpful to X?

_____ **10.** Do you make excuses, openly or mentally, for X?

_____ **11.** Do you do more than your share, that is, work harder than X?

_____ **12.** When X is unsure or uncomfortable about doing something, do you do it for X?

_____ **13.** Do you give up doing things because X wouldn't like it?

_____ **14.** Do you find yourself thinking that you really know what is best for X?

_____ **15.** Do you think X would have grave difficulty getting along without you?

_____ **16.** Do you use the word "we" and then find you don't have X's consent?

_____ **17.** Do you stop yourself by thinking X will feel badly if you say or do something?

_____ **18.** Is it hard for you *not* to respond to anyone who seems hurting or needing help?

_____ **19.** Do you find yourself being resented when you were only trying to be helpful?

_____ **20.** Do you find yourself giving advice that is not welcome or accepted?

_____ *Score.* More than 10 points, rescuing is possible; more than 20 points, rescuing is probable.

listening, you should be an expert at it by now. If you are, though, you are the rare exception. Most people listen passively, because they consider speaking to be the active component of communication. But that is because they confuse listening with hearing.

Apply this idea to the enjoyment of music. As background sound in a workplace it serves to set a mood and perhaps create greater relaxation. But rarely will you attend to the lyrics, or dance to the rhythm. You hear the music, but you are not really listening. Contrast this with your behavior when you go to a concert, symphony, or a dance. Your body is turned in the direction of the band or orchestra. You experience an emotional "rush" as you allow it to move you. You may surrender your body to it and let it direct your movements as you dance. At the conclusion you will clap, or whistle approval, or stand up and yell. You are listening—and it is a dynamic process.

Dynamic listening, sometimes called active listening, needs to be developed by all of us, since we generally allow much of what we hear to go in one ear and out the other. The semanticist, S.I. Hayakawa, gives this example of poor listening:

"Jones says something, Smith gives a heated response to what he mistakenly believes Jones said, and Jones tries to refute what he mistakenly believes Smith meant."[7]

This enormous energy waste is easily remedied by using a very simple technique called "reflecting back." After Jones has spoken, Smith would recount what he understood Jones to be saying. If Jones agrees, Smith would then continue

When you listen to me without interruption or anything that feels like a judgment, you allow me the time and space to get more in touch with the many facets of me

Thank you for never playing with my words, getting a laugh or recognition at my expense.

When you allow me to revise or restructure what I have said, I feel that you are truly committed to understanding me and what I'm about.

Thank you for not feeling that you necessarily have to do something about what I share.

When you listen, I feel that you are listening not only to my words but the feelings behind them.

Bless you for being you and thereby assisting me in my journey.

—Bennett Kilpack, M.F.C.C.

with his remarks. If Jones disagrees, he can restate his case in another way that leaves less room for misinterpretation. Smith then reports what he has heard. The exchange continues on this level until Jones is satisfied that he has been understood. The conversation might go like this:

Jones: The records in your department are terribly confusing to interpret.
Smith: Are you saying that I keep bad records?
Jones: No, not at all. I'm saying that the complexity of your work makes reporting a difficult task. I'm impressed by what you've done, but I need help understanding it.
Smith: Thanks for the compliment. So you need someone to work with you when you look them over?

Jones: That's exactly it! Any suggestions?

This technique can become ridiculous if used all the time, in talking about the weather, for instance:

Jones: What's the weather like outside?
Smith: Am I correct in assuming that you are asking for my knowledge about the current temperature, humidity, and rate of precipitation?

But it is an invaluable tool to use when taking directions or instructions, when discussing matters which might put the participants on the defensive, or when dealing with problems in a close relationship. For example:

Tom: The children have really been unruly lately. I'm getting fed up.

. . . . *Exercise* . . . .

Listening: The Non-Building Blocks

In a very interesting book entitled *The Art of Listening**, *Jud Morris lists what he calls the "Ten Non-Building Blocks of Listening." These are:*

1. *Evaluation, Judgment:* We are so busy planning our attack, or criticizing the other's message that we often do not really hear what is being said.

2. *Jumping to Conclusions:* We jump to conclusions, filling in our own details before the other has had a chance to explain himself/herself.

3. *"We're all the same":* We assume that other people think as we do.

4. *Attitude, the Closed Mind:* We "tune out" people with whom we don't agree.

5. *Lack of Attention:* We let our minds wander, giving in to other external noises or distractions.

6. *Wishful Hearing:* We tend to hear just what we want to hear, or expect to hear.

7. *Excessive Talking:* We interrupt or dominate the conversation so that the other doesn't get a chance to adequately express his/her ideas.

8. *Unclear Words:* We fail to find out what the other means by the particular words he/she chooses.

9. *Lack of Humility:* We feel that we must express our superiority by speaking or contradicting the other.

10. *Fear:* We avoid listening with understanding because we are afraid that the other may challenge some long-held belief. We are afraid to be threatened by a new idea.

   If these are the Non-Building Blocks—what are the Building Blocks?
   List some here:

   _____

   _____

   _____

   _____

. . . .

Terri: You are really frustrated by their behavior.

Tom: Yes—do you think it's just me, or have you noticed it too?

The next time you find yourself embroiled in a heated debate why not try this "reflecting" strategy. You just might find that there really was no disagreement in the first place. If there is, at least you'll have a clearer understanding of what the problem stems from.

Learning to listen brings tremendous, and often immediate, rewards which contribute to health and happiness on all sides. We relieve stress, we meet the other on a common ground and provide them with affirming strokes. To be listened to is to be acknowledged as a worthwhile human being—and that's the best "medicine" there is.

Carl Rogers defined communication in this way: "Real communication occurs . . . when we listen with understanding. What does this mean? It means to see the expressed idea and attitude from the other person's point of view, to sense how it feels to him, to achieve his frame of reference in regard to the thing he is talking about . . . If I can really understand how he hates his father or hates the university or hates communists—if I can catch the flavor of his fear of insanity, or his fear of atom bombs, or of Russia—it will be the greatest help to him in altering these very hatreds and fears and in establishing realistic and harmonious relationships with the very people and situations toward which he has felt hatred and fear."[9, 10, 11]

The Final Goal

Aiming at total agreement as the goal of communication sets you up for failure. You can't win at that game. But if you aim at understanding and mutual respect, everybody can win. Actually communication effectiveness has a direct relationship to the degree of trust that exists between two individuals.

In order to trust others we need to allow trust for ourselves. We nourish trust for ourselves by taking responsibility for our own lives, and living with love and compassion. By now, you recognize these attitudes as the chief supports of wellness, too.

Beyond Human Communication

Humankind has long been intrigued with the idea of contacting and communicating with other intelligences. Elaborate systems have been devised to probe outer space

---

Asserting Your Right To Wellness

People often feel timid about questioning "experts," and this is particularly true in the doctor-patient relationship. Here are some suggestions that may help you assert your rights to wellness.

1. Ask your doctor to explain fully your condition and what exactly is going on in your body. Ask for illustrations if necessary.

2. Ask if there are ways, other than drugs or surgery, to deal with your problem.

3. Ask about possible side-effects of drugs prescribed.

4. Ask for a second, or third opinion. Or investigate alternatives for yourself.

5. Ask for a "generic" drug prescription which is usually less expensive than a brand name.

6. Ask for a full description of a procedure suggested before it is used.

7. Ask for a lead shield to cover other parts of body (particularly ovaries or testes) when X-rays are being taken.

8. State your displeasure and inconvenience at being made to wait.

9. Ask for anything which will provide you with greater privacy or comfort.

10. Ask for a fee-schedule before you make an appointment.

11. Ask about your doctor's previous experience in dealing with a condition similar to your own.

12. Refuse treatment if your questions are not answered adequately.

13. Tell your doctor what *you* think is wrong or right with you.[12]

---

for signals that might be coming to us, and plaques have been designed to identify our space probes to other intelligences. As for more earthly concerns, many studies have been made and are being made on communication in species other than humans, particularly in the higher forms of life such as apes, dolphins, and whales, in an effort to crack their codes and to set up communication with them. Only rudimentary lines of communication have been established so far, and as yet no signals from

outer space have been received. However, in trying to solve these theoretical problems we have learned more about our *own* communication processes and thought mechanisms.

There is the distinct possibility that we would have much to learn from extra-terrestrial beings, and much to learn from the species that share this planet with us, if we only knew how to communicate with them. In a remarkable series of studies that spanned a decade, John Lilly, M.D., set out to do just that

. . . . *Exercise* . . . .

The Inner Dialogue

When was the last time you eavesdropped on yourself? Whether you are aware of it or not, there is an inner dialogue going on in your head all the time. These conversations can seriously undermine your peace of mind. They color your world view. They are the source of your problems, but they can be the source for the solutions, too. They literally run your life! Listening in on yourself will help you get in touch with yourself.

1. Set aside a few short periods each day in which you simply listen to your inner dialogue. Stop yourself now and then throughout the day, especially when you're confronted with a question or problem, and tune in to yourself.

2. After you've done this for at least several days, pose some specific topics to yourself, such as "colds," "old age," "death," and listen to what is being said.

3. Try writing out these "dialogues" as we have suggested in many previous exercises.

4. Assume the role of an objective third party and merely listen, attempting not to get involved.

5. Make a list of the negative messages you frequently hear yourself making. Realize how these are affecting the ways in which you view the world.

6. Make a list of positive counterarguments—start plugging them in.

. . . .

with dolphins.[13] He chose dolphins primarily because the dolphin brain is similar to the human brain in both size and complexity and he felt they would be the logical first choice for trying to establish interspecies communication.

Dolphins communicate almost solely by sonic transmissions. They use sonic and ultrasonic waves to scan their surroundings and to identify objects by shape and distance, and seem to be able to transmit information to each other. Lilly attempted to analyze and codify their underwater sounds in search of patterns that might indicate language. In another series of experiments, he studied the ability of dolphins to mimic human sounds (dolphins are able to vocalize out of

the water). He thought that if dolphins could learn to communicate in the human mode, while at the same time we learned to understand theirs, there would be a greater possibility for finding common ground.

After a lapse of several years, Lilly returned to his research, this time using a computer as a language interface. But the work raised deeper questions. Most recently, he has abandoned his experiments with cetaceans because, he says, "I just didn't want to run a concentration camp for highly developed beings . . ."[14]

Lilly's work invites us to speculate on our own modes of communication. We humans receive at least 80% of our input *visually*, and

then in order to communicate, must translate our experience into words, which we then generally convey orally. For dolphins, the major input is *aural* so they need not translate their experiences from one medium to another in order to communicate. Their communication is more efficient and accurate than ours, and less information is lost in process. If we could communicate as directly as dolphins do, there would be much less misunderstanding and a greater degree of intimacy than we usually experience in our exchanges with each other. It would probably resemble those rare moments of contact we share with someone when minds seem to be joined and words are unnecessary.

Super-organisms

Consider now another level of communication, a level where individual units transcend their separateness and join to form a new unit. This new super-organism then functions with a life of its own. Lewis Thomas in his *Lives of a Cell*[15] gives the example of ants as a group of "individuals" combining to create a larger "individual." The colony becomes the new organism, taking a shape to which it is automatically restored if it is disturbed, and having long tentacles which reach out to the surrounding area, gathering food and materials to support it. When fish form schools, they are also so closely integrated they function as a great multi-fish organism. A certain type of slug is "created" by the union of separate slime-mold cells; to complete its life cycle, the slug produces more slime-mold cells which form the next generation.

These examples point to uncommon modes of communication and extraordinary levels of intimacy and cooperation. This level of communication is not yet well understood even though it can be said to apply to everything from the creation of a single cell to the operation of the entire universe. Complex interactions of many separate organisms of these cells permit you to function as a human being. The town you live in is a collection of human beings; through organization, the town functions as a unit, too. The chain is endless.

Communication and the Planet

By expanding our concept of communication, we can see how entire super-organisms can result from

Dolphins

It seems to me that the life of a dolphin is superior to ours in many ways. We humans often equate happiness with progress, and expend much of our time and energy worrying about the past or future rather than in living in the moment. We continue to kill each other with violence and war, and perpetuate our misery. Those moments of experiencing love and peace are, for many of us, all too rare. Despite mammoth advances in technology, medicine and material welfare, man appears to be little happier than his ancestors of "less civilized" eras.

Without the distractions of a technological society, dolphins and other cetaceans seem to live fully in the present and exhibit much more of what we humans might call love. I believe these enviable qualities they so readily exhibit may in part be due to an ability to communicate with each other in a more advanced manner than do we of the human species. Dolphins have a much wider vocal range than humans and can apparently converse with several different vocal apparatus at the same time.

When I first heard John Lilly talk about dolphins, my whole concept of communication was expanded immensely. Lilly has made several fascinating conjectures about the mode in which dolphins communicate. Imagining what it is like for them is difficult, but I would like to share my understanding with you.

The sonar dolphins use to "see" with passes easily through soft tissue, so when one dolphin "looks at" another it really "looks through" the other. It can see, as an X-ray picture would, any undigested dinner still in the other's stomach, as well as observe the heart rate and other physiologic functions. Lilly reasoned that if one dolphin were to try to lie to another, the physiologic signs of lying, such as increased pulse rate and respiration, would be easily visible. Imagine what your relationships would be like if you too were always completely honest in your communications. To be that transparent is a feeling I would like to experience. This form of communication could well explain the highly ethical behavior for which dolphins have been noted. The fact that the temporal portion of the brain (associated with ethics in human beings) is rather large in dolphins, lends additional credence to this hypothesis.

It appears that we are sharing the planet with a sentient species from which we have much to learn. Were we to communicate with them, we may find this to be as valuable to us as contact with extraterrestrials.

—J.W.T.

intimate contact and cooperation. This then provides a basis for considering that perhaps our entire planet is a single organism.

The hypothesis that the planet is a single organism was first suggested by Johannes Kepler hundreds of years ago. It was most recently expounded by James Lovelock in *The Gaia Hypothesis*.[16] (Gaia, in Greek mythology, was the earth goddess.) Observing that the planet, Gaia, has systems that can regulate temperature, oxygen concentration, and other variables, he reasoned that the earth is much more than a hunk of rock with different species of plants and animals living on it, that it is a whole system made up of many smaller systems, including humankind.

As with any organism, earth's life depends on the integrated functioning of all her elements. There are many signs that all is not well, that the planet is sick. The recent upsurge of volcanic action, earthquakes, and unusual weather patterns may well be messages from Gaia, calling us to pay attention to her needs. If we continue to ignore her communications, there may be even harsher outbursts as Gaia is forced to take more drastic action to regain balance. Our survival may depend upon our understanding the message.

Suggested Reading*

Alberti, R., and Emmons, M. *Your Perfect Right.* San Luis Obispo, CA: Impact Publishers, 1970.

Bach, G., and Goldberg, H. *Creative Aggression.* New York, NY: Avon Books, 1976.

*This is only a representative sampling. Many excellent books have been omitted. At the bookstore or library, look over the whole section and choose according to your judgment.

Berne, E. *Games People Play.* New York, NY: Grove Press, 1964.

Bolton, R. *People Skills.* Englewood Cliffs, NJ: Prentice-Hall, 1977.

Emery, S. *Actualizations: You Don't Have to Rehearse to Be Yourself.* New York, NY: Doubleday, 1978.

Fensterheim, H., and Baer, J. *Don't Say Yes When You Want to Say No.* New York, NY: Dell, 1975.

Gordon, T. *Parent Effectiveness Training.* New York, NY: New American Library, 1975.

Howe, R. *The Miracle of Dialogue.* New York, NY: The Seabury Press, 1963.

Jongeward, D., and Scott, D. *Women As Winners: Transactional Analysis for Personal Growth.* Reading, MA: Addison-Wesley, 1976.

Jourard, S. *The Transparent Self.* New York, NY: D. Van Nostrand-Reinhold Co., 1964.

Lovelock, J. *Gaia: A New Look at Life on Earth.* New York, NY: Oxford University Press, 1979.

McKay, M., et al. *Messages: The Communication Skills Book.* Oakland, CA: New Harbinger Publishers, 1983.

Miller, S., et al. *Straight Talk.* New York, NY: New American Library, 1982.

Powell, J. *Why Am I Afraid to Tell You Who I Am?* Chicago, IL: Peacock Books, 1969.

Prather, H. *Notes to Myself.* Moab, UT: Real People Press, 1970.

Rogers, C. *On Becoming a Person.* Boston, MA: Houghton-Mifflin, 1961.

Reusch, J. *Therapeutic Communication.* New York, NY: W.W. Norton, 1961.

Sanford, J.A. *Communicating One-to-One.* New York, NY: Paulist Press, 1982.

Thomas, L. *The Lives of a Cell.* New York, NY: Bantam Books, 1975.

———. *The Medusa and the Snail.* New York, NY: Bantam Books, 1980.

Notes

1. For more on "dialogue" see:

Howe, R. *The Miracle of Dialogue.* New York, NY: The Seabury Press, 1963.

Powell, J. *Why Am I Afraid to Tell You Who I Am?* Chicago, IL: Peacock Books, 1969.

Johannesen. R. "The Emerging Concept of Communication as Dialogue." *Quarterly Journal of Speech*, LVIII (December 1971), pp. 373–82.

2. We suggest the following books on assertiveness:

Alberti, R., and Emmons, M. *Stand Up, Speak Out, Talk Back!* New York, NY: Pocket Books. 1976.

Alberti, R., and Emmons, M. *Your Perfect Right.* San Luis Obispo, CA. Impact Publishers, 1970.

Bower, G., and Bower, S. *Asserting Your Self.* Reading, MA: Addison-Wesley Publishing, 1976.

Butler, P. *Self-Assertion for Women.* New York, NY: Harper and Row, 1976.

Fensterheim, H., and Baer, J. *Don't Say Yes When You Want to Say No.* New York, NY. Dell, 1975.

Jongeward, D., and Scott, D. *Women as Winners.* Reading, MA. Addison-Wesley, 1976.

3. These books on general semantics are recommended:

Hayakawa, S.I. *Language in Thought and Action.* (4th ed.) New York, NY: Harcourt Brace Jovanovich, 1978.

Berman, S. *How to Lessen Misunderstandings.* San Francisco, CA: The International Society for General Semantics, 1969.

Johnson, W. *People in Quandaries.* New York, NY: Harper and Brothers, 1946.

Fabun, D. *Communications: The Transfer of Meaning.* Encino, CA: The Glencoe Press, 1965.

4. For more on "Games" from Transactional Analysis see:

Berne, E. *Games People Play.* New York, NY: Grove Press, 1964.

James, M., and Jongeward, D. *Born to Win*. Reading, MA: Addison-Wesley, 1971.

5. For more on rescuing and helping see:

James, M., and Jongeward, D. *Born to Win*. Reading, MA: Addison-Wesley, 1971, pp. 85–89.

Wyckoff, H. *Solving Women's Problems*. New York, NY: Grove Press, 1977, pp. 90–99.

6. Baute, P., and Lankford, V., from "The Transactional Checklist." More information from: Institute for Human Responsiveness, Inc., 6200 Winchester Blvd., Lexington, KY 40511. Used with permission.

7. Hayakawa, S.I. *Through the Communication Barrier*. New York, NY: Harper and Row, 1979, p. 73.

8. Adapted from: Morris, J. *The Art of Listening*. Boston, MA: Industrial Education Institute, 1968.

9. Quotation is from:

Rogers, C. "Communication: Its Blocking and Its Facilitation." *ETC*. Vol. 9, Winter 1952, p. 84.

10. For more on openness in communication see:

Gibb, J. "Defensive Communication." *Journal of Communication*, Vol. XI, 1961, pp. 141–48.

Gibb, J. *TRUST*. Los Angeles, CA: Guild of Tutors Press, 1978.

11. Another classic in good communications is:

Gordon. T. *Parent Effectiveness Training*. New York, NY: New American Library, 1975.

12. For a discussion of "patient's lib" see:

Samuel, M., and Bennet, H. *The Well Body Book*. New York, NY, and Berkeley, CA: Random House/Bookworks, 1973, pp. 302–07.

13. Lilly, J. *Lilly on Dolphins*. Garden City, NY: Anchor Books, 1975.

14. Lilly, J. "John Lilly on Satori." *Magical Blend Magazine*. No. 16, pp. 8–9.

15. Thomas, L. *The Lives of a Cell*. New York, NY: Bantam, 1975.

16. Lovelock, J. *Gaia: A New Look at Life on Earth*. New York, NY: Oxford University Press, 1979.

Wellness and Sex

THE SO-CALLED sexual revolution has certainly had many positive effects on the social climate. It has paved the way for more frank and open discussion of sex and sexual problems, has made it easier to get needed information on sexual matters, and has fostered a more tolerant attitude towards behaviors that in previous times would have been condemned as unhealthy, deviant, or criminal. Unfortunately, this new openness has not solved all our problems. In fact, it has created a few new ones.

A quick glance at the newspaper, an overheard conversation, discussions with friends, perhaps an examination of your own thoughts, will reveal that problems, misconceptions, and fears about sex still abound. Here are a few typical statements:

"Before we got married we did it all the time. Now s/he just doesn't seem to have any interest in sex. What's wrong?"

Sex is the vital life force, the *elan vital*, or in Eastern philosophy, the *Ki* or *Chi*. It is the energy of our aliveness. Sex is also about the preservation of life—a type of communication in which the entire organism attempts to unify itself with another. It depends dynamically upon the input sources (breath, sensation, food/fuel) for its complete expression, and is strongly modified by the other energy outputs such as thoughts, feelings, and messages. Sex may also serve to open one to new levels of meaning in life, as well as provide experiences of transcendence.

"I must be abnormal. I've never had an orgasm at the same time as my partner."

"If only I _____, then I could please my partner sexually."

"He says he really loves me. So why do I feel like a sex object?"

The basic problem remains—that, rather than living sex as a total body-mind experience, we have learned to block off sexual energy or to confine it to our genital organs. It is here that we get "turned on," and here that we hold our guilt, our confusion, our fear. As noted in the section on touch in chapter 3, the needs for caring, and tenderness, and total body involvement are unmet when the focus of sex becomes intercourse alone. The result is disappointment, frustration, and damage to the self-concept.

. . . .

What we're born with, what we experience all through infancy and childhood is a sexuality that isn't concentrated on the genitals: it's a sexuality diffused through the whole organism. That's the paradise we inherit. But the paradise gets lost as the child grows up.

—ALDOUS HUXLEY,
FROM *ISLAND*

. . . .

The "sexual revolution" has had no small part in narrowing our focus. Check the latest offerings on the local magazine rack, take a critical look at advertisements, examine the contents of the average TV serial . . . they all underline the preoccupation with sex.

This exaggerated importance assigned to sex has led us in search of the multiple orgasm to prove our potency. It has contributed to the pressures and tensions which many experience in connection with sex. It has led us to develop unrealistic expectations of how great sex is supposed to be, of how it will solve all our problems. When sex is defined in terms of flawless physical bodies, in terms of power and prestige and ecstasy, we are bound to feel inadequate when our own experiences fall short.

To add to the confusion, vestiges of the puritanical past still linger. Many people still consider sex dirty, part of the "lower" nature, something to be feared, earned, or supplied dutifully, still consider the body secondary to the mind, a thing you attend to when necessary and keep carefully covered up. Few of us have escaped contamination from the fear, the embarrassment, the confusion, and the anger which surrounded sex in the thoughts and words and behaviors of our parents, teachers, ministers, and friends. The relationship of sex with all of life is hard to discover when it can't be talked about in school, or in church, or in polite company.

All the fuss and furor, and guilt, and secretiveness about masturbation testify to a fear of the body in general, and of pleasure in particular. The myths that have

. . . . *Regina's Journal* . . . .

At the age of 27, after spending eight years as a nun in a convent, Regina underwent a total hysterectomy. It was necessary because of a seriously complicated condition in her ovaries. She is convinced that years of fear and sexual repression were responsible.

I was a terrifically sensitive child, and a bright one, but I was grossly ignorant about my body in general and about sex in particular. The nuns told us that it was a sin to "touch yourself," and in the same breath declared that the body was good, the temple of the Holy Spirit. The priests told us it was a sin to have "impure thoughts," but it was OK as long as we didn't "consent" to them. My friends told me it was a sin to "go all the way," but they talked and acted as if they knew "the way" very well. Was I the only one who didn't? To put it mildly I was confused.

As an adolescent I was terrified by the notion of sex. I wasn't really sure of the details but I knew it had something to do with being naked and that thought was absolutely disgusting to me. I had never even seen my parents or sisters undressed.

I shook my head and washed my hands when sexual images arose in my mind. I went to confession every week. I prayed for help and at last resigned myself to a life of struggle and tension. I had to keep myself in control.

As I moved into my twenties I continued to suffer from extreme

. . . .

long surrounded this subject have presented it as abnormal, unnatural, anti-social and harmful:

"you'll go insane . . ."

"you'll go blind . . ."

"you'll get warts . . ."

"you'll go to hell . . ."

There is no evidence to support that masturbation impairs mental or physical health, but for many, the guilt learned in childhood endures.[1] Why self-initiated pleasure is held inferior remains a mystery. Perhaps it has to do with a work ethic which attaches a price to pleasure, or that presents it as a reward

for service. Some of us harbor guilt in experiencing joy and other good feelings.

The result of all this confusion is the contamination or blockage of our sexual energy channels, leading to a whole range of problems which include:

impotence or frigidity

compulsiveness

broken relationships

rape

diseases, especially in the reproductive organs

physical and emotional pain

cramps during my menstrual periods. I gained weight in my upper thighs and buttocks; and began to visit doctors regularly for a variety of stress-related ailments.

My body was a battlefield.

As a nun I was safe. Dressed in black and vowed to chastity, I assumed my asexual identity with relief. God, I affirmed, would forgive my sins as long as I remained one of his chosen brides.

Looking back, I realize how the blocking of energy in my sexual organs contributed to the manifestation of disease there. I have learned some hard lessons but can also view the problems as invitations—for self-knowledge and further self-exploration. What I saw was the need to accept my humanness which in this case meant my physicalness. Sex is a natural and normal human process and should be celebrated as such. I needed, moreover, to re-own my own body, to reacquaint myself with the messages it was giving me, day to day. I needed to trust myself. I had to let go of the diseased attitudes of the so-called "experts" whom I had listened to previously, and assume responsibility for my own life and health. And I needed to strike a balance within myself to express my gentleness as well as my strength, my vulnerability as well as my power, my maleness with my femaleness. I needed to integrate, to unify, and to love my wholeness.

"Well-Sex"

Having taken this long look at the darker side, let's now take a look at the brighter side. For those who are troubled, there are ways to attack the problems. For those who are not particularly troubled by the role sex plays in their lives, there are ways to *enhance* the flow of sexual energy. In both cases, the key word is *integration*.

"Well-sex" demands the integration of body, mind, and spirit. If you want an example of integrated sexuality just look at a baby. The infant's body is fully alive; every cell is dancing. If we could capture this energy in motion on film, we would see rivers of energy sparkling all over, and swirling all around. The body would appear as a sea of light. The child responds with pleasure to the stroking of its fingers and toes. Here is a clear, unblocked channel. Sexual energy flows throughout every part, head to toe.

"Well-sex" also demands the integrated flow of all the energies discussed in the preceding chapters. In the adult, sex is a complex activity involving much more than the genital organs and the physical act of intercourse, to repeat the point. It is bound up with feelings and emotions, it involves free use of all the senses, it is a form of play

or recreation. But more than anything else, it is influenced by your inner thoughts, and by your ability to communicate with yourself and with your partner.

In sex, we experience communion with another human being. At least temporarily we are assuaged of our loneliness, we are touched and held securely; we feel unified. So we look to sex for stroking and for integration. Lovemaking, in general, and the moments of orgasm, in particular, allow us a temporary respite from the judging, anticipating, and questioning of our rational minds. Sex provides us with a powerful experience of NOWNESS—full awareness of all that is happening at the moment.

Sexual Awareness

Awareness is body trust. In sexuality, body trust specifically means attending to its cues as to what it likes and needs to be "turned on" sensually and erotically. The primary question becomes "What feels good to me?"

Sex is the only experience which could justify living, draw me back from an abstract future to a present of palpable skin.

—ALLEN WHEELIS

As a child you easily played with your body, you enjoyed the freedom of nakedness, and you delighted in being held against the bodies of others, stroked and tickled. There was no shame or fear attached to any of these activities until uncomfortable others began to give you messages to the con-

. . . . *Exercise* . . . .

Sex Is . . .

Look over this list of words (add more, if you like). Star the five that best reflect what sex is for you now. Put an X by the five that you would never associate with sex. Finally, put two stars by words that describe what you would like to experience most.

If you are sharing sex regularly, have your partner do this exercise. Use your responses as a topic for discussion with each other. Talking freely about your feelings is the first step in making sex what you want it to be.

Sex is:	generous	active	cruel	too short
natural	caring	passive	painful	bothersome
normal	responsible	skillful	embarrassing	pressured
healthy	conscious	delicate	sorrowful	preoccupied
fun	pleasant	erotic	hard	meaningful
freeing	patient	boring	performance-	easy
exciting	slow	ordinary	oriented	spiritual
necessary	fast	compulsive	sickening	silly
beautiful	mellow	scary	guilty	tedious
graceful	gentle	tense	fearful	hurried
flowing	unifying	frightening	angry	
expansive	respectful	demeaning	violent	
inspiring	enjoyable	disgusting	too long	

. . . .

trary. As the sole inhabitant of your body, you knew what felt good to you, and you did it. But at some point you gave up on yourself, and began to believe that what was natural and normal for you was not acceptable.

Reclaiming this realization of freedom—of the goodness of the body, is the first step in body trust, and the basis for the living of wellness.

To say "yes" to the body is to say "yes" to pleasure—and sex can be one of the most pleasant experiences you can have. Pleasure is your reward, not for doing something, but simply for being alive. The fact that you inhabit a body which is soft, and pliable, and cov-ered with sensitive nerve endings, and requires touch for survival, presents a strong case for allowing yourself to accept pleasure, for celebrating the magnificent creation which your body is.

Self-touch, or massage, is an invaluable aid in learning about the unique sensitivies of your body. Often the concentration on genital involvement leaves vast areas of pleasure and arousal unexplored. Many approaches to sexual therapy include a recommendation that individuals and couples deliberately avoid stimulating the genitals for a period of time in order that the sensations in other body parts be appreciated.[2] Masturbation in a non-pressured environment is one way of developing your own sexual awareness.

The next step in awareness is the realization that the most potent sexual organ in your body is very likely your brain. For many, reading erotic literature, or watching sexually explicit films, can be extremely provocative. Sexual fantasies, once considered to be unhealthy, are now being recommended for the powerful effects which they can have on the body.[3] Allowing yourself to experiment in these areas may be as beneficial as allowing your own touch.

On the other hand, the brain can turn you off as readily as it can turn you on. Listen as you "talk" to yourself before, during, and after

. . . . *Exercise* . . . .

Movement Exercises—Releasing Tension:

Tanya, who teaches belly-dancing, instructs her students in a variety of exercises which serve to release tensions in sexual areas of the body. When blocks are broken up, the fullness of sexual energy is free to flow. Try these:

1. Stand with feet about shoulder width apart. Distribute weight evenly on both feet. Unlock the knees. Relax the muscles in the anus. Now rotate the pelvis forward, and then in clockwise circles, keeping the anus open. Reverse the motion, moving the pelvis in a counterclockwise direction. Do each series of rotations at least ten times. Then direct the pelvis in a figure eight pattern. Do this easily, making small 8's, then larger 8's, then smaller 8's. Stop. Lie down on your back and rest, breathe deeply.

2. Lie flat on your back on the floor. Draw your knees up, placing feet flat on the floor. Keeping buttocks on the ground, inhale and arch your lower back. As you exhale, press lower back into the floor. Continue doing this for one full minute. Remember to keep muscles around anus and genitals relaxed, so that energy can flow into them. Rest.

3. Stand up again. Feet shoulder width apart, arms at your sides, anal and genital muscles relaxed, abdomen relaxed. Now bend knees slightly. Keeping the balls of your feet in contact with the ground, begin to bounce your heels up and down. Allow your legs to help in the bouncing. You'll know when you're doing it right when you can feel the fat in your buttocks rippling as you bounce. Do this for at least one minute. Stop, lie down and rest. Breathe deeply and note sensations occurring throughout the body.

. . . .

sex, and you will gain important insights about how your thoughts are creating your reality:

- Since your thoughts assign meaning to sex, your body will follow suit.

- Preoccupations with performance and expectations take you out of the "here and now" and build tensions.

- Your fears can freeze you.

- Your guilt and anxiety can stifle your pleasure.

- Your judgments can easily lead to dissatisfaction.

You can use your brain in the service of sex, as you have in other areas of wellness. As you become aware of the "voices" (your own or others') which fill your head, they can serve as cues to come back to

"Well-Sex" Is

- Freely chosen
- Conscious of consequences
- Respectful
- Erotic
- Playful
- Expansive
- Unifying

the "here and now," to focus on the part of the body being touched, to breathe deeply and allow sexual feelings to carry through your whole body, to open all your sensory pathways to increase your pleasure many times over.

Throughout the process of developing or enhancing awareness, remember to love yourself and to be compassionate. Take small, slow steps and celebrate each new awakening.

The scope of this book does not allow more than a brief presentation of possibilities for your consideration. Programs abound which deal specifically with sexual attitude restructuring, heightening awareness and sensitivity, and coping with sexual blocks or physical problems. If sex is a conflict area for you, you can take the next step by reading some of the resources listed with this chapter, and seeking the support of others in the programs available.[4] Self-responsibility means never staying stuck!

Self-Responsible Sex

Self-responsible sex means accepting that you, and only you, are the "expert" about yourself. Just as you may be tempted to give up personal power and deny your own experience in other aspects of wellness, when it comes to sex you may allow yourself to be confused, if not persuaded, by the opinions of others—your friends, the media, the poll-takers.

In observing self-responsibility here, you need to examine who and what you are listening to, and question who or what you are believing. This youth-oriented culture is inclined to capitalize on appearances. In so doing it often overlooks the needs of the elderly, the incarcerated, the mentally and physically handicapped, for whom sex is a right and a privilege as much as it is for the young. Because the media use sex to sell everything from toothpaste to tractors, they frequently present a distorted image of the whole subject. Popular magazines inform you of the statistics regarding sexual preferences, and frequency of expression, and may lead you to believe that you are not quite normal if you fall outside the mean. The fact that, as some of these surveys report, married couples in the U.S. average X acts of intercourse per month merely indicates that some do it all

Dr. Anita on Sex and Touch

Our friend Dr. Anita, mentioned on p. 192, also happens to be a sexologist, a therapist who deals primarily with sex-related issues. We asked her about what she has learned, especially in the past few years, that she would like to see expressed in this chapter. This is a sample of what she had to say:

If there's one misunderstanding I fight day after day it is that people say "sex" and immediately think "intercourse." Real sexual liberation can only happen when it is fully understood that the two need not be the same! The sex act is something we do—our thinking, our communication, our work and play, our sense of meaning, our spirituality.

I see myself more as a "touch therapist" than almost anything else. When I give people the permission to touch or to consciously refuse touch, help them understand the necessity of touching for health and wellness, encourage them to explore the pleasures of touch, alone and with a partner (with or without genital involvement), real miracles happen.

The media's recent exposure of the magnitude of sexual abuse has been necessary and long-overdue.

And, I see people pulling away in fear from all touch because they are afraid they may be misinterpreted. This is exactly the wrong way to approach the problem. Isolation causes more violence. Our fear of being considered a molester may cause us to either deny or to overreact. We must work within ourselves and together to find the place of balance.

We need to listen to our children more, instruct them about their rights to refuse uncomfortable touch, warn them of potential dangers, gain their confidence so that they will confide in us. But unless we are "stretching our own comfort zones" about sexuality, i.e., facing head-on our fears and misinformation, we may only be increasing the same all around.

Sexuality needs to be freed to grow and change. It is a never ending process, not a goal. Relax and enjoy the process. It takes a real commitment to yourself to explore your sexuality positively because whether you believe it or not, we still live in a sex-negative society.

We can't be whole persons if we cut off our genitals, yet we are cutting them off emotionally and spiritually every day, and that is causing us much pain and suffering in all aspects of our lives.

the time and others only on their anniversaries. Statistics can be very misleading unless you approach them with an understanding of how they are gathered and realize that they are never meant to "prove."

The research of Kinsey, Masters and Johnson, Hite, and others serves to underline the need to

trust your own experience.[5] Their findings demonstrate that individual differences in sexual practice are truly amazing. In fact, there seems to be a wider range of human sexual appetite, capacity, and behavior than of almost any other human trait. Sexual practice often varies as widely as the number of subjects questioned.

Anything which leads you to question if you are "normal" should be held highly suspect—there simply is no such animal. Virginia admits that she feels inadequate because she does not have the same desires for sex that her friend Claudia does. Her guilt serves only to block her free sexual expression. The question "Why don't I enjoy sex, or do it as frequently, as Claudia does?" is the wrong question. There will never be an answer unless the real issue which underlies the question is first addressed. The real issue is: "Why inadequate? Why guilt for being who I am?"

Sex is self-responsible when it is conscious and when it is self-assertive. To be conscious about sex means that it be freely entered into, not coerced or manipulated to prove power, or to get favors, or to keep the other from leaving. Unconscious sex can be compulsive or even raping. It may show little or no regard for the integrity of the body or mind of the other.

When sex is conscious it is informed. This means adequate preparation and protection for disease prevention and birth control. It is surprising how misinformed so many of us are about the sexual functioning of our bodies. Recently, after her second abortion, Glenna remarked that she was really never sure exactly when she was "safe" during her menstrual cycle. Deardre, at thirty-four, guessed that she was sterile simply because she had never conceived, and hence used no birth control. The epidemic proportions of venereal disease reflect this same unconsciousness in sexuality.

While we may speak frankly about sex in general, there is still an unromantic aura attached to straight talk about preferred methods of birth control, and the health aspects of intercourse. The responsibility cannot be laid at the feet of either partner—("She's a liberated woman; she must have taken precautions.")—but requires the joint consciousness of both or all concerned.[6] Far from diminishing the excitement of sex, this kind of communication can actually serve to bring the partners closer together, increasing mutual respect and engendering a deeper tenderness.

Finally, sex is conscious when the rest of life is conscious. What we eat or drink, how we breathe, the exercise we take, the thoughts we program—all will affect our ability for and enjoyment of sex. Les reports that his jogging program did wonders for his sex-life.[7] The increased flexibility, improved muscle-tone, the controlled use of the breath that comes with exercise will enhance sexual vigor. The improved self-concept which exercise encourages is a strong foundation for a healthy sex-concept. And vice versa. When people feel good about their sexuality and the expression of it, they are more inclined to want to care for their bodies, and maybe even their minds and hearts, too.

Self-assertive sex means allowing yourself permission to say YES to what you want, and NO to what you don't.

"Yes" implies:

"I know what I want, what feels good to me, and how best to achieve it." Liberating yourself sexually allows you to guide your partner. Do not assume that the other can read your mind, or your body. Placing sole responsibility for your sexual gratification on your partner is one sure way of leaving the encounter dissatisfied. Learning what feels good, what works for you, may mean practice and experimentation on your own. Self massage and masturbation skills are being taught by many sex educators and therapists today to aid in helping both men and women to rediscover their sensuality and to unlock pleasure centers throughout the body.

"No" means:

Allowing yourself to set limits, to say "no" to any techniques, or to the whole process if you no longer enjoy it or feel good about it. Many times your discomfort is a shared one, and your courage in calling a halt to the proceedings may be a great gift to your partner as well. When people care about each other, they respect each other's limits. Otherwise the encounter can quickly become tense, superficial, or faked. Anger and resentment build when you feel taken advantage of. Intimacy and trust flourish when you accept the other as unique and special. If you find yourself questioning "Will he/she respect me in the morning?" realize that you are really asking: "Will I be able to accept myself?" Your ability to integrate, to feel OK about your sexual interaction should be your guiding principle.

Sex as Communion

In sexual intercourse we have a brilliant symbol for what it is we all seek—integration, union, communion. We seek this with others, we also look for it in ourselves.

Regina's experience, described earlier, resulted in an energy block which developed into disease. Her "cure" was not found in *having* sex, but in accepting and "marrying" the dynamic forces which were at war within her.

The concept of androgyny means that each individual is composed of both "male" and "female" energy.[8] Typically, we associate the outgoing, thrusting, rationally-involved aspects of our nature with "maleness," and the inward-looking, nurturing, intuitive elements with the "femaleness." A whole, balanced person is one who has incorporated the two in one harmonious dance. If there is a definition of healthy sexuality—this is it. The integrated being channels all of life energy.

From this place of wholeness, of personal integrity, one approaches another person out of a desire for *sharing* energy, rather than a need for *taking* what is lacking in oneself. So, if there is any magical formula to be used, or first step to be taken in establishing satisfying relationships with others, it is the realization that you already have within yourself everything that you need for your happiness.

Anita is just such an integrated being. She is a strong and gentle woman. Her power sparkles in her sensitivity. She is happy in living and working alone for weeks, even months at a time. She is happy in living and working with family and friends. She cries as easily as she laughs. She writes poetry with one hand, and a research paper with the other. Her sexuality exudes from every pore and is contagious. She can be celibate for six months of the year without pain. She can make love every night of the week with pleasure. She is a living example of the union of sexuality and wellness.

. . . .

Once we discover that love is the way it is, we are no longer threatened by the possibility of the absence of love, because we recognize that the absence of love is no more than an illusion.

—STEWART EMERY[9]

. . . .

Sex and Love

For too long we have relegated love to a commodity to be earned or won; something that must be held tight. We have guarded it, guessing that there was just so much of it to go around. We have assumed that in loving you, I therefore diminish the quantity of love I have to give others. If any notion needs liberation—this one does.

The great lovers, the great humanitarians of the world loved and were loved by hundreds of people. They flourished with it. They were all the more energized for it. They tasted the reality that love is the energy of life, the breath of God, the ground of being. They realized that everything they did, every decision they made either enhanced their capacity to experience love, or diminished it.

The old problem of "charity begins at home" . . . or the idea that "I can't love you until I can love myself" . . . were never considerations for them. They often spent long periods of time, sometimes years, in contemplation. But their looking within brought them in touch with the place where everything was connected. They found no difference between themselves and us. In loving us, they loved themselves. In loving themselves, they loved us.

So if love is as natural as

Celibacy: A Viable Alternative

Most people are actually celibate most of the time. When this is "involuntary" it is often a great source of preoccupation and frustration. When celibacy is embraced "voluntarily" it can be a powerful means of self-understanding and even spiritual expression.

Today, many therapists who specialize in human sexuality are actually suggesting periods of voluntary celibacy to their clients as a way of revitalizing sexual energy, and to help them in discovering how their sexuality fits in the whole context of their lives. A period of celibacy is one way of challenging old limits—mental programs which say that "I can't be happy and fulfilled unless I have a sexual partner." Actually, what people are learning is that sexuality is so much more than a sex act!

In her valuable book, *The New Celibacy* (New York, NY: McGraw-Hill Book Co., 1980), Gabrielle Brown writes:

"Celibacy can create a wholeness in mind-body functioning that contributes to a more equitable balance of physical, mental and emotional functions . . . . Being celibate is an alternate way to love, even to make love. One can learn to touch nonpossessively without a future goal and to make love nonsexually, unmotivated by the need for sexual gratification. . . . When you stop being celibate, sex will have something new to offer you. Not only because you've been away, but because you are more settled within yourself . . . "

breathing, and eating, and working, and playing, it is as natural as "sexing" besides. If love becomes our "life-support system," then every decision we make, sex included, will be guided by it. We will choose to have sex with one another if it enhances our experience of unification with all that is. We will love each other anyway, whether we have sex or not. We will celebrate the abundance of love that is always available to us if we keep ourselves open channels for the flow of life energy.

Sex and the Planet

As we look at our world today we see only too clearly that integrated sexuality is the exception rather than the rule. People who touch their wholeness, who appreciate their own integrity and their union with everything else, do not ravage their own bodies or the body of the earth. Yet this is commonly what we find.

The word "rape" has been justly applied to our dealings with the land. We have stripped our forests and fields, robbed our soil of its fertility through wasteful overuse and poisoning with chemical substances, and erected hard, cold structures anywhere and everywhere at will.

Personal impotency will often show itself in cruel power tactics towards those whom we perceive to be weaker than ourselves. We often seek our own affirmation at the expense of another. In our attempts to experience a sense of our personal power, we have set out to dominate and control nature. Instead of marrying the earth, or establishing an on-going love relationship with her—we have used her to suit our pleasure, denying her cries for help, disregarding her needs for tenderness and caring.

In war we do the same to a race or nation of people. The enemy becomes an "it"—objectified as evil. Were we to look into their eyes we could not kill them. So the strategy of war demands that the enemy remain faceless, nameless, different from us. War can't work if we remember that we're all one family; that we breathe the same air, that we share the same energy.

During the Vietnam era we of-

Sensuous Sex

The following is a list of activities used by different couples which have helped in increasing their sensual experiences and pleasure in sex.

1. Bathing or showering together. Washing each other, shampooing and massaging scalp. Playing in water—the ocean, a pool, a hot tub, or Jacuzzi.

2. Massaging each other—whole body or just head or face, feet or hands. Deliberately refraining from intercourse for extended periods (several days or weeks) in order to explore sensuous touch.

3. Viewing an X-rated movie together. Reading erotic literature aloud, or writing your own in the form of letters to one another. Some suggest doing this by telephone as well.

4. Enjoying a slow, luxurious meal together in a sensual environment. Feeding each other. Weather permitting, private outdoor picnics can be wonderful.

5. Enjoying music together. Dancing, moving spontaneously, provocatively. Removing clothing slowly as the dance progresses.

6. Trying different environments. The possibilities here are limitless.

7. Describing what you want, what you would like to do for your partner, what feels good, and how it feels.

8. Sharing fantasies and playing them out together.

9. Doing the unexpected, or the unusual—use your imagination.

10. Wearing provocative clothing. Catalogs are readily available; or design and create your own.

11. Using satin sheets, vibrators, fur blankets, etc.

12. Experimenting with tantric practices—meditating, visualizing, breathing together; sustaining peaks without climax.

Arms are for hugging

ten heard: "Make love—not war." The juxtaposition of these two activities expresses a powerful truth. You won't kill if you really love. To love your enemy is to cease to view them, or "it," as enemy. To love is to desire that others fulfill their highest potential. To love is to leave others free to determine their own lives. It is to revere and celebrate their bodies, their minds, their souls. If we experience the free, unimpeded movement of our sexual energy within, not only shall we not make war without, we shall also not make the ornaments of war, or monuments to our greed, or playgrounds of waste, or furnish for ourselves apartments in a city of death. Rather we will kiss the earth, and touch the sky, and clothe our planet in beauty. We will truly love ourselves, and in so doing, revere our primal lover—the Earth.

Suggested Reading*

GENERAL

Barbach, L. *For Each Other: Sharing Sexual Intimacy.* Garden City, NY: Doubleday, 1982.

Boston Women's Health Book Collective. *The New Our Bodies, Ourselves.* New York, NY: Simon and Schuster, 1984.

Brown, G. *The New Celibacy.* New York, NY: McGraw-Hill, 1980.

Bullough, V., and Bullough B. *Sin, Sickness and Sanity.* Los Angeles, CA: Meridian, 1972.

*This is only a representative sampling. Many excellent books have been omitted. At the bookstore or library, look over the whole section and choose according to your judgment.

Sex is my chance to revel in the
  fact of my incarnation
my opportunity to celebrate
  that which has been my only home.
It involves me nakedly in the
  birth canal of my primal experience.
It reconnects me with the mother.
In sex I allow myself to express
  what is common to and feared by
all—the sense of vulnerability.
When I am naked I can be bruised.
  When we are naked together in
  sharing pleasure—I am freed.
I look my fear in the face
  go through it, and exhaust myself
in the thrill of riding the crest
  of the wave, of skiing the edge of
the mountain.

—Regina

Cassell, C. *Swept Away: Why Women Fear Their Own Sexuality.* New York, NY: Simon and Schuster, 1984.

Chang, J. *The Tao of Love and Sex.* New York, NY: E.P. Dutton, 1977.

Chesser, C. *Love without Fear.* New York, NY: New American Library, 1973.

Colton, H. *The Gift of Touch.* New York, NY: G.P. Putnam's Sons, 1983.

Downing, G. *The Massage Book.* Westminster, MD: Random House, 1972.

Doyle, J.A., *The Male Experience.* Dubuque, IA: New American Library, 1980.

Fromm, E. *The Art of Loving.* New York, NY: Bantam Books, 1956.

Goldberg, H. *The New Male.* New York, NY: New American Library, 1980.

Gunther, B. *Neo-Tantra: Bhagwan Shree Rajneesh on Sex, Love, Prayer and Transcendence.* New York, NY: Harper and Row, 1980.

Hite, S. *The Hite Report: A Nationwide Study of Female Sexuality.* New York, NY: Macmillan Publishing Co., 1976.

———. *The Hite Report on Male Sexuality.* New York, NY: Alfred A. Knopf, 1981.

Huxley, A. *Island.* New York, NY: Harper and Row, 1972.

Inkeles, G., and Todris, M. *The Art of Sensual Massage.* San Francisco, CA: Straight Arrow, 1972.

National Sex Forum. *SAR Guide for a Better Sex Life.* Multi-Media Resource Center, 1525

Franklin St., San Francisco, CA 94109.

Nelson, J.B. *Embodiment: An Approach to Sexuality and Christian Theology.* Philadelphia, PA: Pilgrim Press, 1978.

Rajneesh, Bhagwan Shree. *Tantra, Spirituality and Sex.* San Francisco, CA: Rainbow Bridge, 1977.

Zilbergeld, B. *Male Sexuality.* New York, NY: Bantam Books, 1980.

FOR OLDER PEOPLE:

Brechner, E.M., and the editors of Consumer Reports Books. *Love, Sex, and Aging.* Boston, MA: Little, Brown and Co., 1983.

Scheingold, L.D., and Wagner, N.N. Sound Sex and the Aging Heart. New York, NY: Human Services Press, 1974.

FOR THE DISABLED:

Sex and Disability Project. *Who Cares? A Handbook on Sex Education and Counseling Services for Disabled People.* 1828 L St. NW, Suite 704, Washington, DC 20036, 1979.

FOR PARENTS AND CHILDREN:

Bell, R., and Wildflower, L.Z. *Talking with Your Teenager.* New York, NY: Random House, 1984.

Calderone, M.S., and Johnson, E.W. *The Family Book about Sexuality.* New York, NY: Harper and Row, 1981.

LESBIAN/GAY SEXUALITY

Berzon, B., and Leighton, R. *Positively Gay.* Studio City, CA: Mediamix, 1984.

Clark, D., *Loving Someone Gay.* Berkeley, CA: Celestial Arts, 1977, 1987.

Silverstein, C., and White, E. *The Joy of Gay Sex.* Hamden, CT: Fireside Press, 1978.

Sisley, E.L., and Harris, B. *The Joy of Lesbian Sex.* New York, NY: Delacorte Press, 1977.

Walker, M., *Men Loving Men.* Berkeley, CA: Book People, 1977.

Notes

1. See:

Dodson, B. *Liberating Masturbation.* New York, NY: Bodysex Designs, 1975.

Barbach, L. *For Yourself: The Fulfillment of Female Sexuality.* New York, NY: Doubleday/Anchor, 1975.

Zilbergeld, B. *Male Sexuality.* New York, NY: Bantam Books, 1980.

2. Masters, W., and Johnson, V. *The Pleasure Bond.* New York, NY: Bantam Books, 1976.

McCarthy, B.; Ryan, M.; and Johnson, F. *Sexual Awareness: A Practical Approach.* San Francisco, CA: Boyd and Fraser Publishing Co., 1975.

3. Friday, N. *My Secret Garden: Women's Sexual Fantasies.* New York, NY: Pocket Books, 1973.

———. *Men in Love.* New York, NY: Delacorte Press, 1980.

Kronhausen, P., and Kronhausen, E. *Erotic Fantasies.* New York, NY: Grove Press, 1969.

4. For information on available programs contact:

The National Sex Forum
1523 Franklin Street
San Francisco, CA 94109

Reproductive Biology Research Foundation
William Masters, M.D. and Virginia Johnson
4910 Forest Park Blvd.
St. Louis, MO 63108

Dr. Albert Ellis
Institute for Advanced Study in Rational Psychotherapy
45 E. 65th St.
New York, NY 10021

5. Masters, W., and Johnson, V. *Human Sexual Response.* Boston, MA: Little, Brown and Co., 1966.

Kinsey, A.; Pomeroy, W.; and Martin, C. *Sexual Behavior in the Human Male.* Philadelphia, PA: Saunders, 1948.

———. *Sexual Behavior in the Human Female.* Philadelphia, PA: Saunders, 1953.

Hite, S. *The Hite Report: A Nationwide Study of Female Sexuality.* New York, NY: Macmillan Publishing Co., 1976.

———. *The Hite Report on Male Sexuality.* New York, NY: Alfred A. Knopf, 1981.

6. For intelligent information about birth control contact any local office of Planned Parenthood, or write:

Planned Parenthood Federation of America, Inc.
810 Seventh Ave.
New York, NY 10019

7. See chapter 2—"Fitness for a Better Sex Life," in:

Kuntzleman, C. *The Exerciser's Handbook.* New York, NY: David McKay Co., 1978, pp. 17–24.

For a good laugh read: Smith, R. *The Dieter's Guide to Weight Loss During Sex.* New York, NY: Workman Publishing, 1978.

8. Singer, J. *Androgyny: Toward a New Theory of Sexuality.* New York, NY: Doubleday, 1977.

9. Emery, S. *Actualizations: You Don't Have to Rehearse to Be Yourself.* New York, NY: Doubleday, 1978.

Eleven

Wellness
and Finding Meaning

GENERALLY SPEAKING, the meanings we assign to our lives flow out of our relationships with those close to us, the jobs we do, the roles we play, and our religious beliefs. When significant changes take place in our lives—graduation, retirement, divorce, the death of a loved one, the last child leaving home—we lose a piece of our identity. We may even feel that we have lost our reason for being. Such periods of change are often periods of great stress, anxiety, and unhappiness.

Feelings of uneasiness arise because we are being forced to face those big questions that have formed the basis of philosophy throughout the ages, namely *Is life worth living? Who am I? What's it all about?* And we are being forced to face ourselves, and the fact of our mortality.

A certain amount of worry and fear is built into the process of adjusting to change and the process of working it all out. It is when we

---

The search for meaning is a complex energy output that involves all previous energy forms. It involves the basic questions: Who am I? Why am I here? Where am I going? What do I want? What is real? What is true? Regardless of whether these questions are conscious or unconscious, all life activity, all other energy expressions, are colored by them. Addressing these questions to some satisfaction encourages a balanced life, and provides the individual with a focal point toward which to direct energy.

---

become stuck in delaying and evading tactics that problems arise. Some people are thrown into deep depression or are beset with feelings of uselessness, emptiness, boredom. Other people launch themselves on a series of feverish activities, anxiously keeping themselves occupied at all times. Others play Russian Roulette with high risk behaviors such as over-eating, drinking to excess, or taking drugs. And for some, the ultimate solu-

---

tion is suicide. (It is interesting to note that late adolescence is the time when questions of purpose first become important, and that suicide is one of the major causes of death in that age group.[1])

. . . .

The Work is with you and in you in such a way that once you find it in yourself, where it always is, you have it always, wherever you may be, on land or sea.

—ATTRIBUTED TO
HERMES
TRISMEGISTUS

. . . .

Finding meaning is probably the most personal and most difficult issue anyone can address because it requires looking inward and self-searching, which are frightening prospects for most people. And they are not something another person can do for

. . . . *Exercise* . . . .

Your Big Question

Not everyone can relate to the same Big Question about life-purpose. Some people have worded theirs this way:

What's life all about?

Why am I here?

What am I doing with my life?

Why did God make me?

How can I find happiness?

What about you? How do you express your Big Question? Spend a moment or two reflecting, and write it down here:

_____

_____

_____

_____

_____

. . . .

you. Because finding meaning is a process, however, there are some guidelines you can follow that may help you.

1. Learn to look within and begin to trust what you find there. Listen to your own inner voice, your own wisdom.

2. Focus on what *is* instead of living for future breaks or living in the past.

3. Strive for greater honesty and clarity in your relationships with other people; *be just who you are*, not what you think you are *supposed to be*.

4. Make friends with death and pain rather than running from them and awarding fear an unwarranted place in steering your life.

Living well and fully experiencing life means squarely facing the question of purpose and meaning. As Socrates has said, "The unexamined life is not worth living." On the other hand, it is important to see a balance and not get deadly serious about the whole matter, for as Marcel has said, "Life is a mystery to be lived, not a problem to be solved," and that, too, is a wise statement.

So go ahead and ask the questions, examine motivations, read the lives of other people, meditate on the ultimate purpose of things, but at the same time live with your questions if they can't be answered in black and white; relax, laugh, and play when things get too heavy and realize that you'll never be finished with learning, changing, and growing.

Where Do Meanings Come From Anyway?

Meanings are made up in human minds. They vary with your need, or mood, or what you ate for breakfast. You *give* meanings to things. But in and of themselves— things simply are!

Look at something near you right now—a lamp, a chair, a diamond ring, a scratch on your finger. What does it mean?

For you—the lamp may simply mean something to light your page. For the antique dealer it may mean a profitable sale. For the child it may mean something pretty to play with. For your mother it may mean a recollection of the old homestead where it first stood. Each person will treasure, discard, or ignore the lamp based on the meaning they have assigned it.

When Barbara broke her leg recently parachuting from an airplane, she was grounded for several months. Sometimes this experience meant pain and frustration. At other times, it meant much needed rest, the chance to get to know herself again, or an opportunity to pray.

Meaning in life comes from *you*, too. Since meaning comes from inside of you, finding meaning will be a process of going to the source—*yourself*. This may be a good time to repeat the Who Are You Anyway? exercise on page 167, or for a reflective conversation with yourself.

Meanings Are Found in the Present

The meaning you assign to something can change from one moment to the next. The ring that you wear today and treasure as the sign of eternal fidelity or friendship may tarnish in the back of your drawer next year. Meanings change because people's lives change.

Looking to the future for happiness or living on past glories is a sure set-up for disappointment. Ultimately, we have no assurance of anything beyond this present moment. There really is no future or past—just a continuous progression of NOW moments.

The question then becomes: What are you to *do* in the NOW in order to experience meaning? The answer is: Do just what you are doing, but do it with awareness. Be just who you are, but be it intensely. Look long and lovingly at what is real *right now*. This is the secret of happiness shared by great mystics throughout the ages.

What the Frog Taught Us

Today the biology teacher brought a frog, fresh from the neighborhood lake, into the lab. We were going to learn about what makes frogs work—how they digest, eliminate, breathe, reproduce—to discover the essence of "frogginess."

The frightened little thing moved nervously in the teacher's hand, hopped onto the table, gazed wonderingly in all directions, gave an occasional "croak" to the amusement of the class. We were excited. All eyes following the movements, delighted by how closely it resembled the cartoon frogs of our TV experience. We "OOHED" and "AHHED" and giggled and screamed. Occasionally there was even a moment of reverent silence when one of our crowd, talking quietly, seemed to have established an instant of rapport. The movements of our hands, our bodies, mimicked our tiny subject. We were animated, questioning, intrigued.

But then something changed all that. Under the skillful knife of our instructor, we watched the life force, with the sticky frog-blood, oozing from our victim. The time had come to get down to the real business at hand—to dissect, to label, to describe, to preserve tiny frog-heart in clear, liquid solutions. We had to watch carefully because tomorrow we would have to do the same. But somehow, we really didn't care. This was not a frog. In pulling back its familiar warty skin it became an objectified mass, a lump of slime. No longer were we amused. This was messy business and the fun had left.

We left the class with a neat list of drawings, a rack full of samples adequately preserved, a full page of notes to be transcribed into our workbooks. But we also carried away a funny taste in our mouths, a tension behind our eyes, and a feeling of sadness that in seeking to understand the parts, we had lost life in the whole.

Frank Young

On Goals and Meaning

Before you can have any real sense of getting somewhere, it's helpful to know where you're starting from, and where you want to go. Goal-setting, evaluation, and redirection are one set of dynamic tools for creating a greater harmony with the current of life, rather than allowing yourself to be washed down the stream.

Many of us resist setting goals. As a result, we often take whatever comes along in life with half-hearted resignation, making "the best" of a situation rather than risk frustration when our plans and expectations fail. And then we wonder why a once technicolored world is now only a blur of greys. Too bad.

Admitting our tendency towards resignation is a quantum

. . . .

We stake our lives on our purposeful programs and projects, our serious jobs and endeavors. But doesn't the really important part of our lives unfold "after hours"—singing and dancing, music and painting, prayer and lovemaking, or just fooling around?

—FATHER WILLIAM
McNAMARA

. . . .

leap in changing a wishy-washy approach to life. It takes courage to call into question some of our most basic life scripts. Working at the process of goal setting heightens this awareness, and that is often uncomfortable. Nonetheless, we have found that it is well worth the effort, regardless of the pain involved. Even if we don't accomplish all the goals we initially set for ourselves, the very process involved in formulating them is energizing and life-affirming. It says to the deeper self, "I'm worth it." Such a declaration flies in the face of passivity, of submitting to the status quo, of seeing life as a struggle or a problem, rather than a possibility or a dance.

We recommend a simple exercise that never ceases to surprise us, no matter how many times we do it. To start, you take four blank sheets of paper. On the first you write: "Where/How I Want to Be Five Years from Today." On the next: "Where/How I Want My Life to Be Two Years from Today." Then on the third: ". . . Six Months from Today." On the fourth paper you write: "How I Would Spend the Next Six Months of My Life If I Knew for Sure They Would Be My Last." Give yourself a time

limit, say no more than fifteen minutes to work on each sheet, beginning with the five-year projection, and moving down to the last six months. As you complete each page, cover it, and do the next one without referring to the previous ones. They may connect, or they may be totally different. This exercise is all about generating lots of data which you will later work over in a variety of ways.

To provide this exercise with a wellness perspective, recall now that a whole life is an integration of body, mind, and spiritual components. Then look back at your lists and note if you have included goals that reflect all of these aspects of

---

At this moment if you set the alarm to get up at 3:47 this morning and when the alarm rings and you get up and turn it off and say: What time is it?

You say: Now.

Where am I?: Here. Then go back to sleep. Get up at 9:00 tomorrow.

Where am I? Here!

Try 4:32 three weeks from next Thursday.

By God

It is—there's no getting away from it—that's the way it is

    that's the Eternal Present

You finally figure out that it's only the clock that's going around . . .

It's doing its thing but you—you're sitting

    Here

    Right Now

    Always.

—Ram Dass[2]

---

being. Perhaps you recorded lots of things about new tasks to be accomplished in a job, or different types of relationships you want to establish, but have written nothing about your state of physical health, your lifestyle habits, or your desires for enhanced emotional well-being. Now is the time to add those. Take two or three minutes to rework each sheet, including these newly-remembered aspects. (If you are using a Personal Wellness Journal—see Appendix B—record these observations in your journal.)

Read over what you have written and look for things that are repeated or strongly expressed. Note patterns that are emerging. As you write, listen to your internal self-talk which may be undermining the process, saying: "But that can never happen." Or: "I don't have the money [or courage or time] to do that." Keep moving ahead despite these self-defeating messages.

Put this exercise aside for at least a day, and do it again tomorrow, or next weekend. Compare and contrast the results of the two experiments, and keep asking yourself, "What would I have/do/ be if I had no limitations [like time, money, children, etc.]?" So often we use our imagined limitations as defenses against clearly asserting and then setting out after what we really want. The difference between a life of greatness and a life of mediocrity is that the great move ahead with their limitations, while the mediocre stay stuck in them.

The next step is to focus on one or more of your strongest goals, and to draw a road map or time line with actions or steps that will begin to bring your dream into form. For instance, if you've always wanted to run your own school, you can start today with a trip to the library to find every book available on innovative education. You can make three phone calls and talk to people involved in a similar venture, sign up for an adult education course in administration, and so on. Many people testify to the power of "magnet maps" (see chapter 7 on Affirmations), colorful collages that depict your dreams as accomplished realities. These maps are placed somewhere where they can be seen regularly and serve to keep your vision alive.

It is beyond the scope of this book to outline a full-blown course in goal setting, and besides, others have already done it so much better than we could. Refer to Alan Lakein's *How to Get Control of Your Time and Your Life* (New York, NY: Peter A. Weyden, 1973), Richard Bolles's *The Three Boxes of Life and How to Get Out of Them* (Berkeley, CA: Ten Speed Press, 1978), and a real treasure called *Wishcraft*, by Barbara Sher (New York, NY: Ballantine Books, 1983), and start using goals today to create and enhance meaning in your life.

Facing Death and Finding Meaning

Paradoxically, for those who seek to understand it, death is a highly creative force and a meaning-filled fact of life. The highest spiritual values of life can originate from the thought and study of death. But, before we can use the confrontation with loss, separation, or death as a way of finding meaning, we will need to repudiate the connection between death and failure. We

> The past
> is dead
> The future
>   is imaginary
> Happiness
>   can only be
> in the Eternal
>   Now
>   Moment

The meaning of here and now is beautifully illustrated by a Zen story of a monk who was being chased by two tigers. He came to the edge of a cliff. He looked back—the tigers were almost upon him. Noticing a vine leading over the cliff, he quickly crawled over the edge and began to let himself down by the vine. Then as he checked below, he saw two tigers waiting for him at the bottom of the cliff. He looked up and observed that two mice were gnawing away at the vine. just then, he saw a beautiful strawberry within arm's reach. He picked it and enjoyed the best tasting strawberry in his whole life!

Although only minutes from death, the monk could enjoy the here and now. Our life continually sends us "tigers" and it continually sends us "strawberries," But do we let ourselves enjoy the strawberries? Or do we use our valuable consciousness worrying about the tigers?

Reprinted with permission from *The Handbook to Higher Consciousness* by Ken Keyes.

need to replace death within its rightful context if we are to use it to find meaning in life.

The culture in which we live has emphasized the prolonging of life—often supporting its *quantity* above its quality.

A recent cartoon in a major magazine depicted a hospital bed surrounded by monstrous electronic devices attached to a sad-faced patient. One weak arm emerged from under the covers holding a tiny white flag. The nurse turning to the attending doctor remarked—"Everything is working, doctor, but Mr. Jones doesn't want to cooperate."

Mr. Jones had had it! He was ready to give up, to surrender rather than to be subject to any more life-supporting technological "miracles." His response causes us to chuckle grimly because we relate to stories of people being kept alive at any cost. And cost it does! In his book *Medical Nemesis* Ivan Illich reports that the average daily rates for intensive care in U.S. hospitals range from $500 to $2000.[3]

Hospitals are established for the handling of disease and accident and trauma, for remediating conditions and then releasing patients once they can stand on their own. Doctors are committed to keeping us alive—as an inherent value. Consequently, when death occurs it means failure. It's that simple.

But, death is not the ultimate enemy, the terminal disease to wage war against, to be eliminated at all costs. Nevertheless, this attitude subtly underlies so many approaches to health and well-being. As if by doing the right things—eating the proper foods, taking our exercise programs seriously, keeping infection at bay, improving surgical techniques—death, like the smallpox virus, could be wiped out.

We delude ourselves in believing that medical research will dis-

. . . . *Regina's Journal* . . . .

What Death Teaches About Meaning

In the midst of my writing, a friend and her eight-year-old daughter died in a car accident coming home from Christmas vacation. Their deaths brought me closer to this reality than any of my previous life experiences. The questions raised were questions of deep meaning. Finding meaning in life can only be achieved by finding meaning in death. I want to share what I learned with you.

The span of one human life, even if it be 80 or 100 years, is but the twinkling of an eye in the history of humanity. Everything is transitory. Everything dies. In every moment I am being born and in every moment I am dying. On the inhalation I take in the spirit, on the exhalation I let it go—I expire.

I have no guarantee that there will be any more than there is right now. Nevertheless, I live my life as if I have forever. And in reality I do—but certainly not in this particular manifestation of the physical body—for no one will hold this form forever. All is movement, all is change, all is passing away, all is resurrecting in this moment. To look at death is to look at life. To live with the presence of death is to live with the presence of life. Not in the sense of eat, drink, and be merry, but in the sense of "dayenu"—a Hebrew word meaning "it is enough," i.e., all in this moment is sufficient. If there is no next moment, I leave freely, happily, with deep appreciation for all that has been and is.

. . . .

cover a cure for death.

The fact is that people who watch their diets, exercise, and enjoy satisfying relationships *do* live longer. Nevertheless, *we are all terminal* and *death is our natural inheritance.*

We may speak easily of the cycle of life, the food chain, the ecological balance when we are talking about plants and animals, yet we often retract in horror from the stark reality that we humans are also a part of this. My body will return to the earth to nourish it, to feed my children's children. My thoughts and accomplishments build a foundation which will support the growth of future genera-

tions. It is the way of nature. Death is an energy-transforming process, thus fighting it is a wasteful and irrelevant effort. Relaxing enhances its smooth progression.

The poet Gibran writes of life and death as one,[4] and says that in every moment of life you are dying, and in dying you are preparing the way for new life. You experience living and dying in every instant in small ways. Your baby teeth must fall out in order that your adult teeth may emerge. Skin cells constantly die and are sloughed off so that new cells may take their place. To take a new job means death to a previous one. To

grow means death to old patterns of belief.

In each event there is a dying which precedes a rebirth, for death and life are one. As we become increasingly aware of dying and being born in every situation then the experience of the death which occurs at the culmination of life becomes one more familiar transformation to be embraced and accepted. If each small death has meant a small transformation, a new life, why should the "Big Death" be any different?

Looking squarely at any of our fears about death can supply us with meaningful information about what holds us back from the full experience of life.

Many people claim that they don't fear death. When questioned further they are quick to add:

" . . . but I don't like to think of the sorrow it will cause my family, or children."

" . . . but I'm not ready for it to happen for a long while yet."

" . . . but I want to go quickly."

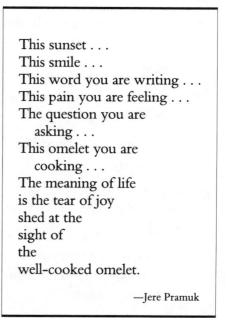

This sunset . . .
This smile . . .
This word you are writing . . .
This pain you are feeling . . .
The question you are
    asking . . .
This omelet you are
    cooking . . .
The meaning of life
is the tear of joy
shed at the
sight of
the
well-cooked omelet.

—Jere Pramuk

"... but I don't want to be laid out in a funeral parlor."

As reasonable as they sound, these statements imply a fear of sorts. Few people express no uneasiness at all about the subject of death.

If you fear death because you fear the unknown, chances are this is the way you approach life—with fear, avoiding change, minimizing risk, keeping yourself secure in known routines.

To face death consciously, you must face life consciously—embracing your fears, kissing your monsters.

What do *you* fear about death?

• the unknown that follows

• the judgment of God, the possible condemnation to hell

• the idea that my physical body will corrupt

• the unendingness of eternity

• the experience of nothingness

• the humiliation of giving up control

• the loss of bodily functions

• the separation from family and friends

• the pain

• the sorrow and hardship to family and friends

• the surprise, not knowing the time or place

• the sense of incompleteness, that you didn't do all you intended to do

• the sense of meaninglessness, that you never found out your purpose in being?[5]

. . . . *Regina's Journal* . . . .

The Connection Between Death and Wellness

For the past three years, I have taught two different classes at the community college level. One is High-Level Wellness, the other is Death and Dying. My experience has been they continually overlay each other. In talking about illness as a positive force in the wellness class, I express my belief that death is a friend to be learned from. In dealing with how to handle grief, I spend a great deal of time in explaining the value of expressing emotions as a way of opening up channels to life energy. I present death as being one more energy-transformation process and that is precisely the way John and I view wellness.

—RSR

. . . .

. . . .

One Who Found Meaning—One Who Didn't

From their graves, the spirits of Lucinda Matlock and George Gray, characters in *The Spoon River Anthology* by Edgar Lee Masters, share with us about the question of meaning.

Lucinda—Finds Meaning

I went to dances at Chandlerville,
And played snap-out at Winchester.
One time we changed partners,
Driving home in the moonlight of middle June,
And then I found Davis.
We were married and lived together for seventy years,
Enjoying, working, raising the twelve children,
Eight of whom we lost
Ere I had reached the age of sixty.
I spun, I wove, I kept the house, I nursed the sick,
I made the garden, and for holiday
Rambled over the fields where sang the larks,
And by Spoon River gathering many a shell,
And many a flower and medicinal weed—
Shouting to the wooded hills, singing to the green valleys.
At ninety-six I had lived enough, that is all,
And passed to a sweet repose.

. . . .

Now look back over the fears of death which you have identified. Ask yourself—How do these reflect upon the ways in which I live, or fail to live, my life right now? What do fears of death tell me about my real fears of life?

Then, have a dialogue with yourself about each fear in turn.

Dying Well

Sooner or later we will all face death. You can take greater responsibility for your death right now. The large part of this entails taking responsibility for your life. There are many facets unique to the death experience which allow you to maintain your personal power and enable to you embrace death with conscious awareness. First of all, face it. This takes courage, but the alternative is fear and withdrawal which block energy needed for living fully. Secondly, make some choices about it, now. Do you currently have a will? (It doesn't matter if you are twenty or eighty, you have no assurance of living beyond this very moment.) How do you prefer to die? Do you wish to be hospitalized in your last days? What alternatives exist for your care outside of a hospital? Do you know about Hospice programs for

Hospice

Hospice represents an interdisciplinary, holistic approach to caring for people with a life-threatening illness, either in the patient's home or in a facility. The patient and family together are considered a single unit of care. Hospice combines the skills of physicians, nurses, clergy, psychotherapists, social workers, and volunteers who, together with the family, design and implement the care plan. Care continues for the family after the patient's death.[6]

home treatment of the terminally ill? Assuming that you wish to die with the greatest amount of dignity possible, what decisions have you communicated to loved ones about your wishes for life-support systems, for surgeries, for pain medication, for the presence of clergy? Will you donate your eyes or other organs to organ banks? Have you ever considered willing your body to a medical school for research? What kind of funeral ceremony do you want? Are you aware of the costs of burial and all that goes with it? What about cremation? Who do you entrust with making choices for you when, or if, you can no longer make them for yourself?

Finally—accept your weaknesses, as well as your strengths as you confront death and go through it. Knowing that death is a transformation, allow your darkness to surface with your light. Be fearful, or angry, or overcome with deep sadness. These are all a part of who

What is this I hear of sorrow and weariness,
Anger, discontent, and drooping hopes'
Degenerate sons and daughters,
Life is too strong for you —
It takes life to love life.

George—Doesn't:

I have studied many times
The marble which was chiseled for me
A boat with a furled sail at rest in a harbor.
In truth it pictures not my destination
But my life.
For love was offered me, and I shrank from its disillusionment;
Sorrow knocked at my door, but I was afraid;
Ambition called to me, but I dreaded the chances.
Yet all the while I hungered for meaning in my life
And now I know that we must lift the sail
And catch the winds of destiny
Wherever they drive the boat.
To put meaning in one's life may end in madness,
But life without meaning is the torture
Of restlessness and vague desire—
It is a boat longing for the sea and yet afraid.

What's Important?

By looking at our values today we catch a glimpse of what is most meaningful to us. Supposing that you needed to escape from where you presently live, and could take along only ten things which you currently have, what would they be?

1. _____   5. _____   8. _____

2. _____   6. _____   9. _____

3. _____   7. _____   10. _____

4. _____

What will be important to you at the moment of your death? What will it take, by way of accomplishment, or attitudes, or possessions, to allow you to die satisfied? Spend a few moments in quiet reflection and then write about that here.

Now write your own epitaph—one sentence that sums up your life, its meaning and purpose.

R.I.P.

For example:

R.I.P
Regina Sara Ryan
1945–2045
She hungered after God and Truth.
They found her first and ate her up.
Yum!

R.I.P
John Walton Travis
1943–2038
He finally learned it was OK
If it didn't all get done,
As long as he had a good time
Doing it.

you are as a fully functioning, alive and aware human being. Give yourself permission to express the emotions that are real for you. Flow with and love yourself. Let go. The body, mind and spirit know when it is time to move on. Trust yourself—trust the process.

What Death-Bed and After-Life Experience Teach Us

In her many years of study with dying people, Elisabeth Kubler-Ross found that almost everyone reaches a stage of resignation and acceptance prior to death. There is a growing body of literature collected from people who have "died" and continue to live; people who have gone "beyond and back." The tremendous popularity of such books as Raymond Moody's *Life After Life*[7] indicates a widespread curiosity about what happens after death. A book of this nature has as much to say about living as it does about dying. De-

* * * * * * *

I have been able to function as a catalyst, trying to bring to our awareness that we can only truly live and enjoy and appreciate life if we realize at all times that we are finite. Needless to say I have learned these lessons from my dying patients—who in their suffering and dying realized that we have only NOW—"so have it fully and find what turns you on, because no one can do this for you!"

—ELISABETH
KUBLER-ROSS

* * * * * * *

* * * * * * *

Also, there is the fear that there is an afterlife but no one will know where it's being held.

—WOODY ALLEN

* * * * * * *

spite differing descriptions of what was found on the "other side," almost every report was consistent in recounting the lessons brought back from these close encounters with death. And what were the lessons? Simply, that life is given to us in order that we may learn from everything.

In learning, we can grow in love for, and acceptance of, all that exists. Learning and loving are the attitudes and behaviors that give meaning to life. These are the things which will endure.

Suggested Reading*

Bach, R. *Illusions*. New York, NY: Delacorte Press, 1977.

Cousins, N. *Human Options*. New York, NY: W.W. Norton & Co., 1981.

Dass, R. *Be Here Now*. New York, NY: Crown Publishing Co. 1971.

Fields, R., et al. *Chop Wood, Carry Water*. Los Angeles, CA: J.P. Tarcher, 1985.

Frankl, V. *Man's Search for Meaning*. New York, NY: Pocket Books, 1963.

Da Free, J. *Scientific Proof of the Existence of God Will Soon Be Announced by the White House!* Clearlake, CA: The Dawn Horse Press, 1980.

This is only a representative sampling. Many excellent books have been omitted. At the bookstore or library, look over the whole selection and choose according to your judgment.

———. *Easy Death*. Clearlake, CA: The Dawn Horse Press. 1983.

Gibran, K. *The Prophet*. New York, NY: Alfred A. Knopf, 1923.

Golas, T. *The Lazy Man's Guide to Enlightenment*. Palo Alto, CA: The Seed Center, 1972.

Keyes, K. *The Handbook to Higher Consciousness*. Coos Bay, OR: Living Love Publications, 1975.

Krishnamurti, J. *Think on These Things*. New York, NY: Harper and Row, Perennial Library, 1964.

Kubler-Ross, E. *Death, the Final Stage of Growth*. Englewood Cliffs, NJ: Prentice Hall, 1975.

Levine, S. *Who Dies?* Garden City, NY: Anchor Books, 1982.

Lozowick, L. *Living God Blues*. Prescott Valley, AZ: Hohm Press, 1984.

———. *Laughter of the Stones*. Prescott Valley, AZ: Hohm Press.

———. *The Cheating Buddha*. Prescott Valley, AZ: Hohm Press, 1980.

Neale, R. *The Art of Dying*. New York, NY: Harper and Row, 1973.

Moody, R. *Life After Life*. New York, NY: Bantam Books, 1975.

Peck, M.S. *The Road Less Travelled*. New York, NY: Simon and Schuster, 1978.

Pirsig, R. *Zen and the Art of Motorcycle Maintenance: An Inquiry into Values*. New York, NY: William Morrow, 1974.

Rajneesh, B. *Journey Towards the Heart: Discourses on the Sufi Way*. New York, NY: Harper and Row, 1976.

Simon, S.; Howe, L.; and Kirschenbaum, H. *Values Clarification*.

New York, NY: Hart Publishing Co., 1972. Tillich, P. *The Meaning of Health*. Richmond, CA: North Atlantic Books, 1981.

Trungpa, C. *The Myth of Freedom and the Way of Meditation*. Boston, MA: Shambhala, 1976.

Notes

1. See:

Cantor, P. "The Effects of Youthful Suicide on the Family," *Psychiatric Opinion*. Vol. 12, 1975, pp. 6–13.

Shneidman, E. "The College Student and Death," in *New Meanings of Death*. Feifel, H., ed. New York, NY: McGraw-Hill, 1977, pp. 67–88.

2. Dass, R. *Be Here Now*. New York, NY: Crown Publishing Co., 1971.

3. Illich, I. *Medical Nemesis*. New York, NY: Bantam Books, 1976, p. 95.

4. Gibran, K. *The Prophet*. New York, NY: Alfred A. Knopf, 1976 (94th printing), pp. 80–96.

5. A brilliant treatment of the relationship between fears of living and fears of dying is found in:

Neale, R. *The Art of Dying*. New York, NY: Harper and Row, 1973, pp. 24–45.

6. See:

R.W. Buckingham. *The Complete Hospice Guide*. New York, NY: Harper and Row, 1983.

Or write: The National Hospice Organization, 1901 North Fort Myer Dr., Suite 402, Arlington, VA 22209, 703-242-5900

7. Moody, R. *Life After Life*. New York, NY: Bantam Books, 1975.

———. *Reflections on Life After Life*. New York, NY: Bantam Books, 1977.

Also see:

Ring, K. *Heading Toward Omega: In Search of the Meaning of the Near Death Experience*. New York, NY: William Morrow and Co., 1984.

. . . .*Exercise*. . . . .

A Living Will

To My Family, My Physician, My Lawyer and All Others Whom It May Concern

Death is as much a reality as birth, growth, maturity and old age—it is the one certainty of life. If the time comes when I can no longer take part in decisions for my own future, let this statement stand as an expression of my wishes and directions, while I am still of sound mind.

If at such a time the situation should arise in which there is no reasonable expectation of my recovery from extreme physical or mental disability, I direct that I be allowed to die and not be kept alive by medications, artificial means or "heroic measures." I do, however, ask that medication be mercifully administered to me to alleviate suffering even though this may shorten my remaining life.

This statement is made after careful consideration and is in accordance with my strong convictions and beliefs. I want the wishes and directions here expressed carried out to the extent permitted by law. Insofar as they are not legally enforceable, I hope that those to whom this Will is addressed will regard themselves as morally bound by these provisions.

Signed _____   Date _____

Witness _____   Witness _____

Copies of this request have been given to   _____
_____
_____

Twelve

Wellness and Transcending

> Transcending is the movement in which all energies, once experienced as separate types and in individual contexts, are appreciated as one. Put another way, we come to know that we are one with all that is . . . and that "one" that we are is Energy. This knowledge inspires both love and self-responsibility, which takes us full circle in the never-ending spiral of wellness.

A T SOME TIME or other, each of us has experienced moments of transcendence—moments when the body-mind leaps beyond its ordinary limits, moments of supreme joy, of enlightenment, of gazing into the face of God. You may simply be looking across the kitchen table at your children and be momentarily overwhelmed with joy. Or you may experience it as the ecstatic high following sex. For a brief time all problems, all worries disappear. You feel more "together" than you've ever felt before. There are many other examples:

- watching the waves at the ocean and losing your sense of time and space

- pushing your body to the limit in dancing or running a race; breaking through the "wall of pain," and then feeling like you could go on forever

- the simultaneous breathlessness, excitement, and peace when a realization of unconditional love melts through you

- total absorption in a piece of music, or blending with the dancers or actors on a stage

- the joyful after-glow of giving birth

- the "aha" moment when the solution to a problem you've long wrestled with spontaneously pops into your head.

Such moments of transcendence leave us changed— sometimes only for a brief time, occasionally forever. They supply us with new energy, joyfulness, and motivation about this business of living. They open us to previously untapped possibilities, expanding horizons, creating new options. They often put us in touch with our truest, most peaceful and balanced selves. They show us glimpses of the connectedness, the oneness of all things.

. . . . . .

The most beautiful experience we can have is the mysterious.

—ALBERT EINSTEIN

. . . .

Most of us are quite busy handling daily routines and the immediate problems of life. And most of us are quite comfortable within the confines of the world as we know it. So we do not feel the need to reach beyond, to peek through the cracks in the cosmos. The aim of this chapter is to pique your curiosity, to help you break through conventional ways of thinking when you are ready for it. This chapter

Then your window is clear, and as you pitch over, getting near horizontal, you catch the first glimpse out the window of the Earth from space. And it's a beautiful sight . . . And you realize from that perspective that you've changed, that there's something new there, that the relationship is no longer what it was.

—RUSSEL SCHWEICKART
CREW OF APOLLO 9
MARCH, 1969

Love the world as your own self; then you can truly care for all things.

—LAO TSU,
TAO TE CHING

deals with many of the spiritual dimensions of well-being. For some people, spiritual wellness is experienced primarily in participation in an organized religion. For others, the agnostics among us, "spiritual" is synonymous with the unknown or mysterious. The material presented here is for everyone. Hopefully it will stretch your mind and heart, and even inspire you to take a longer and deeper look.

Peeking Through the Cracks

History is filled with accounts of people who held fast to dreams—even when they contradicted the consensus of society. Often these dreams came in a state of awareness other than the normal waking consciousness. They have occurred in sleep, or in a state induced by trance, or after ingesting drugs, or running for fifteen miles, or in looking at the earth from the surface of the moon, or in prayer. What the dreamers shared afterwards was a new vision of the way things worked, or a new realization of connectedness with all things and everyone.

Mystical revelation and scientific insight from generations of dreamers point to alternate ways of looking at the world. The Hermetic philosophers saw thoughts as vibrational levels—energy exchanges which could change the physical universe. Christ challenged the pervasive myopia when

Self–Responsibility Theory

- all things are connected because everything is one energy

- we create our own reality and are therefore responsible for our own lives

- life is a process in which we are significant agents of change

- falling apart may be only one stage preparatory to a falling together

Traditional "Wisdom"

- everything can be evaluated on a continuum bounded by opposites

- reality is objective; its component parts can be dissected, studied, and described; things happen *to* us

- some things never change: e.g., hunger is inevitable, war is unavoidable

- things fall apart because of some inherent weakness

he taught that God was Father, that all human beings were "Sons" of this Father, that the "Kingdom" was within. The shaman in widely scattered cultures saw illness as a result of disharmony in the sick person's world. Pythagoras developed a mysticism based on his vision that "all things are numbers." Anaximander described the universe as one large organism supported by the cosmic breath.

Religion only seems different if you're dealing with a retailer. If you deal with a wholesaler, they all get it from the same distributor.

—STEVE GASKIN

If history teaches anything, it teaches that the consensus reality, in almost any age, has been woefully inadequate; that those whose minds were open to alternate visions of "the way things are" have

been our greatest teachers, our most powerful agents of change. The hard and fast view of reality held by contemporaries of Copernicus, Galileo, Pasteur, and Mesmer, led them to discount and ridicule the dreams these great thinkers revealed.

Perhaps you are ready now to make your own break with consensus reality. The box above contains four theories which break with traditional thinking. These theories are not really new ideas . . . they have been part and parcel of mystical thinking for ages. What is new is that today they are receiving support from the research of scientists, notably physicists, psychologists, and medical doctors. All are related in some way to the transcendental experience and have implications for wellness.

Everything Is Related

In chapter 7, Wellness and Thinking, it was observed that we live in

. . . . *Exercise* . . . .

When Have You Transcended?

Can you recall a moment in your life when this experience of seeing the big picture, or feeling that all was connected and everything was right happened to you?

What happened?

Were you changed as a result?

How?

a predominantly left-brain oriented culture, one that values the logical, linear, mathematical approach to life, accepting C as the result of adding A and B. Unless the causal connection can be established between things, we all too often dismiss them as coincidental and hence meaningless.

Carl Jung, M.D., the Swiss psychiatrist, popularized the term *synchronicity* to describe the occurrence of two events, in close proximity of time, which have no causal relationship yet appear related.[1] For instance, you are thinking about a friend you haven't seen in ages at the very moment that she calls. Or, you are humming a tune to yourself as you turn on the car radio, and are amazed to hear the same tune playing back at you. Or, you

dial a wrong number only to discover that the person on the other end is a long-lost acquaintance.

Jung found that such coincidences happen far more often than would be expected by random chance, and increase in frequency for those who are open to them. In teaching psychology for many years, Regina notes that some of her students start "seeing" these connections soon after they learn about the concept of synchronicity.

The idea of synchronicity gets strong "scientific" support from Bell's theorem. Proposed in 1964 and verified in 1972, it was pronounced "the most profound discovery in science" by physicist Henry Stapp in a 1975 federal report. Bell's theorem (anticipated by Einstein in 1935, who was too un-

comfortable with it to accept it), proposes that everything in the universe is connected as an indivisible whole. In experiments based on Bell's theorem, it was demonstrated that if paired and identically charged particles "fly apart," and the polarity of one is changed by an experimenter, the other changes instantaneously. They remain mysteriously connected.[2]

What this implies is that, as Gary Zukav puts it, "There is no such thing as separate parts. All of the parts of the universe are connected in an intimate and immediate way previously claimed only by mystics and other scientifically objectionable people."[3]

If Bell's theorem is correct, and most experiments do bear it out, it helps to explain many previously

All Is One—All Is Right

Everything in the Universe is connected, somehow. Everything is all right! There is no need to be afraid of anything—even death. I know this surely, so deeply —and it brings utter peacefulness and real understanding.

The moment of awareness, which I only later learned to label a "peak experience"—happened to me in 1968 when I was an Air Force pilot in Vietnam. I was returning to the airfield in my single-person aircraft. It was sunset. On this particular evening, the sun was setting directly into the horizon at the end of the runway. As I lined up to make my final approach, I was momentarily concerned. Flying directly into the sun, it was difficult to see. That was my last conscious thought before "it happened."

Words fail to adequately communicate what next took place. The best I can tell you is that I merged totally with the sun—I was one with the light. There was no longer any sense of "me." There was no separation between Bob and everything that exists. All personal boundaries were completely dissolved.

Nothing mattered. There was no fear. There was no sense of time—no sense of space.

All was One and all was Right.

My next awareness was that I was on the ground, moving in a perfectly straight path down the runway. "I" had been "gone"—but yet "I" had made a textbook landing.

I knew I was completely safe. I had no sense that I had gone crazy. There was simply nothing to fear.

Despite the fact that this happening was totally outside the realm of everything I had ever known, I never doubted it, I never questioned it. I just *knew* it.

I walked away feeling that something exciting and powerful had taken place. Yet I felt no compulsion to do anything about it. No sense of "mission" to go out and change myself or anyone else.

Nor has there been any need to seek out some way, some means, to bring it about again.

It was complete.

I was complete.

All I know is that I can say with total clarity:

I no longer fear death.

From a conversation with
Bob Arnold
Loveland, Colorado
Educational/Aeronautics
Consultant

questioned psychic occurrences. It doesn't seem logical that a parent will "hear" his/her child crying when the child is 500 miles away; or that I could know what your home looks like when I have never been there or talked to you about it; or that Jim would develop a boil on his knee on the same day that his dad injured his knee on the job; or that psychic healer Olga Worral could diagnose an illness of a person she has never met, or cause a tumor to disappear simply by placing her hands on it; or that psychic Ingo Swann can significantly raise the temperature in a graphite cube by simply concentrating on it.

There is no question that there is an unseen world. The problem is how far is it from midtown and how late is it open.

—WOODY ALLEN

If, despite their distance, or lack of apparent logical relationship, event A is connected to event B at the sub-atomic level—is it too difficult to make the leap in saying that ESP, psychokinesis, distant viewing, psychic healing, and "miracles" are merely everyday manifestations of an underlying connectedness? The skeptics among us may dismiss these happenings as mere coincidence. For others, they are meaningful indications that everything is somehow related.

Rupert Sheldrake, a plant physiologist from England, has proposed a testable hypothesis that will be as important as Darwin's theory of evolution, if it proves true. His "Hypothesis of Formative Causation," described in a book by the same name, proposes that all entities, living organisms and inert substances as well, are each part of a "field" that connects them in some way with every other member of their species or type. He calls these fields "morphogenetic," which literally means "giving rise to structure or form." Morphogenetic fields do not obey the laws of thermodynamics, and operate irrespective of distances. Here's how they work. Suppose a mouse in England learns to run a maze. This mouse, in effect, creates a morphogenetic field for the solution of the maze, and therefore sets up a "form or structure" which allows mice all over the world to run the same maze with greater ease. The field becomes stronger with each mouse that completes the maze. This model explains the existence of instincts and habits, which have never been adequately understood, and once again reinforces the appreciation of our connectedness with everything in creation.

. . . .

At the heart of each of us, whatever our imperfections, there exists a silent pulse of perfect rhythm, a complex of wave forms and resonances, which is absolutely individual and unique, and yet which connects us to everything in the universe.

—GEORGE LEONARD
THE SILENT PULSE

. . . . . .

If you accept this relatedness you are immediately presented with alternatives that may significantly affect your life and health. In the early 1970s, neurosurgeon Norman Shealy, M.D., began documenting cases in which psychic healing methods succeeded in both

John's License Plate Games

Many pre-1980 California license plates have three letters and three numbers. Some of the three-letter combinations hint at pronounceable or meaningful words, like 916-EZY or 621-XON.

I've found I can use them to assess my unconscious process by saying the first word that comes to mind when I see three letters together, e.g., MDR = murder; SLP = slap; HDE = hide. After hearing myself say six such words in a row that involved violence, I might suspect I am suppressing anger about something. If the words I say have as a common theme being isolated or separated, I might get the idea I need a break or a vacation.

One evening as I was reading *New Realities* magazine, I saw a picture of a California license plate with an accompanying story about a woman who had seen that plate and noticed that it was the phone number of a friend in New York City, with whom she hadn't talked for a long time. This prompted her to call the friend, only to learn that the friend had been trying to reach her!

Carl Jung called such events, which are related and occur together but have no apparent cause-effect relationship, "synchronistic." I was aware that my life was, and still is, filled with synchronistic events. I began noticing that license plates would suggest words which would solve a problem I was thinking about, or remind me to do something I had forgotten.

One day, I was thinking of my friend, Jutta (pronounced YUTTA), and, in fact was saying her name out loud when I saw the plate JYU immediately followed by another car with TTA on the plates! These events seem to become more commonplace the more I expect them to happen.

diagnosis and treatment where traditional medical practice had failed.

Irving Oyle, D.O., in his book *The Healing Mind*, describes methods of helping his patients achieve an altered state of consciousness. In this state they "talk" with their "inner guides" to aid in diagnosing and treating a health-related problem.

Physicians, such as Brugh Joy, M.D., and Richard Moss, M.D., have trained thousands of health professionals to sense body-energy fields, and to use a method somewhat like a "laying on of hands," along with powerful music, to alter these fields, and thus effect healing.[4]

These examples suggest that numerous "illogical" alternatives often succeed where logical approaches have failed.

We Mold Our Own Reality

Throughout this book the connection between the thoughts that we

. . . . *Exercise* . . . .

A Bit of Magic

Find a key, and tie one end of a 20″ (50cm) length of thread through the hole. Copy the pattern below on a single sheet of paper, and lay it on a table top. Now sit in front of the paper, resting your elbow on the table for support, and with your hand dangle the key over the center of the design. Keep the tip of the key close to the crossing lines, *without actually touching them.*

When the key has come to rest, without closing your eyes, visualize or imagine it swinging back and forth along one of the straight lines. It may just barely move, or it may swing quite strongly, even though you are not aware of moving your hand. Once the key has begun swinging visualize it swinging along the other straight line. After a few moments, it will probably begin swinging along that line. Then visualize it swinging in a circular motion clockwise around the circle.

If you have trouble getting the results described above you may be trying too hard. Just let it happen. While the key may be seeming to move as if by magic, what is actually happening is that the muscles of your arm are moving imperceptibly, and the key on the length of thread acts as an amplifier, making the effects of those small muscle movements visible. This illustrates a level of mind–body connection outside of our conscious awareness.

A further application of this principle is in using it to gain access to information from your subconscious mind. You can ask yourself a question, and obtain a yes or no answer, depending on which way the key swings. You must define beforehand that a swinging along one line means yes, and along the other means no. This allows you to bypass the censoring of your rational/logical mind, and obtain information directly from a deeper part of yourself that knows what's really true for you.

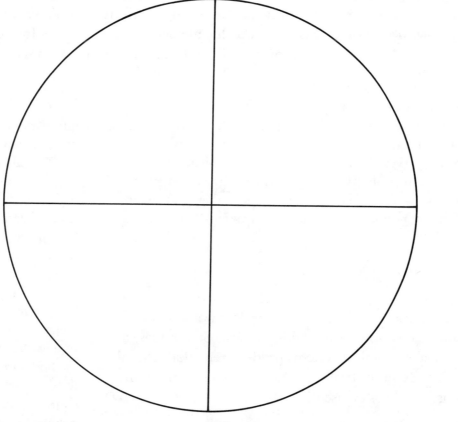

create in our minds and the conditions that manifest in the body has been stressed. In the chapter on thinking (chapter 7) the issue of the reality-molding power of our thoughts was developed.

This premise receives strong support from the most unlikely quarters—the laboratories of the sub-atomic particle physicists. From them we are finding out that our old concepts of a hard and fast, objective reality are simply not true.

According to Einstein's model of the universe, time actually slows down as your speed increases, and light travels in curves! The new physics of quantum mechanics demonstrates that a sub-atomic particle emitted when an atom is split is not even a "thing"—it is merely a "tendency to exist"—and that it is not possible to observe reality without changing it.

Heisenberg has said that the term "happens" is restricted to the observation. What he means by this is that there is *no reality* apart from our observations, evaluations, and judgments about it. "A" doesn't strike "B" in a void. It strikes B within the awareness of an observer—otherwise we would not know about it. Furthermore, not only does the observer's skill, computer programming ability, and visual or auditory acuity affect the report—his/her *very presence* has

Pendulums, Ouija Boards, and Other Weirdnesses

There are many "unexplainable" techniques used for healing and for diagnostic purposes—hypnosis, acupuncture, laetrile, visualization, ouija boards, astrology, etc. There is a diagnostic technique using a crystal hanging from a thread, much like the swinging key exercise— "A Bit of Magic." The person holding the crystal asks questions about problems the "patient" is having. For instance, "Is the problem in the kidneys?" or "Should this person be taking vitamin B6?" or "Should this person avoid sugar?" The answer is reflected in how the crystal pendulum swings.

I dismissed this technique for several years. Then I realized that it often actually worked, and that many other illogical, unconventional techniques worked too. At the same time, I was beginning to develop a belief that each of us has an inner spirit self or being which knows all there is to know. Out of this, I constructed a "logical" explanation for these various phenomena.

I think that through various non-logical modes, such as the swing of a pendulum, we are able to tap into a higher level of consciousness, a Universal Mind, and bypass the logical parts of our mind which is always seeking answers from the outside. The mode will only be successful, however, if we believe that it will work. It is a manifestation of the placebo effect. In other words, if you believe the drug you are taking is effective, you'll start feeling better; if you believe allopathic medicine is the best way for you, then it will be best for you; if you believe laetrile (or a crystal pendulum, or whatever) will work, then it will.

—JWT

an impact on the process. The observer's energy field is interacting with (and thus changing) the energy field of the whole system. It follows, then, that you are more than a bystander. You have a definite part in structuring your own life, in creating your own reality.

This altered view that our energy patterns influence reality, and that our thoughts actually create reality has been incorporated into the medical practice and educational approach of many highly reputable and courageous professionals. The whole field of biofeedback training is based upon using mental imagery and verbal suggestion to change a stress condition in the body. In Pacific Palisades, California, Carl Simonton, M.D., encourages his cancer patients to meditate three times a day, and to

I believe it is not helpful to analyze everything. It is not always necessary to find out exactly how or why things work. Sometimes, the most unconventional or illogical systems produce remarkable results. Your belief seems to be the critical factor at play in all of it. So, my recommendations—if it works, use it!

—JWT

image healthy cells destroying the cancerous ones.[5] And he is getting results! In Denver, Colorado, educator Marty Belknap teaches visualization to children and finds that it not only relaxes them, but stimulates their creativity.[6] Gerald Jampolsky, M.D., at the Center for Attitudinal Healing in Tiburon, California, works with children with leukemia and other life-threatening diseases. His methods center around guiding children in letting go of fear, in changing their thinking about their illness, in helping them to break with previously limiting ways of viewing their disease and the world. Such words as *impossible, can't, should, if only* are eliminated from the vocabulary. Jampolsky has seen time and again that it is love that heals— and that it is primarily our fear thoughts, our attack thoughts, that keep us stuck in illness.[7]

Change your perspective and once again the options multiply.

Everything Is in Process

As the Greek philosopher Heraclitus said centuries ago, "You can't step twice into the same river." Everything in the universe is in the constant process of changing. All you can do is watch what is happening, and observe what you're left with afterwards. Even modern physics is a science of *process*.

Arthur Young, the inventor of the Bell helicopter, in his book *The Reflexive Universe*,[8] presents his own "process" model. He proposes that the universe is not a thing. Rather it is a continual state of evolution from photons of light, through atoms, molecules, minerals, plants, animals . . . to conscious beings such as dolphins and humans.

· · · · · · ·

Reality is what we take to be true. What we take to be true is what we believe. What we believe is based upon our perceptions. What we perceive depends upon what we look for. What we look for depends upon what we think. What we think depends upon what we perceive. What we perceive determines what we believe. What we take to be true is our reality.

—GARY ZUKAV
*THE DANCING
WU LI MASTERS*

· · · · · · ·

These conscious beings are also in process towards more advanced states of development—which brings us back to where we started in chapter 1. Wellness is a never-ending *process* of moving towards the living of your highest potential. It also brings us back to Ilya Prigogene, who was mentioned in chapter 1, and his theory of dissipative structures, and how these structures change. Prigogene's theory has much to teach us about wellness.

Dissipative structures are open systems, which take in energy from the environment, transform it, and then return ("dissipate") energy to the outside world. An important property of dissipative structures is that they are able to resist (dampen) small fluctuations or changes in the energy field around them. For instance, a healthy body (an open system) is able to maintain its equilibrium in the face of minor alterations in diet, exercise, and level of stress.

When these fluctuations or changes reach a certain critical in-

Life After Life, After Life, After Life

Psychiatrist Elisabeth Kubler-Ross, the primary catalyst for the systematic study of death and dying, has had profound experiences which convince her that death does not terminate an individual's existence.[9]

Psychologist Helen Wambach uses hypnosis to take people back past birth. Often they report "living" other lives. She has found that data they recall about themselves can be verified by courthouse records and gravestones.[10]

Ian Stevenson, a medical doctor at the University of Virginia School of Medicine, published a paper in 1977 in the *Journal of Nervous and Mental Diseases* entitled "The Explanatory Value of the Idea of Reincarnation." For over twenty years he has been gathering and documenting data from children in many cultures who report having lived before.[11]

These findings inform us of new ways of explaining the process of life. They ground us in the awareness that, as the mystics have long told us, we are "more than our physical bodies." We also have a spirit which survives bodily death.

tensity, however, the dissipative structure alters drastically—in some cases completely reordering itself to a higher level of complexity—and a transformation takes place. For instance, when pushed to its limits with strenuous exercise, such as long-distance running, the body will switch from glucose usage for energy to eating up its own fat reserves. This reordering can mean significant changes in the shape of the physical body.

Solid forms or structures (closed systems, like a rock) can remain relatively stable or unchanged over extended periods of time. Open systems, on the other hand, always possess the ability to change because they constantly channel energy. They are structures in process! Each open-system, then, has within it the *potential* for change into a more complex, often more beautiful, more elaborate, structure.

. . . .

What the caterpillar calls the end of the world, the master calls a butterfly.

—RICHARD BACH

. . . .

When transformation occurs it often appears as if things are falling apart. The cocoon that shields the caterpillar looks like a tomb—a dead thing. But within, a magical regeneration is taking place. Far from falling apart, this apparent death signals a falling together—a restructuring, a transformation.[12]

This same breaking down as a prelude to a higher state of evolution is frequently observed in human beings faced with serious illness and even death. Sickness in the body, disease in the mind, the disintegration of a relationship, can be transforming experiences. At one level they bring us face to face with deep questions of personal value, of the meaning of life. They frequently cause a reordering of priorities—a change of job, a dramatic resolution of an alcohol or drug addiction, a lifestyle altera-

Reincarnation???

Over the years, as I have studied self-responsibility in wellness, I have gradually been "forced" into expanding my world view to include a reality wherein something like reincarnation is at work. I think it's rather more complex than the idea that we live one life after another, coming back to learn new lessons. It's probably more like the holographic model of the universe in which everything is connected, but at this point in my understanding, it is more an intuition than a definite knowing.

What seems to be true, and is a part of the perennial philosophy, is that we all originate from some spirit nature that transcends our physical limitations. Further, as Jung suggests in his theory of the collective unconscious, I believe that at some deep level, if we are open to it, we can access information/experience that seems to come from other people, often in other periods of history.

Many people who have had near-death experiences (NDE's) report that they no longer fear death and know that "something greater" is at work in their lives. Perhaps some "part" of us chooses to be born into a particular time, and to a certain set of parents. Of course we would have to forget all about this process, or it would spoil the fun. (Ian Stevenson, M.D., finds that children between ages three and six often can remember experiences that seem to originate from other lifetimes—perhaps because they first become verbal enough to express these thoughts at three and learn that it's not socially acceptable to do so by age six.)

tion. On another level they may unlock doors that have been closed to us for years:

- Stress reduction techniques that were used to deal with an ulcer, become daily practice and result in a changed perception of the world in general.

- Massage, deep tissue work such as Rolfing, realignment systems such as the Feldenkrais technique, undertaken as forms of physical therapy, at the same time facilitate the release of long-held emotional trauma stored in the muscles of the body.

- Adverse reactions to drug treatment have led people to the investigation of hypnosis for pain control, mental visualization for treatment of cancer, and significant diet changes as an alternative to unsuccessful traditional therapy.

- Chronic back pain has led many to the practice of yoga; and yoga has then become a way of life.

The examples multiply. The options increase and so do the possibilities for wellness.

The transcendent view of life as a *process* is the basis for recommen-

If reincarnation, and choice of life circumstances and parents, is indeed true, then we are in charge of our lives a great deal more than we usually imagine. It means that we are not the helpless victims of chance in a random, uncaring universe. It means that each of us is equally powerful and responsible, even if we have chosen ways that do not appear to be so on the surface (by being born disabled, dying at an early age, etc.). This idea is very upsetting to most people's egos and often generates violent opposition from some quarters—especially from "hard-core" victims. I know this position well because I feel like a victim more often than I like to admit. It has taken time and a healthy dose of courage for me to even consider the possible truth of these ideas. Because it is so common for people (myself included) to confuse self-responsibility with blame, beliefs in reincarnation and total choice are particularly hard to swallow. (See chapter 1.)

As I live out these beliefs in my daily life, I find that they encourage me to resist pity for people. Rather, I am committed to supporting others with respect, honoring their right to change in their own way, at their own pace, or not at all if they so choose. (See section on rescuing in chapter 9.) I am even learning to give myself the same freedom.

We may never be able to prove what is true, but my experience verifies to me that people who live their lives as though they are primarily responsible are usually more empowered and happier than those who don't.

—JWT

Awakening to God is often conceived of as a victory because of the illusion that there is something to attain, that there is a battle to be won. Actually, enlightenment is a defeat because all one does is become ordinary.

—LEE LOZOWICK

dations that we allow the body the freedom to do what it does best. It allows us the healing attitude of compassion as we examine and reassess every aspect of our lives. Realizing that we are in process lets us relax with mistakes, enjoy the paradoxes which life proposes to us every day, and give ourselves permission to be just who and what we are at the moment. And finally, it serves to excite us with the realization that we will never be finished—that there will always be new ways to grow, new doors to open, new cracks to explore in the cosmos.

Transpersonal Psychology and Wellness

A field of inquiry in psychology has emerged called the fourth force. (The first was Freudian psychoanalysis; the second—Behavioral psychology; the third—Humanistic psychology; and now the fourth—Transpersonal psychology.) Transpersonal psychology seeks to incorporate the spiritual into the therapeutic process. It grows out of this expanding realization that energy is one, that there are multiple, or alternate, realities which many of us have touched in our transcending experiences; that ancient, religious, and mystical traditions have much to say to the condition of twentieth century woman and man; that a transformation is taking place.

Do I contradict myself? Very well then I contradict myself, I am large, I contain multitudes.

—WALT WHITMAN

Investigators in this realm are examining such matters as astrology, psychic inspiration, dreams, and altered states of consciousness and how they relate to body and mind processes. Indeed, the existence of fourth force psychology testifies to a growing need for help in explaining, handling, and using such "mystical" transcendent/transformational experiences.

Two of these areas, dream analysis and meditation, are accessible to all of us. They require no elaborate equipment, charts, or intermediaries. You can explore them yourself and reap whatever benefits you can from them.

Dreams

Dreams are particularly useful tools for developing self-understanding and self-awareness. Because they happen in sleep, in an altered state of consciousness, they often give us the side of the story which is out-voted when the rational, word-oriented brain is in control. Thus, they become a way of looking at a neglected part of ourselves.

There is a universal fascination with the content and meaning of dreams. We know their power because we have all awakened in terror, exhilaration, or sexual excitement as a result of one. Supermarket booklets of dream symbols offer elementary equations (for instance, an ocean means you want to take a trip) which generally leave the seeker dissatisfied. Since dreams are such highly personal experiences, simple explanations will not apply to everybody.

. . . .

A dream which is not understood is like a letter which is not opened.

—TALMUD

. . . .

Theories regarding the meaning of dreams range from mechanistic (the mind is categorizing and filing the information of the day), to psychoanalytic (dreams express hidden desires which the conscious mind is afraid to face), to psychic (dreams are modes of spirit-travel and ways of predicting the future). All of which are probably partially true.

A dream is like a movie, written, directed, and acted out by a whole range of characters in your personal consciousness. The parts you will remember the most vividly are the parts that have something to say to you at the moment. You can, therefore, use them to great advantage.

A number of years ago, Regina was at the point of going back to

A Transformation

A recent trip through the eastern United States, at which time I gave presentations in five states, convinced me we are entering a period of *transformation* in thinking and lifestyles. I saw that more and more individuals are accepting greater responsibility for their own health, welfare, environment, education, and spiritual direction. More and more "ordinary" people are interested in learning, growing, and in living wellness. What seemed to have been a passing fad in 1975 now seems to me to be a major mass movement, a true transformation.

—J.W.T.

. . . .

school to pursue her doctoral studies. She had a dream in which she needed to get to the airport to catch a plane for a very important meeting. The details she remembers most clearly are:

The plane would not take a direct route. To get to Seattle (her destination) she would have to go first from Denver to New Orleans (quite a circuit!).

The taxi to the airport never arrived so she had to rely on hitchhiking. And her bags were not packed. As she opened her suitcase she found it filled with religious objects—rosary beads, prayerbooks, long black dresses, like the habits she had worn as a nun.

The dream had a powerful impact on her. In writing it down and telling it to her friends, she became aware of how many times she said things like:

"I feel pressured."

"I'll be late."

"Why do I have to take such a roundabout route to my destination?"

"I'm not ready."

"I have to get rid of this old junk before I can put in my new stuff."

The more she dealt with these reactions, the clearer it became to her that these were the same feelings she had in planning for graduate school. One week after this dream, she withdrew her application for admission—and breathed a sigh of relief.

You can interpret your own dreams. Carl Jung speaks of the "aha" experience which accompanies dealing with dream content. "Aha" means "Yes that feels good to me," or "That applies to my life now," or "That's just the piece of the puzzle I've been looking for." While experienced analysts can prove helpful, you are the only one who can generate "aha" about your dreams. *So become your own expert.*

A Dream Journal

Everybody dreams, every night. We know this because sleep researchers have shown that rapid eye movements (REM) correlate with

. . . . *Exercise* . . . .

Working With a Dream

Dreams not only provide us with information about ourselves, but can also serve as creative inspiration for poems or stories, or paintings or inventions.

10 Ways to Grow With Dreaming:

1. Paint your dream.

2. Write your dream in a three-line poem, capturing its essence.

3. Compose a short story, or an essay detailing your dream.

4. Dialogue with your dream characters—one at a time.

5. Dialogue with your dream symbols.

6. Play with the notion that all the dream characters and dream symbols are all different parts, different aspects of yourself. Ah, what then?

7. Daydream and finish an unfinished dream in any way you would like it to turn out. Or re-dream a total dream, changing whatever you want to change.

8. Write down your ideal dream. What would it be about? What elements would it include?

9. Talk your dream out loud. Listen to the words you use, especially the phrases you may repeat. Listen for emotions as well as content. Ask yourself to what situation in your present life do those same phrases and emotions relate?

10. Follow up on the intuitions you tap in dreams. Write a letter to the old friend you dreamed about. Call your mother on the phone when you dream about her. Wear a red shirt on the morning after a red dream. Look for connections all day long.

Happy Dreaming.

. . . .

the state of dreaming. We may not remember our dreams, but since we all experience REM during sleep, we all dream.

You can train yourself to remember your dreams in a number of different ways. The first and most effective is to give yourself the suggestion at night that you will recall your dreams in the morning. Placing pencil and paper (or a tape recorder) beside your bed, will allow you to note even a few details which may bring back the fuller context the next day. The intention to work with dreams is often all it takes to begin to remember them. Do not become discouraged. For some, this intention and practice takes several weeks. But in our experience, it usually involves no more than a few days. When all else fails Regina suggests eating an anchovy pizza just before retiring. While it won't make you dream any more, you may wake up repeatedly throughout the night, and remember your dreams better as a result.

Here are some practical suggestions:

1. Pick out a special notebook and pen to use for your dream journal.

2. Keep the pen and notebook in

· · · · · · · · · · · · · · · · · · · *Exercise* · · · · · · · · · · · · · ·

Finding Center

This exercise is designed to help you find the place of "center" within yourself. Ask someone to read these questions to you, one at a time, giving you plenty of time to touch each "center" in answer to the question. It may help you to close your eyes and breathe quietly before beginning.

1. If you imagine that your "soul" exists at some place in your body, where would it be?

2. Imagine that your body is a building, and that in one, tiny room there is a spot where you feel most relaxed and at home. Where is that place located?

3. Pretend that you are trying to balance your physical body on a fulcrum. Where is the point of contact?

4. Take a few slow and very deep breaths. From what place does the breath originate? What place does the deepest breath reach?

5. Say "I am me" several times as you point to yourself. Where do you point? Which place feels truest?

You may have found several different places which felt like your "center," your "home." As you practice some of the techniques suggested in this book, you may find that one "center" becomes more and more true for you.

· ·

a clear space, next to your bed. Put it in the same place each night.

3. Date the page at the top. Do this at night just before you turn out the light. Let it be a reminder to you: "I am going to remember my dreams."

4. Record dreams whenever you awake, during the night or in the morning. Don't wait.

5. Write down anything you remember, even one word, or a disconnected fragment, a color, a feeling which the dream generated.

6. Write in the first person, in the present tense. For example: "I am in my house and the water is running in the kitchen . . ."

7. Describe the dream, and the feelings it gave you, but avoid writing your interpretations at this time. That can come later.

8. See books on dreams in the reading list.

Transformation Through Meditation

The stress of living in the twentieth century on planet Earth requires the programming of safety valves to keep us healthy and happy. From every direction we are bombarded with forces that tend to draw us away from ourselves. The media tell us what we should like and dislike. Pressured jobs preoccupy us and can disturb our necessary sleep. Noises in the environment continually distract us from the task at hand. We can be left feeling like a battered boat in an angry sea—losing touch with what we really want, really believe, ultimately with who we *really* are. A variety of meditation forms have become popular because they work to help us in relaxing, concentrating, and attuning to the deeper, spiritual, creative self.

· · · · · · · ·

To love is to approach each other center to center.

—PIERRE TEILHARD
DE CHARDIN

· · · · · · · ·

When we discussed Prigogene's theory earlier we learned that it is the critical fluctuations which provoke a shift into a higher level of restructuring. Meditation and other altered states of consciousness can cause just such critical fluctuations. Normal states of awareness show up on EEG machines as small rapid brain waves. They look something like this:

When people meditate, or move inward by other means, their brain waves slow down, but also become larger. Like this:

In other words, larger waves mean larger fluctuations affecting the structure. Such states, then, break traditional patterns and in so doing, open the system to the possibility of a new shift—a leap in consciousness, even a transformation.[13] This might take the form of a more gentle approach to life, the ability to flow with contradictions rather than to be overwhelmed by them. Or it may mean the opening of a new creative potential, since it has been demonstrated that meditation-like techniques enhance personal creativity.

Meditation, from the Sanskrit *medha*, literally means "doing the wisdom." It is a process of locating your center, your temple of inner wisdom, your truest self.

There are many different methods of meditating, ranging from drumming to chanting to breathing to simply sitting. Should you decide to explore some of them, there are general guidelines that apply to any type of meditation practice. They are presented here to help you on your way.

1. *Make this your express intention.* Set aside the time (perhaps ten or twenty minutes each morning and each evening) and prepare a quiet, private place for yourself.

2. *Eliminate side trips.* Meditation is an exercise of the right brain, the intuitive, spiritual, spontaneous side of you. As you meditate, the logical left brain will be busy trying to distract you. ("Remember to call Harry tonight." "This is a waste of time." "I wonder what the kids are doing now.") You will need to learn to set these distractions aside.

3. *Select a centering device.* Each meditational practice makes use of some centering device to keep you on course. Sometimes it is a sound which is repeated, a word or song. It can be an object, like a candle or picture. It can be a repeated bodily movement.

4. *Ask for help.* In many cities and on campuses around the country there are groups and organizations devoted to the teaching of meditation technique. While it is not essential, joining such a group can be very helpful. Moreover, there is an intensified energy which develops when people meditate together.

Finding a center, a home, a place of balance, makes anything possible. The universe, from this perspective, is viewed as friendly, and our place in it is experienced as blessed. Life energy emanates from the center, and all that shares this energy is found there as well. Being there means being in harmony with ourselves, with our brothers and sisters, with our environment, our planet, our universe.

. . . .

The more faithfully you listen to the voice within you, the better you will hear what is sounding outside.

—DAG
HAMMERSKJOLD

. . . .

If these ideas seem remote to you, please don't feel left out. Our orientation betrays years of spiritual searching, for better or worse. Transcending need not be "cosmic" or "spiritual" at all. In fact, ageless wisdom supports that only when we are experiencing the simple and ordinary of life as the simple and ordinary of life, are we truly in harmony. Transcending is really about moving from complexity to greater and greater simplicity. Therefore, each time you make even a tiny step in eliminating "excess baggage" from your environment, from your diet, from your mind, you are moving towards greater wellness. Each time you pose a new question, open a new door, willingly challenge any limit you have placed upon yourself, you are transcending.

................................*Exercise*..

Approaches to Meditation

A Candle Meditation

Light a candle in a semi-darkened room. Place it about 18 inches from you, at eye level. Look at it. Become absorbed with it. As thoughts arise bring your attention back to the awareness of the candle and flame. Try not to verbally analyze or describe what is taking place. Simply be with it.

Close your eyes and find the image imprinted on your eyelids. Stay with it. As it fades, open your eyes again and see the candle again. Do this for 15 or 20 minutes.

Yantra

The picture on the next page is a type of Hindu symbol called a yantra. This one, the Sri Yantra, represents the entire cosmos. The center design is formed by two sets of triangles—four pointing up, representing the feminine principle in the universe, five pointing down, representing the masculine principle. Pictures of this kind were used to help student meditators realize their unity with all life.

Experiment with it as a centering device for yourself. Look at it softly, with eyes only partially open. Each time you realize that your mind is wandering, draw your attention back to the picture, allowing your thoughts to pass.

Why not make a copy of the yantra. Color it. Put it on a wall where you will see it often. Each time you do, let it remind you to "center in" once again.

Walking Meditation

You can do this at any time—either spontaneously as you walk to work, or formally in your room or garden—either barefoot or with shoes on.

Simply concentrate as fully as possible on the sensation of walking. Feel your heel contact the ground. Then attend to the ball of your foot and your toes as they come into play. Realize the motion involved in lifting your foot and preparing it for the next step.

You may wish to add the use of a word, or phrase, or affirmation so that you walk in step with an established inner rhythm.

Chants..

Using your voice to repeat a song or chant is a doubly effective way to center yourself. Even greater is the effect when several people together chant the same sounds. If you don't know any chants try making up your own refrains for these:

Peace, peace, peace, peace,
    May peace fill up my heart.

All is One, All is One
    All is One, All is One.

Truth and beauty are now
living in the temple of my soul.

I am light, I am light
    I am light, I am light.

See Appendix A for some beautiful recordings of chants and music for meditation.

Suggested Reading*

Benson, R. *The Relaxation Response*. New York, NY: Avon Books, 1975.

Bentov, I. *Stalking the Wild Pendulum*. New York, NY: E.P. Dutton, 1977.

Dossey, L. *Space, Time and Medicine*. Boulder, CO: Shambhala, 1982.

Drury, N., ed. *Inner Health: The Health Benefits of Relaxation, Meditation and Visualization*. San Leandro, CA: Prism Press, 1985.

Faraday, A. *The Dream Game*. New York, NY: Harper and Row, 1974.

Foundation for Inner Peace. *A Course in Miracles*. Tiburon, CA: 1975.

Head, J., and Cranston, S.L., eds. *Reincarnation in World Thought*. New York, NY: Julian Press, 1967.

Jampolsky, G. *There Is a Rainbow Behind Every Dark Cloud*. Center for Attitudinal Healing, 21 Main St., Tiburon, CA 94920. 1977.

Jung, C. *Man and His Symbols*. New York, NY: Dell Publishing Co., 1964.

Leonard, G. *The Transformation*. New York, NY: Delta Books/ Dell Publishing Co., 1972.

———. *The Silent Pulse*. New York, NY: E.P. Dutton, 1979.

LeShan, L. *How to Meditate*. New York, NY: Bantam Books, 1974.

Lilly, J. *The Center of the Cyclone*. New York, NY: Bantam Books, 1979.

Mishlove, J. *Roots of Consciousness*. New York, NY, and Berkeley, CA: Random House/ Bookworks, 1975.

Moss, R. *The I That Is We*. Berkeley, CA: Celestial Arts, 1981.

Oyle, I. *The Healing Mind*. Berkeley, CA: Celestial Arts, 1979.

Shealy, C. N. *Occult Medicine Can Save Your Life*. New York, NY: Dial Press, 1975.

Sheldrake, R. *A New Science of Life: The Hypothesis of Formative Causation*. Los Angeles, CA: J.P. Tarcher, 1983.

Stevenson, I. *Twenty Cases Suggestive of Reincarnation*. New York, NY: American Society for Psychical Research, 1966.

Vaugn, F. *Awakening Intuition*. Garden City, NY: Anchor Press/ Doubleday, 1979.

Wambach, H. *Reliving Past Lives*. New York, NY: Bantam Books, 1978.

———. *Life Before Life*. New York, NY: Bantam Books, 1979.

Wilber, K. *No Boundary: Eastern and Western Approaches to Personal Growth*. Boston, MA: Shambhala, 1981.

Wilson, R.A. *The Cosmic Trigger*. New York, NY: Pocket Books, 1977.

Worrall, A., and Worrall, O. *The Gift of Healing*. New York, NY: Harper and Row, 1976.

Young, A. *The Reflexive Universe*. New York, NY: Delacorte Press, 1976.

Zukav, G. *The Dancing Wu Li Masters*. New York, NY: William Morrow and Co., 1979.

Notes

1. Jung, C. *Synchronicity: An Acausal Connecting Principle*, in the *Collected Works*, Vol. 8, *The Structure and Dynamics of the Psyche*.

Princeton, NJ: Princeton University Press, 1969, Par. 816–997.

2. Ferguson, M. *The Aquarian Conspiracy*. Los Angeles, CA: J.P. Tarcher/St. Martin's Press, 1980, p. 171.

3. Zukav, G. *The Dancing Wu Li Masters*. New York, NY: William Morrow and Co., 1979, p. 272.

4. See:

Moss, R. *The I That Is We*. Berkeley, CA: Celestial Arts, 1981.

Joy, W.B. *Joy's Way*. Los Angeles, CA: J.P. Tarcher, 1979.

5. Simonton, C.; Matthews-Simonton, S.; and Creighton, J. *Getting Well Again*. Los Angeles, CA: J.P. Tarcher, 1978. Contact: Simonton Cancer Center, 875 Via de la Paz, Pacific Palisades, CA 90272.

6. Marty Belknap is a private educational consultant, and the author of *Taming Your Dragons*, practical exercises for stress reduction and creativity for children. For more about her work write to her at: Salina Star Route/Gold Hill, Boulder, CO 80302.

7. See:

Mary, A. "Coping with Sickness through Love," *New Realities*, Vol. II, No. 44 (February 1979), pp. 448–53.

Jampolsky, G. *Goodbye to Guilt: Releasing Fear Through Forgiveness*. New York, NY: Bantam Books, 1985.

Contact: Dr. Gerald Jampolsky, Center for Attitudinal Healing, 21 Main St., Tiburon, CA 94920.

8. Young, A. *The Reflexive Universe*. New York, NY: Delacorte Press, 1976.

9. See:

"Commentary: The Ineffable and the Incredible, Elisabeth Kubler-Ross . . ." *Brain-Mind Bulletin*, Vol. I, No. 21A.

10. Wambach, H. "Past Life Recall," *Psychic*, Vol. 7, No. 5, (November/ December, 1976), pp. 56–61.

———. *Reliving Past Lives*. New York, NY: Bantam Books, 1978.

———. *Life Before Life*. New York, NY: Bantam Books, 1979.

11. Stevenson, I. "The Explanatory Value of the Idea of Reincarnation," *Journal of Nervous and Mental Disease*. May, 1977. See also:

———. *Twenty Cases Suggestive of Reincarnation*. New York: American Society for Psychical Research, 1966.

12. See: Ferguson, M. *The Aquarian Conspiracy*.

13. Ferguson, M., pp 168–69.

---

*This is only a representative sampling. Many excellent books have been omitted. At the bookstore or library, look over the whole section and choose according to your judgment.

Afterword

IF YOU HAVE been frustrated because you have not found any clear and simple answers in this book, then paradoxically, you have really understood the message. For there are no answers other than the ones that come from you. And because you are growing and changing even those answers may not be true tomorrow. If you have been puzzled or taken aback at some of the unconventional ideas that have been presented here, again, you have understood the message. For it is by stretching yourself, by expanding your vision that you enable yourself to make the continual changes, the continual growth toward high-level wellness.

These ideas can help you understand that you are not a helpless victim struggling in life's ocean, tossed by every wave, that you are essentially in complete control of your own life and health, that you are a powerful channel of an energy that connects everything. You are capable of changing your own body and the world by changing your way of thinking and by opening yourself to the flow of all the energies of the body/mind. You can love yourself in the process. You can live well.

The book ends here, but your journey will never be over.

DISCOGRAPHY OF NEW AGE AND RELATED MUSIC

There is an abundance of music now available that is collectively known as "New-Age Music." This is music that has the power to relax and calm the listener while producing a positive, stimulating and peaceful experience.

This is music to "get inside of" which can be equally useful for active listening or background flavorings. At its best, this is today's classical music, reflecting the moods and melodies and desires that are part of our lives. Take the time to listen and explore; use your heart and your body and your imagination as you listen with your ears.

This annotated bibliography of personal favorites and currently popular recordings is compiled by our good friend, Lloyd Barde, the owner of BACKROADS DISTRIBUTORS, which carries these and over 800 other titles of New Age Music.

Request the free 20-page *Heartbeats* catalog published three times yearly. Write: Backroads Distributors, 417 Tamal Plaza, Corte Madera, CA 94925, or call (415) 924-4848, or (800) 825-4848.

PIANO MUSIC

George Winston. "Autumn": Windham Hill label. Lyrical and transcendent music. Winston paints pictures and tells stories at the keyboard. We recommend anything by Winston, and the same for the recording company.

Spencer Brewer. "Shadow Dancer": Willow Rose #1006. A masterfully conceived and performed work. Includes Spencer playing four different synthesizers, as well as bells and gongs. Very beautiful music.

Jim Chappell. "Tender Ritual": Unspeakable Freedom #101. Just when you think you've heard enough solo piano music, along comes a great surprise. This is it. Images of the sea and fantasy excursions are expressed through many emotions on this tape of quality.

GUITAR MUSIC

William Ackerman. "Past Light": Windham Hill #1028. Ackerman is the founder of the Windham Hill label and a brilliant musician. The selections on this album are all new. One solo piece plus works with other Windham Hill artists create a musical feast with many delicious courses. Treat yourself to this, or anything else that bears his name.

Michael Hedges. "Aerial Boundaries": Windham Hill #1032. Hedges has become one of our favorite guitarists because of his incredible virtuosity and fluidity as well as the humanness that comes across in his music. It's amazing how one person with a guitar can produce such a full sound. Obviously he has four hands!

HARP MUSIC

Georgia Kelly. "Seapeace": Heru #101, #104, #107. This is Georgia's classic first album. It contains meditations and etudes for the harp. The four pieces perfectly convey the variety of style and tone that a harpist can conjure. Contemplative, gentle, compassionate, and above all, transcendentally beautiful music. Newer releases of note include: "The Sound of Spirit" and "Harp and Soul."

Andreas Vollenweider. "Behind the Garden": Columbia #37793, #37827. This music is bound to make you smile. Very original. Electronic harp which is bouncy and jazzy, and flows from the heart. This plus his album "Caverna Magica" will make a wonderful addition to your music library. Recommended for playful, light dancing or exercising, as well as simple listening pleasure.

Patrick Ball. "Celtic Harp" and "From a Distant Time, Vol. 2": Fortuna #005, #011. If you haven't been introduced to the Celtic harp, this is the place to start. Ball's music is crystal clear. Albums contain pieces from the timeless folk tradition, as well as spirited modern performances by this master of the instrument.

FLUTE MUSIC

Larkin. "O'cean": Sona Gaia #131. An exquisite blend of Larkin's flute with ocean sounds, songs of the humpback whales and synthesizer chords. A classic.

James Newton. "Echo Canyon": Celestial Harmonies #012. This is one of the finest solo flute recordings we've ever heard. Set in a magical canyon in New Mexico, Newton plays the C-flute, bass flute and wood flute. The result is nothing less than majestic.

MEDITATIVE MUSIC

Mike Rowland. "The Fairy Ring": Sona Gaia #136. There is nothing quite like it. This tape touches people in a deep place and brings a positive and tranquil response. The simplicity of the music, performed on piano and gentle synthesized strings, is utterly profound.

Rob Whitesides-Woo. "Miracles": Search for Serenity #101. Gorgeous harp, strings and wind instruments will penetrate your soul. Inspired by the book *A Course In Miracles*. Exceedingly powerful.

Tony Scott. "Music for Zen Meditation": Verve #8634. A 15-year-old classic that is responsible for bringing the traditional flavor of the East into full Western exposure. It is what it says it is.

Wolff and Hennings. "Tibetan Bells II": Celestial Harmonies #005. Pure, timeless, and unearthly. This recording utilizes the finest high-frequency techniques known, and has captured the exquisite tonalities of the Tibetan bells. An extraordinary musical voyage.

Steven Halpern. "Spectrum Suite": Grammavision #770. Halpern is the founder of "Anti-Frantic Alternative" music and a true pioneer. His music calms and clears the body/mind. In his most popular recording, he relates the seven notes of the musical octave to the seven colors of the visual spectrum, and the seven energy centers of the body. Powerful.

GUIDED TAPES WITH MUSIC

Emmett Miller, M.D. "Healing Journey," "Letting Go of Stress," or "Rainbow Butterfly": Source #16, #23, #11. The deep, reassuring voice of Dr. Miller combines with exquisite musical compositions by masterful artists like Georgia Kelly and Stephen Halpern. For self-healing, relaxation, and creative imagination development. Highly recommended

Jon Shore (with Frank Smith). "Meditation 1/Meditation 2" Light Unlimited. Guided meditations about listening to your own "inner voice." With music that is sweet and gentle and ocean sounds providing the space to return to the here and now.

ENVIRONMENTAL SOUNDS

Environment Series. "Ultimate Thunderstorm," "Slow Ocean," "English Meadow": Syntonic. Exactly what they say—and nothing else. Great for relaxation, for background sound, for insomniacs.

Aiki Domo. "Sunrise Walk Along a Tahitian Seashore": Invincible #1004. A South Pacific environment filled with the sounds of the seashore and the distant barrier reef. The ocean's majesty and power are so well expressed you may leave everything behind. Some musical accompaniment.

Bearns and Dexter. "The Golden Voyage, Vol. 1": Awakening Productions. This is our top of the line, timeless, galactic exploration through celestial harmonics. Uses the sounds of nature blended with flutes, bells, piano, guitar and electronic sounds to create a unique and magical experience for the listener. Very visual, and highest quality.

ELECTRONIC WEAVINGS

Ray Lynch. "Deep Breakfast": Ray Lynch Productions. This tape is a perfect balance of electronic "space" music and deeply lyrical emotional music. Superb synthesizer orchestrations with additional viola, flute and piano. Regina's all-time favorite for movement, dance, and "bliss."

Kitaro. "Silk Road": Kuckuck #51–52. This master sound creator from Japan lives quietly in the foothills of Mt. Fuji. Here he produces some of the world's finest music. This one is perhaps his best. An abundant two volume masterpiece blending the sounds of East and West.

Deuter. "Ecstasy": Kuckuck #044. This is the most popular album of this renowned artist. Filled with images of nature and the heavens. Like "new classical" music, the power is in the beauty of the music, the joy and the balance. A true gem! We highly recommend anything by Deuter or Kitaro.

RHYTHMIC OR JAZZY

Tri Atma with Klaus Netzle. "Yearning and Harmony": Fortuna #016. A delightful, effervescent fusion of buoyant Eastern rhythms and electronic popular music. Light, but grounded, with some vocal additions and an intertwining of sound and cultures you're sure to enjoy. Very popular.

Patrick O'Hearn. "Ancient Dreams": Private Music #1201. One of Lloyd's favorites. Very modern, visual music performed on synthesizers and percussion creating an aural landscape of new rhythms and enticing sound—from thundering and majestic to cool and elegant.

Paul Winter. "Canyon": Living Music #6. It's hard to put this one in any category, for fear of limiting its reception. Recorded in both the Grand Canyon and in St. John's Cathedral in New York City. Paul has brought together a team of the finest musicians for this special journey. His own soprano sax has never sounded better.

VOCAL FRIENDS

Kate Wolf. "Poet's Heart": Kaleidoscope #24. Her sixth album—Kate at her very best. Her music is the perfect blend of folk, country and New Age Music; in the lyrics she will touch your heart. You'll want her for your friends too. We recommend anything she's done.

David Tate. "Love Will Have Its Way": Lion #1. A gentle and sensitive blend of sound, rhythm and heart. A blessing for the vocal world. The title cut contains sufficient wisdom to last a lifetime.

CLASSICAL MASTERPIECES

"The Pachelbel Canon." By Maurice Angre and the Jean- Francois Paillard Chamber Orchestra: RCA #5468. This is generally considered to be the finest recording of this very classical piece.

"Andante—Collection of Chamber Music Classics": Decca #16.35186. Features 20 different selections of Bach, Haydn, Schumann, Beethoven, Brahms, Schubert, Mozart, Debussy and others. The performances are by some of the world's finest musicians and quintets. This double album is a treasure to own.

CHANTS AND DEVOTIONAL SONGS AND SOUNDS

"A Few Good Friends—Songs of the Abode": Abode. Simple heartfelt songs from the Sufi community (The Abode of the Message) in upstate New York. Wonderful harmonies and voices. Inspiring. Regina's special recommendation.

Evan Hodkins. "The Heart Is the Vessel": School of Alchemy Chorus and Orchestra. From Boulder, Colorado, comes this heartfelt collection of chants from various religious cultures. Repetitive, mantra-like phrases. A fine musical backing. Deep and magical.

David Hykes and Harmonic Choir. "Current Circulation": Celestial Harmonies #010. This music extends the boundaries of traditional and sacred or contemporary spiritual music. The seven-member choir chants a fundamental tone and one or more higher harmonics or overtones of it simultaneously. Mystical, eerie, captivating, and potent.

..... Appendix B.....

A PERSONAL WELLNESS JOURNAL

WHAT IS IT?

The Personal Wellness Journal is a notebook/diary/scrapbook. It is personal because it is private and confidential. It is a wellness journal because it is used in conjunction with this workbook, or separately, as a means of enhancing your health and overall well-being. It is a journal because it is a dated, written record.

WHAT SHOULD THE JOURNAL BE USED FOR?

Anything and everything you wish, and specifically to respond to exercises suggested and questions raised in the Wellness Workbook. For instance, my friends and students and I have used the Journal:

- To keep notes from lectures or workshops attended.

- To summarize books or articles read.

- To record memorable quotes. Like: "The missing nutrient in the diets of most people is love." —John W. Travis, M.D.

- To list the hundreds and thousands of questions about wellness that occur every day.

- As a scrapbook, in which to tape special articles, cartoons, pictures, etc., that pertain to wellness.

- For poetry writing.

- As a dream diary.

- As a sketchbook, to "draw your feelings" about someone, or something that is important to you.

- To chart an exercise schedule, and performance (as suggested in chapter 5).

- To keep track of how various foods, meals, times of eating and quantities affect overall energy and mental clarity (as suggested in chapter 4).

- To record goals, inspirations, and prayers.

- To write out dialogues, i.e., conversations, with imaginary guides, or parts of the self, as a way of gaining new insights.

- And more . . .

WHAT TYPE OF BOOK SHOULD I USE FOR MY JOURNAL?

One that feels comfortable to you. Basically, you should choose a book that suits your taste, your personality. I suggest a book that is special in some way rather than a plain notebook, but it's up to you. A bound book is sometimes helpful in the process because you will be less likely to tear out or discard pages too quickly. It happens that a page of doodles drawn one day serves to inspire a new creation a month or so later. The page size of your journal should be large enough to allow you to write a complete letter, or draw a bold picture. I recommend that it be at least 8 inches by 8 inches.

IS THERE A STANDARD WAY TO KEEP A JOURNAL?

Yes.

First—Be honest. Dare to admit to your journal what you are afraid to admit to someone else. "Talk" to yourself as a most trusted friend. Address yourself by name if you care to: "Now Henry, you know that's a lie. . . ."

Second—Work quickly, and avoid reading over your work until you feel complete. This is to discourage self-editing and self-judgment as you write or create. Most people are amazed at how easily and prolifically they can express themselves when they put the critic to rest for a while.

Third—Challenge yourself with different modes of expression. If you only write in poetry, draw with crayons for a few days. If you generally use descriptive writing, try writing your feelings/thoughts as a dialogue between two people, two different aspects of yourself.

Fourth—Date all your work. I always find it so interesting to chart my progress. At the same time I am constantly amazed to realize that nothing much changes.

ARE THERE BOOKS THAT CAN HELP IN THE JOURNAL-KEEPING PROCESS?

YES. I recommend: *The New Diary: How to Use a Journal for Self-guidance and Expanded Creativity*. By Tristine Rainer. Los Angeles, CA: J.P. Tarcher Press, 1978.

The Creative Journal: The Art of Finding Yourself. By Lucia Capacchione. Athens, OH: Ohio University Press, 1979.

And now for a very special treat, get yourself a copy of: *The Castle of the Pearl* by Christopher Biffle, NY: Barnes and Noble Books, 1983. This gem of a book is a ready-made journal, complete with fascinating imaginary journeys and intriguing questions about life, and particularly your relationships. You'll love it!

Good Luck,

Regina

Index

Abdominal breathing exercise, 96
Acceptance, exercise, 18–19
Accident reports, to insurance companies, 157
Accidents, as a reward, 14, 17
Acupressure, and touch, 49–50
Adapted Child, 149–150
Additives
    in food, 76–77
    and food labeling, 79–81
Aerobics, 94–95
Affirmations, 142–143
After-life experience, 205
Air conditioning, and health, 53
Air pollution
    and breathing problems, 27
    diseases caused by, 38
    lawsuits about, 38
    pollutant standards index (PSI) values, 39
Allen, Robert F., xx
Altered states of consciousness, and exercise, 102–103
Amara Association of Health Professionals, 23 (note 6)
American consumption
    of chemical additives, 77
    of food, 76
Amino acids, 66
Anger, 118–121
Anorexia, 73–74
Assertive Bill of Rights, 172
Assertiveness, and communication, 172–173

Asthma
    and emotions, 27
    and tension, 28
Attack and defense, and thinking, 146
Automobiles, and pollution, 107
Awareness
    and breathing, 29–31
    and eating, 82–88
    and feeling, 122–125
    and sex, 187–190

Baby food, and sugar, 83
Backroads Distributors, 228
Ballet, in water, 103
Balloon walk, 106
Bates, William, 54
Bathing, 47–49
Bell's theorem, 212–213
Bentov, Itzhak, 91
Berne, Eric, on strokes, 111
Beyond War, 140
Biofeedback, 32
    and lowering blood pressure, 138
Blood pressure
    lowering with biofeedback, 138
    and salt, 68–69
Blood sugar levels
    and caffeine, 79
    and headaches, 83
Body roll exercise, 97
Boredom
    and eating, 72–73
    and exercise, 105

Brain
    feeling and thinking parts, 110
    right brain/left brain, 134, 136
Brainstorming, and thinking, 140–143
Breast cancer, and dietary fat, 77
Breastfeeding, and bottle-feeding, 72
Breathing
    and activity, 35
    amount of air breathed each day, 26
    awareness and, 29–31
    disease, 27
    and emotional release, 29
    exercises, 27, 31, 33, 34, 35, 36
    and healing, 35–37
    input and output of, 25–26
    and posture, 28–29
    process of, 26–27
    and relaxation, 32–34
    and tension, 28
    and the work environment, 35
Bulimia, 73–74
Burn-out
    among physicians, 5
    prevention of, 159

Caffeine, and blood sugar levels, 79
Calories, and nutrient types, 66
Cancer, and dietary fat, 77
Cancerphobia, 132
Capricorn Incident, 118
Carbohydrates, 67–68
    consumption guidelines, 78
    fiber sources, 77
Cardiovascular exercise. *See* aerobics

Castaneda, Carlos, 75
Celibacy, 192
Centering exercise, 222
Chanting, 60
    recordings of, 230
Charles, Ray, 17
Chi, 185
Childbirth, and controlled breathing, 35
Childhood illness, exercise, 11
Children
    and food dye consumption, 76
    "getting to know" exercise, 112–113
Choking, death from, 75
Cholesterol
    consumption guidelines, 78
    and protein consumption, 78
Classical music, 230
Clean Air Act of 1970, 38
Clothing
    and breathing, 29
    and skin health, 47
Cobra movement, 99
Colon cancer, and dietary fat, 77
Color, and health, 56–57
Color televisions, X-rays emitted by, 56
Communication
    assertiveness, 172–173
    beyond human communication,
        180–182
    "cornering" questions, 173
    exercises, 167, 170, 174, 177, 179
    games and, 175–176
    interpersonal, 169–176
    intrapersonal, 165–168
    judgments and rigidity, 173–174
    listening, 176, 178–180
    monologues and dialogues, 171–172
    positive self-concept, 168–169
    rescuing, 176
    and touch, 45–46
    wellness and, 165
Compassion, 14, 17, 20
    and eating, 88
Competition, and play, 150–152
Conduit analogy, and the Wellness
    Energy System, xxiii–xxiv
Conscious selectivity, 132
"Cornering" questions, 173
Coronary heart disease
    and exercise, 92, 94
    and obesity, 77
    risk factors, 94
Cow's milk, personal writing about,
    84–85
Creative imagination exercise, 135
Creative thinking, 139–142
Crying quiz, 117
Cultural norms, xx–xxi
Cycling, in water, 103

Dairy industry, response to McGovern
    committee report, 79

Dancing
    exercise, 93
    in water, 103
Death
    after-life experience, 205
    dying well, 203, 205
    from choking, 75
    grief process and, 116
    and hospice care, 203
    leading causes of, 5
    living will, 207
    and meaning, 200–205
    prescription drugs as cause of, 4
    wellness and, 202
Denial, and grief, 116
Devotional songs and sounds, 230
Dialogues, characteristics of, 171–172
Dietary Goals for the United States, 64
    dairy and livestock industry
        responses, 79
    goals listed, 78–79
    ordering information, 79
Disease care costs, 4
Dissipative structures theory, xxii
Diverticulosis, and lack of fiber, 77
Doctors, and asserting your right to
    wellness, 180
Dolphins, communication and, 180–181,
    182
Drama Triangle, 175
Dreams, 219–222
Duffy, William (*Sugar Blues*), 67
Dyes, in food, 76

Eating
    awareness and self-trust, 82–88
    body image and, 87–88
    boredom and, 72–73
    complex carbohydrates needed, 68
    exercises, 65, 69, 82
    and fasting, 85
    imbalanced dietary patterns and lack
        of wellness, 64–66
    love and compassion, 88
    mealtime atmosphere, 75–76
    metabolic individuality, 81–82
    nutrients described, 66–69
    and self-responsibility, 76
    slowing down, 84–85
    speed-eating, 75
    stress and, 75–76
    vitamin and mineral supplements, 68
    and wellness, 78–81
    See also food
Ego development, and thinking, 129
Electronic weavings, 230
Emotional insulation, and food, 72–75
Emotions, and breathing, 27–28
Emphysema, 27
Energy, xviii
    distortions of flow, xxx–xxxiv

and the Wellness Energy System,
    xxii, xvi
Environmental Protection Agency
    levels of noise, 58, 59, 60
    and pollution, 38
Environmental sounds, 229–230
Erhard, Werner, 145
Exercise
    aerobics, 94–95
    amount of, 100
    and boredom, 105
    designing an environment for,
        105–107
    and heart disease, 92, 94
    heart rate table, 100
    journal for, 101
    joy, 115
    popularity of, 92
    pulse, taking of, 100
    Rescuer's Checklist, 177
    time for, 102
    values, 204
    yoga, 96–99
Exercises
    acceptance, forgiveness and wellness,
        18–19
    anger, 120
    awareness of feelings, 126–127
    bodily symptoms, 10
    body parts, 12, 13
    breath a full breath, 27
    breathing for balance, 33
    breathing for healing, 36
    centering, 222
    child, getting to know, 112–113
    childhood illness, 11
    color your body, 15, 16
    communication formula, 170
    conversation with body part or
        symptom, 13
    creative imagination, 135
    creative self-massage, 46
    crying quiz, 117
    cultural norm questioning, xxii
    dietary pattern, 65
    dreams, 221
    emotional awareness, 124, 125
    eye relaxation, 54
    food additives, 80
    food, messages about, 69
    foot massage, 50
    forgiveness, 18–19, 21
    hand warming, 52
    illness and wellness, 3
    inner dialogue, 181
    internalized messages, 167
    journal for, 101
    learning to be sick, 9
    learning to eat, 82
    listening, 179
    magic, 215
    massage, 45

meaning, 197, 199–200
meditation, 224
meditation and relaxation, 31
natural breathing, 35
nourishment poetry, 158
nutrition journal, 86
"oughtism", 123
physical
 dancing, 93
 tension release, 189
 waking up exercises, 104
 in water, 103
 yoga, 96–99
play report, 150, 156
self-healing and positive thinking,
 133
sex, 188
strokes, 169
touching, 44
transcending, 212
wake up and release tension, 34
"Yes-But" game, 174
Extra-terrestrial communication, 180
Eyes
 poor vision and, 53–54
 relaxation exercise, 54
 See also sight

Fascism, in the holistic health movement,
 xviii
Fast-foods, and mealtime atmosphere,
 75–76
Fasting, 85
Fats, 68
 consumption guidelines, 78
 over consumption of, 77–78
Fear, 121–122
 of cancer, 132
Federal Water Pollution Control Act of
 1972, 38
Feeling
 awareness and, 122–125
 awareness exercise, 126–127
 emotions, 114–122
 good or bad?, 111, 114
 and love, 124–125
 sensation compared to, 109
 support and, 122–125
 Transactional Analysis and, 110–111
 and wellness, 109–110
 working with, 119
Fiber, sources of, 77
"Fight or flight" mechanism, 33
Fishhook pose, 99
Flexibility exercises, 94
Fluorescent lighting, harmful effects of,
 55–56
Flute music, 229
Food
 attitudes about, 69, 72–75
 average American consumption, 76
 dyes in, 76

eating slowly, 84–85
as emotional insulation, 72–75
exercises, 80
faddism, 83
grow your own, 88
hunger and, 72
labels, 79–81
as a pain reliever, 72
processing and chemical additives,
 76–77
as security, 69, 72
See also eating
Foot reflexology, 50–51
Forgiveness, exercise, 18–19, 21
Four-way stretch, 97
Full-spectrum light, 55
 fluorescent tube problems, 63
 (note 19)

Games, and communication, 175–176
GIGO analogy, 132
Glasses (eye), and full spectrum light, 56
Global Wellness Energy System, xviii
Goals, and meaning, 198–200
Grief, 116–117
 personal writing about, 28
Guided tapes with music, 229
Guilt, 122
Guitar music, 228–229

Hand warming exercise, 52
Hare posture, 98
Harp music, 229
Head, self-massage, 45
Headaches, story about, 166
Healing
 and breathing, 35–37
 with touch, 49–51
Health, and cultural norms, xx–xxi
Health care, self-responsibility and, 6–10
Hearing, 58–61
Hearing loss, and noise, 58–59
Heart rate table, 100
Heat, distribution in the body and health,
 51–52
Hospice, 203
Hospitals, intensive care costs, 200
Houses, and noise, 58, 60, 61
Human body
 body temperature and stress, 33
 and breathing, 26
 conversation with, 13
 eating and body image, 87–88
 feeling and thinking parts of the
  brain, 110
 and light, 54–56
 nutrition and listening to your body,
  82–84
 part of, 12
 right brain/left brain, 134, 136
 and self-trust, 10–14
 and temperature, 51–53
 thinking and, 129–130

Humor, 153–154
Hunger
 "mouth" and "stomach" hunger, 72
 See also eating; food
Hunger Project, 87, 145
Hypnotism, and thinking, 131–132
Hypoglycemia, and headaches, 83
Hysterectomy and sexual attitudes,
 186–187

Iatrogenesis, 4
Iceberg Model, xix–xxi
Illness
 cost of, 4
 exercises about, 3, 9–11
 as a reward, 14, 17
 thinking about, 132–134
 traditional treatment of, 4–6
Illness/Wellness Continuum, xv–xviii
Input sources, and the Wellness Energy
 System, xxiii, xxiv
Intensive care costs, in hospitals, 200
Interaction (individual and environment),
 and the Wellness Energy System, xvii
Internal-output, and the Wellness Energy
 System, xxiv
Interpersonal communication, 169–176
Intrapersonal communication, 165–168

Jazz, 230
Jogging, in water, 103
Journal
 dream journal, 220–222
 personal wellness journal, 231–232
Journal entries. *See* personal writings
Joy, 114–116
Jung, Carl, 212, 220
"Junk" food, 76–77

Keller, Helen, 17
Ki, 185
Kubler-Ross, Elisabeth, 116, 217

Labeling of food, 79–81
Lateral thinking, 144
Laughter, healing qualities of, 154–155
Light, 54–56
 color and, 56–57
 light pollution, 57
Lilly, John, 180–181
Livestock industry, 78
 response to McGovern committee
  report, 79
Living will, 207
Love, 124–125
 and compassion, 14, 17, 20
 and eating, 88
 meaning of, 2
 and sex, 192–193
 and wellness, 1–2
Love Project, 146

McGovern, George (Senator), 64
Malnutrition
    of Americans, 64
    "reasons" for, 88–89
Maltz, Maxwell, 87
Massage, 47–48
    foot massage exercise, 50
    head massage, 45
    of self and sex, 188
Masturbation, 188
Mealtime atmosphere, 75–76
Meaning
    death and finding meaning, 200–205
    and dreams, 219–222
    exercise, 197
    finding, 197–198
    goals and, 198–200
    meditation and, 222–224
    the present and, 198
    process, 217–219
    and reality, 214, 216–217
    transpersonal psychology and
        wellness, 219–223
    wellness and, 196–197
Meditation
    and meaning, 222–224
    meditative music, 229
    and relaxation exercise, 31
Mental problems, and noise, 59
Metabolism, individuality of, 81–82
Milk jug movements, 103
Minerals. *See* vitamins and minerals
Monologues, 171
Mosquitoes, 130
Movement
    designing an environment for
        exercise, 105–107
    exercise, 92–102
    mind and emotions, 102
    and religious ritual, 103
    tension releasing exercise, 189
    and wellness, 91–92
Music, "New-Age", 228–230
Mutations, and fluorescent lighting, 56
Mysticism and religion, 211

Natural Child, 149–150, 154
Near-UV controversy, 63 (note 20)
Need-satisfaction, and food, 72
Negative thinking, 132–134
"New-Age Music", 228–230
Noise
    decreasing in the home, 61
    home environment, 58
    levels of, 60
    See also sound
Nutrients
    described, 66–69
    over consumption of fat, 77–78
    U.S. dietary goals, 78–79
Nutrition
    and listening to your body, 82–84

"nutrition addicts", 74–75
nutrition journal, 86

Ott, John N., 55
"Oughtism", 123
Ouija boards, 216
Our Town, 159
Outdoor lighting, increase of, 57
Output, and the Wellness Energy System,
    xxiii, xv

Pain
    and breathing, 37
    food to relieve, 72
Pendulums, 216
Personal wellness journal, 231–232
Personal writings
    affirmations, 142–143
    all is one, 213
    asthma and breathing, 37
    Beyond War, 140
    bulimia, 74
    Capricorn Incident, 118
    communication, 173
    cow's milk, 84–85
    on death and meaning, 201
    death and wellness, 202
    dolphins, 182
    dots, 155
    ego development and thinking, 129
    fear, 121
    forgiveness and self-acceptance, 22
    frog story, 198
    grief, 28
    hearing loss, 59
    Hunger Project, 87, 145
    hysterectomy and sexual attitudes,
        186–187
    jail story, 59
    license plate game, 214
    on medical school and sick care, 8
    mosquitoes, 130
    playing, 149
    reincarnation, 218–219
    school and thinking, 138–139
    self-acceptance, 14, 20
    on touching, 43
    a transformation, 220
    the "unexplainable", 216
    wart removal and visualization, 141
    weight and withholding, 73
Physicians, burn-out among, 5
Piano music, 228
Pill Fairy, 7
Playing
    Child in us, 149–150, 151, 154
    competition and, 150–152
    healing qualities of, 154–155
    humor, 153
    redefining of, 148–149
    report exercise, 156
    seriousness, 152–154

Pollution
    light pollution, 57
    pollutant standards index (PSI)
        values, 39
    and traffic, 107
    See also Air pollution
Positive self-concept, 168–169
Positive thinking, 132–134
Posture, and breathing, 28–29
Prescription drugs
    death caused by, 4
    Pill Fairy, 7
Prigogen, Illya, xxii, 222
Process
    and meaning, 217–219
    of wellness, xvi
Protein, 66–67
    and cholesterol, 78
Psychocybernetics, 87
Psychological/Motivational level, xix
Pulse, taking of, 100

Rapid eye movements (REM), 220–221
RDA, for vitamins and minerals, 70–71
Reality
    and meaning, 214, 216–217
    and thinking, 128–129
Recommended daily amount (RDA), of
    vitamins and minerals, 70–71
Refined carbohydrates, 67
Reincarnation, 218–219
Relaxation
    and breathing, 32–34
    and meditation exercise, 31
Religion, and transcending, 211
Religious ritual, and movement, 103
REMs, 220–221
Rescuing, as a game strategy, 176
Respiratory disease, and breathing, 27
Respiratory system, and weather, 53
Rhythmic music, 230

Sadness, 116–117
Salt, 68–69
    consumption guidelines, 78
Security, and attitudes about food, 72
Sedentary occupations
    consequences of, 35
    and movement, 92
    See also work
Self-acceptance, 14, 20
Self-concept, 168–169
Self-healing, and positive thinking
    exercise, 133
Self-love, and work wellness, 161
Self-nourishment, and play, 154–155
Self-responsibility
    and eating, 76
    for health care, 6–10
    meaning of, 2
    and sex, 190–191
    and transcending, 211

and wellness, 1–2
and work wellness, 160
Self-trust
and the body, 10–14
and eating, 82–88
Selye, Hans, 33
Sensations, distinguished from feelings, 109
Senses
hearing, 58–61
sight, 53–57
smell, 57–58
temperature, 51–53
touch, 42–51
wellness and, 41–42
Seriousness
and play, 152
strategies for breaking, 152–154
Sex
and awareness, 187–190
celibacy and, 192
as communion, 191–192
exercise, 188, 189
and love, 192–193
self-responsible, 190–191
sensuous sex, 193
"sexual revolution", 185, 186
and touch, 190
wellness and, 185–186
"well-sex", 187–192
Sexuality, and smell, 58
Sight
and the body, 54–56
color and, 56–57
light pollution, 57
stress and, 53–54
Silence, 61
Simultaneous monologues, 171
Skin problems, and clothing, 47
Smell, 57–58
Smoking
and emphysema, 27
and exercise, 94
Songs, 230
Sound
creative uses of, 60–61
See also noise
Speed-eating, 75
slowing it down, 84–85
Spiritual/Being/Meaning level, xx, xxi
"Split brain", 136
Sports, and controlled breathing, 35
Stalking the Wild Pendulum, 91
The Stork position, 98
Strength-developing exercises, 94
Stress
eating and, 75–76

and sight, 53–54
stress-management, and breathing, 32
and work wellness, 160
Strokes (stimulation or recognition), 110–111
exercise, 169
Sugar, in baby food, 83
Sugar Blues, 67
Sugar (refined), 67
Sunlight, 55
Super-organisms, and communication, 182
Support, and feeling, 122–125
Swim-a-thon, 103
Symptoms
conversation with, 13
and deeper meaning exercise, 10
Synchronicity, 212

T'ai-chi T'u, 137
Tapes (music), 228–230
T.A. *See* Transactional Analysis
Television, and thinking, 132
Temperature
of the body, 51–53
weather and health, 53
Tension
and breathing, 28, 33
as a necessary component of life, 34
Thinking
affirmations, 142–143
attack and defense, 146
body changes, 129–131
brainstorming, 140–143
creative thinking, 139–142
and ego development, 129
GIGO analogy, 132
and hypnotism, 131–132
lateral thinking, 144
power of, 128
programming illness/wellness, 132–134
and reality, 128–129
right brain/left brain, 134, 136
whole brain wellness, 136–139
Touch
and bathing, 47–49
and clothing, 47
and communication, 45–46
exercises, 44, 45
healing, 49–51
lack of, 42–43
and massage, 47–48
reluctance to, 43, 45
and sex, 190
Transactional Analysis, 110–111
Drama Triangle, 175

and games, 175–177
and play, 149–150, 154
Transcending
mysticism and religion, 211
relatedness of everything, 211–214
self-responsibility and, 211
wellness and, 209, 211
Transpersonal psychology and wellness, 219–223
Triangle Pose, 99

Ultraviolet light, 56
near-UV controversy, 63 (note 20)
Ultraviolet radiation, 55
Unrefined carbohydrates, 67–68
Urban high-rise buildings, and light, 57

Values, exercise about, 204
Vegetarianism, and protein consumption, 78
Video display terminals, and health risks, 56
Vision. *See* sight
Visualization, 142–143
and wart removal, 141
Vita-Lite, 63 (note 19)
Vitamin D, 55
Vitamins and minerals, 68–69
information table, 70–71
Vocals, 230

Water, 69
urban water supply contamination, 79
Weather, and wellness, 52–53
Wellness Antidote, 162–163
Wellness Energy System, xxii–xxx, 1
Wellness journal, 231–232
Wellness Wheel, xxix
"Well-thinking", 134
Whitehead, Alfred North, xxxv
Wilder, Thornton, 159
Win-Win Integrity Game, 160
Work
defining, 157
environment and natural breathing, 35
problems with, 157, 159
wellness and, 159–161
See also sedentary occupations

X-rays, and color televisions, 56

"Yes-But" game, 174
Yin-Yang, 137
Yoga, 96–99

Beyond This Book–Support from Wellness Associates

This book is about personal growth. It is also about changing our existing attitudes and behaviors. Many of our cultural norms subtly reinforce feelings of powerlessness, alienation, or isolation, and often reward illness and non-responsibility. Although you may be excited by many of the ideas and feelings you experienced from reading the book, they will likely have little lasting influence as long as you live your life in an environment where there is little support for these values.

In making life changes, a supportive network of like-minded people is of tremendous value. One highly effective way you can use this workbook is by meeting regularly with a group of friends to share and discuss the ideas and exercises in the book. If you want to join/create such a group, it is important that it be made up of people with whom you feel safe to be yourself and let your rough edges show without fear of judgement by the group.

An optimal wellness environment—where people can experience an atmosphere of openness, trust and honesty—can be created almost anywhere. It may manifest as a support group that meets regularly at someone's house, or at a church. It may be created in a group at your place of work, or it could show up as a whole community working together to understand and respect each other's commonalities and differences.

Supportive environments are so rare that most people don't even know that they are missing them. Either they've never experienced one, or the experience was so fleeting as to be dismissed as a oddity—never considered as a possible norm.

We are convinced that people grow and evolve more readily with regular access to an optimal wellness environment. If you have one, rejoice, and let us know about it! If you don't have a support group to help you in making changes in your life, we urge you to find or create one.

If you need help creating an optimal wellness environment around you, it is a primary mission of Wellness Associates to facilitate you in finding one. We maintain a geographic roster of wellness facilitators we believe are committed to fostering optimal wellness environments in many different settings. Some are in private practice, others work in institutions. Some regularly hold support group meetings which you can join, while others may offer individual counseling or weekend programs.

By our criteria, these wellness facilitators are people who listen, ask questions and support others in exploring their own personal truth. They usually raise more questions than they answer. They are not people who will try to tell you what to do, offer unsolicited advice, or use guilt and fear as a motivator. They will not try to get you to take their brand of supplements or sell you their special gimmick or guru. Likewise they will not do "therapy" on you (unless they are qualified, and you specifically ask for it).

The people we recommend are well-versed in the Wellness Energy System approach, and skilled in most, if not all, of the areas of counseling, stress reduction, nutrition, etc. Most importantly they emphasize the psychological and spiritual aspects of being human, and support people in beginning to consciously take charge of their lifelong personal journey.

At this time (1987), their numbers are small but growing. If you want to find one, or to learn how to become one, write us.

We are also assembling a manual to assist in teaching classes using the *Wellness Workbook*. Write for additional information.

About the Authors

Regina Sara Ryan received a Master's Degree in Communications from Colorado State University in 1973, and has been an educator in the field of wellness since 1975. She is currently doing private consulting, teaching about grief and death, and completing several projects, including a book which deals with the process of recuperation from a wellness perspective.

The main focus of her life and work continues to be the spiritual dimensions of well-being.

Regina lives in Denver, Colorado with her husband, Jere Pramuk.

John W. Travis, MD, MPH, completed his medical training in Boston. In 1972, while a resident in preventive medicine at Johns Hopkins, he was inspired by Dr. Halbert Dunn's 1961 classic *High Level Wellness.* He subsequently gave up the practice of sick care, studied widely in areas of humanistic and transpersonal psychology and launched his pioneering Wellness Resource Center in 1975.

Four years later, he closed the Center to focus on offering consulting and seminars for helping professionals worldwide. From 1980 to 1983 he, and his wife Meryn Callander, lived in the mountains of Costa Rica exploring self sufficiency within the context of a spiritually oriented community. They now live in rural Northern California.

Since the writing of the *Wellness Workbook,* John has co-authored, with his wife, Meryn, *Wellness for Helping Professionals* and has developed a Wellness Resource Kit of materials to support others in the transition to a wellness orientation.

He has developed a computerized Wellness Inventory for home and professional use and expects to interface the computer with video as a means of conveying wellness concepts. Another current interest is in fostering communities wherein wellness facilitators can create spaces where people feel safe to be themselves.

What is Wellness Associates?

Wellness Associates is a nonprofit educational corporation based in California. It is the successor to the Wellness Resource Center founded by John in 1975. It is also a **membership group** consisting of people committed to exploring wellness in greater depth. Available to members are:

Δ The **Wellness Associates Journal** edited by John and his wife, Meryn. Rather than present facts or tips, it shares with characteristic openness, the trials and tribulations of the editors and contributors as they document the personal journeying that is tantamount to wellness.

Δ A **listing** of members who subscribe to the Journal.

Δ Priority status on mailings for **seminars** offered around the US, Canada, Australia and New Zealand. Open to both professional and strongly motivated laypersons, these programs bring together likeminded persons interested in creating a more supportive environment in their life and committed to introducing more life-enhancing norms in the culture. Particular emphasis is placed on developing communication skills, exploring the meaning and purpose in life, nurturing the planet, and experiencing the spiritual (not necessarily religious) aspects of being.

Graduates raduates of these seminars can join our **wellness network.** This network offers:

Δ A **Network Newsletter** and **directory** for, and by, dues-paying network associates.

Δ An **Advanced Studies Program** for helping professionals and strongly motivated laypersons— available to those who have attended introductory programs.

Δ A **Facilitator's Group** wherein people gain experience in creating optimal wellness environments in their own communities or workplaces—offering an alternative to therapists who usually diagnose, prescribe and treat. These facilitators listen non-judgementally to their clients, raise more questions than they answer, and **provide a supportive environment,** usually composed of other similarly oriented persons, to facilitate making life changes that may not yet be supported by the culture at large. Names of graduate **Wellness Facilitators** recommended by Wellness Associates, can be obtained by using the enclosed postcard, or the form at right.

Private consulting and public or in-house presentations are also available for wellness professionals in organizations wishing to enhance communication within their teams, and deepen the scope of their work.

The affiliated Wellness Publications organization offers these additional resources:

Δ The separately bound **Wellness Index** ($2.95) found in this book. (Bulk discounts available.)

Δ An abridged version of the Wellness Index, the **Wellness Inventory** ($1.95). This is designed to be an introduction to wellness and takes about 20 minutes to complete. (Bulk discounts available.)

Δ *Wellness For Helping Professionals* (Travis and Callander, Kendall Hunt, 1988, $24.95)

Δ The **Wellness Resource Kit** which includes the above items, this book, and a compendium of the tools John has found most useful in his 15 years of full time development of the field of wellness.

Δ The **Wellness Inventory—Interactive,** a micro-computer version of the abridged Wellness Index.

Δ A videotape, **Your Health... Who's Responsible?,** which presents the concepts of the Wellness Energy System described in this book, using visual images, music and narration by John & Meryn.

Δ Colorful **bookmarks** listing the definitions of wellness shown on page *xiv* of this book and a one-page-a-day wellness **calendar** of inspirational passages from the book.

Become a Wellness Associate:

Joining Wellness Associates will keep you connected with our work as we continue to explore the questions raised in the latter chapters of the book through the *Wellness Associates Journal*. Wellness is a never ending personal journey and in the journal we document our saga, and those of others exploring the frontiers of wellness in a personal, informal way. Joining will also provide you with mailings on our other offerings and a listing of other members.

- -

Mail to:
Wellness Associates
Box 5433 W
Mill Valley, CA 94942

In Australia:
59 Cratloe Rd.
Mt Waverley, 3149
Victoria, Australia

Please send me 4 issues of the *Wellness Associates Journal* (20-25 pages, 3-4 times/yr.) beginning with the current issue. Includes a geographic listing of subscribers.

__ $25 Regular __ $40 Contributing __ $100 Sponsor

__ Do *not* include my name in the geographical listing.

Tell me more about Wellness Associates!

My interests are:

___ other publications by John Travis or Regina Ryan.
___ computer software based on the *Wellness Workbook*.
___ the Wellness Associates Journal.
___ finding a local support group.
___ becoming a wellness facilitator.
___ other _____

Name _____

Address _____

_____

Occupation _____

___ Keep me on your mailing list.

To speed your reply, please enclose a self-addressed business size envelope with two oz. postage.

Feedback Page

We want this book to be the best possible. Your feedback and information are invaluable.
For future editions, please share your ideas with us.

Thank you,

Regina

John

mail to:
Wellness Associates
Box 5433-W
Mill Valley, CA 94942

. . . .

Dear Regina and John,

Here are some of my thoughts and feelings:

Completing the certificate on the following page acknowledges that you believe yourself to be a Wonderful Person and have awarded yourself the W.P. degree. You may either find six persons to sign it for you or make up names and put them at the bottom yourself. (Copies suitable for framing are available from Wellness Associates.)

GRAND CERTIFICATE

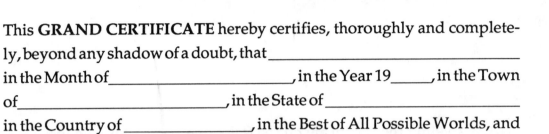

This **GRAND CERTIFICATE** hereby certifies, thoroughly and completely, beyond any shadow of a doubt, that _____ in the Month of _____, in the Year 19____, in the Town of _____, in the State of _____ in the Country of _____, in the Best of All Possible Worlds, and that said _____ thoroughly and completely, beyond any conceivable shadow of a doubt, and beyond any inconceivable shadow of a doubt, with all the Angels and Spirits of the Cosmos attending and watching over benevolently, and with the Higher Intentions of the Universe in harmonious musical and occipital accord with the movements of the planets and all persons pursuant and participant to the above-named and heretofore specified person, beyond any imaginable shadow of a doubt, and beyond any unimaginable shadow of a doubt, blah, blah, in which all inhabitants and participants in the County of yadda yadda to which a testimony of conclusions and the reasons stated and explicit as well as, yet by no means limited to, harmonious physical and physic yuk-yuk and therefore to the **rights, ranks, privileges, insignias**, and yawn, burp to which and to wit, and that we, the undersigned **do recognize you,**

to be a

WONDERBARUS PERSONUS

and hereby entitled to the degree of WONDERFUL PERSON (W.P.),
in all manner, shape, form, and transportation.

_____ W.P.   _____ W.P.

_____ W.P.   _____ W.P.

_____ W.P.   _____ W.P.

©1976, Kenneth Maue, Ph.D.